Radiopharmaceuticals in the Management of Leptomeningeal Metastasis

Franklin C. L. Wong
Editor

Radiopharmaceuticals in the Management of Leptomeningeal Metastasis

Springer

Editor
Franklin C. L. Wong
Dept of Nuclear Med, Unit No 1483
U Texas MD Anderson Cancer Ctr
Houston, TX, USA

ISBN 978-3-031-14290-1 ISBN 978-3-031-14291-8 (eBook)
https://doi.org/10.1007/978-3-031-14291-8

This Springer imprint is published by the registered company Springer Nature Switzerland AG
The registered company address is: Gewerbestrasse 11, 6330 Cham, Switzerland

Preface

When I started learning to treat leptomeningeal metastasis (LM) as a neurology resident physician in Los Angeles during the 1980s, diagnostic tools and therapeutic regimen were hardly available. The next station after cytopathology confirmation of LM in a cancer patient was often the hospice. Since then, I have been privileged to continue studying LM diagnosis and therapy in a cancer center. Today, the grim outlook of LM has improved to some degree and silver linings are ahead. It is my hope to share this collection of chapters to make it easier for trainees and mentors of nuclear medicine, neurology, and oncology to contribute to the care of patients with LM. This book is designed in breath and in depth for audience from scientists in basic medical sciences and clinical practitioners in medicine, specifically neurology, oncology, radiation physics, imaging physics, and radiotherapy.

In fact, human LM has been found with increasing frequency, likely because of longer human life span, increasing cancer incidences, and better diagnostic tools and better diagnostic criteria. The management of LM, nevertheless, has remained challenging with slow progress in therapy. In the meantime, there has been multiple pivotal advancement in molecular imaging schemes (including MRI, radiopharmaceuticals, PET and SPECT in Chaps. 2, 3, and 10) and therapeutic regimens (approved alpha and beta emitters as in Chap. 3) with molecular specificities using conventional and novel radiopharmaceuticals.

This book is a collection of current reviews and original research on human LM on its occurrence, pathophysiology, diagnosis, radiotherapy, systemic therapy, targeted therapy as well as radionuclide interventions using approved and experimental radiopharmaceuticals. Brief reviews of epidemiology, pathophysiology, state-of-the-art neuroimaging, systemic therapy, radiotherapy and electrophysiology, and an original semiquantitative study of CSF flow using In-111 DTA are presented (Chap. 4). Conventional intrathecal therapy (Chap. 5), radiotherapy of human LM (Chap. 6), and electrophysiology monitoring (Chap. 7) are reviewed along with established algorithms and results. Selected intrathecal therapeutic trials using radiopharmaceuticals are reviewed and contrasted (Chap. 8). Radiation dosimetry to CSF compartments and to vital organs is simulated in simplified anthropomorphic models to allow comparison of potential candidate radiopharmaceuticals and for validation of biodistribution assumptions (examples in Chap. 9). Dosimetry imaging schemes are outlined in Chap. 10. Regulatory boundaries of the clinical practice of radionuclide therapy of LM are outlined in Chap. 11. The scientific and logistic frameworks for clinical management of LM and the opportunities in the near future are further illustrated in Chap. 12.

Houston, TX, USA Franklin C. L. Wong

Acknowledgments

I am indebted to the chapter authors and coauthors for their contribution to this book and to teach me on my blind spots. I would like to express my sincere gratitude to Fabiola Josephine and Margaret Moore from Springer for assistance to make the publication possible, in spite of the 3 years of pandemics and all the delays. I must thank my family for putting up with my absence while working on this book, even though the pandemic has quarantined us under the same roof.

The research findings included in Chaps. 4, 8, 9, and 12 were made possible by US federal grant support to me as Principal Investigator from US NIH/NCI (Grants R21-CA89891 and R21-CA97729 for intraventricular and intralumbar trials) as well as US DOD (Breast Cancer Research Idea Grant BC020808 for locoregional radionuclide therapy).

Contents

Contributors

Samantha M. Buszek, MD Department of Radiation Oncology, University of Texas MD Anderson Cancer Center, Houston, TX, USA

T. Linda Chi, MD Department of Neuroradiology, The University of Texas M. D. Anderson Cancer Center, Houston, TX, USA

Caroline Chung, MD Department of Radiation Oncology, University of Texas MD Anderson Cancer Center, Houston, TX, USA

Hannah Culver, MPAS Neuro-Oncology, Texas Oncology, Austin, TX, USA

J. Matthew Debnam, MD Department of Neuroradiology, The University of Texas M. D. Anderson Cancer Center, Houston, TX, USA

Morris D. Groves Jr, MD, JD Neuro-Oncology, Texas Oncology, Austin, TX, USA

Dao Le, Pharm D The University of Texas, MD Anderson Cancer Center, Houston, TX, USA

Ian E. McCutcheon, MD Neurosurgery, The University of Texas M. D. Anderson Cancer Center, Houston, Texas, USA

Rodolfo Núñez, MD Tufts Medical Center, Boston, MA, USA

Richard B. Sparks, PhD, DVM, MBA CDE Dosimetry Service, Inc., Knoxville, TN, USA

Sudhakar Tummula, MD University of Texas M. D. Anderson Cancer Center, Houston, TX, USA

Richard E. Wendt III, PhD, MBA Department of Imaging Physics, The University of Texas MD Anderson Cancer Center, Houston, TX, USA

Brian S. Wong, MD, MPH Department of Radiology, University of Texas Medical Branch, Galveston, TX, USA

Franklin C. L. Wong, MD, PhD, JD, MBA Department of Nuclear Medicine, University of Texas M. D. Anderson Cancer Center, Houston, TX, USA

Chapter 1
Human Leptomeningeal Metastasis (LM): Epidemiology and Challenges

Brian S. Wong and Franklin C. L. Wong

Leptomeningeal Metastasis Frequency of Occurrence/ Incidence

Cancer has remained the second leading cause of death in the USA. Distal metastases beyond the primary cancer site upon staging occur frequently with lymphoma (51%), ovarian cancer (50%), lung cancer (46%), and less often with breast cancer (6%), prostate cancer (7%), or melanoma (5%) [1]. Conversely, leptomeningeal metastasis (LM) involving arachnoid (and rarely the pia) is frequently noted with melanoma, lymphoma, leukemia, and breast cancer in Table 1.1. As one of the insidious cancer complications, LM is often diagnosed late during the course of care.

The LM prevalence is rarely described in the literature because of the lack of sufficient data. Most reports are from institutional experience. Therefore, detailed gender and racial profiles cannot be generalized. Similarly, LM incidence (new cases within a fixed period, typically 1 year) data are not available. Instead, the frequency of occurrence of LM with primary cancers has been reported interchangeably as incidence (in the generic sense). Trends of rising frequency of occurrence (or incidence) have been also reported and likely related to availability of better diagnostic tools (including MRI) and more efficacious therapies of primary as well as secondary cancers [2].

Recent reports of cancers with higher frequency of LM since 2004 [3–7] are listed in Table 1.1, along with frequency of distal metastasis of primary cancer [1].

B. S. Wong (✉)
Department of Radiology, University of Texas Medical Branch, Galveston, TX, USA
e-mail: bswong@utmb.edu

F. C. L. Wong
Department of Nuclear Medicine, University of Texas M. D. Anderson Cancer Center, Houston, TX, USA
e-mail: fwong@mdanderson.org

F. C. L. Wong (ed.), *Radiopharmaceuticals in the Management of Leptomeningeal Metastasis*, https://doi.org/10.1007/978-3-031-14291-8_1

Table 1.1 Reported frequency of occurrence of LM with primary cancers, compared with distal metastasis from CA2022 and 1-year overall survival of patients with LM on therapy

LM	Frequency					Distal mets on CA staging	5-year survival with mets	LM median survival	1-year OS with LM
Author	Wang N	O'Meara W	Jaeckle K	Deangelis L	Elting	Seigel R [1]	Seigel R [1]	[8–12]	
Reporting year	2018	2007	2006	2005	2005	2022	2022		
Cancer type						%	%	Weeks	%
Breast	5% – 8%	5%–25%	27% – 50%	3% – 34%	3%	6	29	16 (15–17)	16
Lung	9% – 25%	10% – 25%	22%– 36%	10% – 26%	11% – 26%	48	6	42.4 (32–52)	44
Melanoma	6% – 18%	15% – 25%	12%	17% – 25%	5% – 11%	5	30	10 (8–14)	10
Lymphoma		2% – 10%		7% – 15%	5% – 30%	51	66	35	38
Leukemia		5% – 15%	5% – 15%	5% – 15%	10% – 30%	–	–	45 – 130	28
Primary CNS lymphoma		15% – 40%			25% – 30%	–	–		
Medulloblastoma		30%			50%	–	–		

Table 1.2 Reported outcome of LM-specific therapeutic trials. Median survival is in unit of weeks

LM	5-year OS with distal mets [1]	Recent LM trial	LM patients	1-year OS range on RX	Median survival on RX
Cancer type	%		*N*	%	Weeks
Breast	29	Niwinska 2018 [9]	67	16–17	16
Lung	6	Yan 2019 [10]	135	20–50	38 – 59
Melanoma	30	Harstad 2008 [8]	110	7–10	8–14
Lymphoma	66	Al Feghali 2021 [12]	20	38	35
Leukemia	–	Kwon 2016 [11]	31	12–28	45 – 130

The ranking of LM frequency and frequency of distal metastasis upon cancer staging is not in the same order and likely owing to the delay of 1.2–2 years for diagnosis of LM from cancer diagnosis [6], different biology of LM, and intervening therapy. Leukemia is a systemic disease and the treatment is mostly directed toward leukemia itself; LM prophylactic intrathecal therapy is a common practice.

Outcomes of LM therapy are pessimistic but slow progresses have been made. Selected recent reports of LM therapy of the top 5 cancer types with LM with survival data are listed in Table 1.2. The shortest median survival of 10 weeks is noted in a US report of 110 melanoma patients with median survival of overall survival of 10% at 1 year and statistically significant hazard ratio of 0.5 (0.4–0.8) for intrathecal therapy [8]. A European study of 187 breast cancer patients has shown median survival of 16 weeks and overall survival of 15–16% in 1 year [9]. A Chinese study of 135 patients with non-small cell lung cancer and LM demonstrated median survival of 42 weeks and 44% overall survival at 1 year [10]. A Korean study found 38 patients with LM (from 775 with acute myeloid leukemia). Whole-brain irradiation improved OS from 10.4 to 29.9 months (and 1 year OS from 10% to 28%) [11] for those patients who had induction therapy and received intrathecal therapy. A US study of 20 patients with LM and diffuse large B-cell lymphoma who had standard lymphoma treatment and radiation therapy found a median survival of 35 weeks (and 1 year survival of 38%) compared with 87 weeks (1 year survival of 69%) for those with localized targetable disease. For comparison with therapy not specifically targeting LM or the brain (including 2 with LM) who were able to undergo stem cell transplant after radiation therapy, the 2 year survival rate is 100% [12]. The different ranking of survival from patient with metastatic disease of different cancer versus survival of patients with LM in Table 1.2 is likely related to specific LM therapy, concurrent therapy of primary cancer as well as lethality of metastasis in other parts of the body. In summary, LM is a lethal cancer complication that is difficult to diagnose and difficult to treat. This is an area of unmet need in the care of oncologic patients. Although LM is one of the cancer complications among others that would cause mortality and morbidity, the importance of treating LM can be illustrated by an earlier radionuclide therapy for LM prophylaxis using Au-198 gold colloid [13]. Median survival was similarly shortened to 5 years for those treated who had bone marrow recurrence or LM recurrence, while median survival for those without LM recurrence was beyond the observation period of 8.5 years.

Challenges of LM Treatment

Limited Knowledge of Meningeal Anatomy, Physiology, and Pathophysiology

Leptomeninges refer to the arachnoids and pia matter which actually lay in the opposite of the subarachnoid space throughout the brain and spinal cord. Subarachnoid spaces are bathed with cerebrospinal fluid produced from the choroid plexus distributed loosely in the roof of the lateral ventricles. The traditional view of cerebrospinal fluid flow is derived from the cardiac pulsation to drive CSF flow through the third ventricle to the fourth ventricle. Portions of the spinal fluid will go up toward the cerebral convexity and other portions go down the posterior aspect of the spinal cord to reach the cauda equina before returning to the anterior aspect of the spinal cord to join the circulation in the basal cistern and then back over the cerebral convexity.

Conventional cisternograms and ventriculograms localize radioactive tracers in the spinal fluid compartments with multiple (3–4) overlapping static images because of the limited field of view of the gamma cameras (25–30 cm) [14, 15]. With 15 min for each static image, each session of static imaging of CSF will take up to 1 h which is the basis of temporal resolution of cisternograms. Cisternograms have been employed to evaluate spinal fluid flow over many hours/days with multiple image sessions in neurologic diseases including LM [16]. Clinical improvement in LM has been correlated with improved CSF flows in patients with LM [17]. Even limited temporal resolution (hour) and inherit low spatial resolution of gamma camera (cm) nevertheless have been sufficient to evaluate gross events of spinal fluid flow such as hydrocephalus, spinal fluid leakage, and blockage.

Recent advances in animal research and high-resolution MRI have enabled investigation of refined fluid movement within the brain substance and among different compartments and within short durations. Glymphatics referred to the perivesicular fluid flow within the brain towards the lymphoid tissues and has been found to contribute substantially to integrity of brain function [18]. It also interacts with spinal fluid flow and may contribute to substantially higher proportions of bulk fluid flow during sleeping. The contribution of CSF flow to brain health includes cushioning of the brain substance and clearing of metabolites and amyloid deposits. Further investigation of crossflow between spinal fluid and glymphatics may allow better understanding of interstitial exposure of intrathecal therapeutic agents and deployment of higher intrathecal therapy efficacy. This type of investigation would require scintigraphic scanning with better spatial and temporal resolution than those of current clinical cameras. Because of ethical concerns most leptomeningeal studies have to rely on animal studies and experimental imaging devices.

Metastases from solid cancer or hematological malignancy usually reside diffusely in the arachnoids to form multiple LM colonies, after they overcome the host resistance. There is difference in abilities of successful establishment of LM deposits from different cancer types. There is also different preference of location to establish LM (spinal cord versus convexity versus cerebellum). It is not clear about the relationship between the seed versus soil both of which are focus of intense investigation to identify biomarkers and targetable entities for diagnosis and intervention.

Limited LM Diagnosis: Cytology, MRI Abnormalities, PET-CT, RANO-LM

Neurologic findings of LM patients are nonspecific. Traditionally, the exclusion of LM diagnosis requires negative cytology of serial spinal fluid sampling because of the relatively low yield of CSF cytology [19]. That certainly involves patient discomfort and delays in diagnosis. Using cytology positivity as the only affirmative criteria to treat LM, many LM patients with negative CSF cytology have been deprived of early entry into therapeutic trials. Neuroimaging modalities have provided suboptimal tools neither. Even with contrast-enhanced MRI, the findings are subject to low sensitivity (~60%) and low specificity (Chap. 2) that would frequently include inflammation from other causes including the procedure of CSF access. At times, meningeal enhancements are noted beyond the lumbar spine level after lumbar puncture [20]. Case reports of positive findings on LM patients have been made on PET-CT using F-18 FDG and C-11 methionine. However, their sensitivity and specificity have not been established. PET-CT will be further discussed in Chap. 3. Partly owing to these difficulties, LM diagnosis is often made 1.2–2 years after initial cancer staging in patients even though they have already had other metastatic sites. A Response Assessment of Neuro-Oncology in Leptomeningeal Metastasis (RANO- LM) has been proposed to incorporate standardized neurological examination, cytology response, and radiologic progression (contrast-enhanced MRI) [21]. For instance, clear progression in MRI findings in the absence of cytology response would still be classified as radiographic progression. The RANO-LM proposal is awaiting validation and is further described and assessed in Chap. 2. Laboratory efforts are ongoing to find the molecular signatures of LM for more effective identification but to date there is no universal serum nor CSF biomarker has been identified that is common to multiple malignancies.

Limited Efficacy of LM Therapy

Intrathecal therapy is usually injected through the intraventricular approach or lumbar puncture. It is more effective via the intraventricular injection approach, typically with an Ommaya reservoir, because this approach assures exposure to all the CSF spaces including the ventricle which is proximal to the spinal CSF space and would not be readily accessible from the lumbar puncture approach. Assurance of spinal fluid flow patency is an important concern because of the dire consequences of a blocked catheter tip resulting in intraparenchymal injection to the brain substance. Alternatively, CSF patency needs to be confirmed before intrathecal treatment when blockage is suspected on ventriculo-peritoneal shunt (VP) shunts attached to an Ommaya reservoir. Scintigraphic confirmation of CSF patency for intrathecal therapy is further described in Chap. 4.

Multiple efficacious systemic therapies for primary cancer treatment have also been found to be effective in treating LM for several cancers. Successful treatment of LM with immunotherapy and cellular therapy has been reported in selected cancers. Nevertheless, intrathecal therapy has remained the mainstay of LM treatment because of the immediately high dose delivery to the meninges. Arachnoiditis has been a concern for intrathecal chemotherapy which typically involves repeated injection of multi-mg of pharmaceuticals. Intrathecal therapeutic agents may be subject to low diffusion across the meninges and intrathecal metabolism such as with Ara-C. The alternative of liposomal ara-C (DepoCyte) has managed to elevate the intrathecal level of the effective form of the drug. The systemic and intrathecal therapy of LM are further described in Chap. 5.

Whole brain and spine irradiation are effective to treat LM. Its efficacy has been further enhanced by image modulation and meticulous dosimetric schemes. However, the brain and spinal cord are inevitably within the radiation field and there is a relatively low dose limit. They are further described in Chap. 6. The effectiveness of LM treatment is typically measured by neurologic assessment, conversion of CSF cytology, and standard oncologic assessment as progression free survival (PFS) and overall survival (OS). However, PFS and OS as measures of LM efficacy are also subject to additional considerations of complications from the primary tumor and other non-LM related morbidity and mortality. More LM-specific measurement of CSF cytology conversion may be subject to low sensitivity. Another possible LM-specific measure in the clinics is neurophysiologic assessment and monitoring schemes that will be reviewed in Chap. 7.

Advantages of Radiopharmaceuticals for Intrathecal Diagnostics and Therapeutics

Radiopharmaceuticals typically involve gamma- or positron-emitting radionuclide with minute amounts of physical material in the range of nanomole. Once injected, they follow blood flow or spinal fluid flow to reach the target and may be retained according to their biochemical property which is often determined by the attached moiety. Sensitive gamma cameras are able to localize radiopharmaceuticals inside the body that is distributed according to their biochemical characteristics. In other words, scintigraphy of radiopharmaceuticals reveals and localizes radiopharmaceuticals according to their biochemical activities.

The main advantage of radiopharmaceuticals is the minute physical mass at sub-nanogram level that does not cause pharmacologic perturbation of the organs while revealing the underlying biochemistry. Since there are many available radiopharmaceuticals, multiple biochemical pathways of the body can be investigated, in a relatively noninvasive manner and without pharmacologic perturbation of ongoing physiologic processes. Radiopharmaceuticals can be readily designed for the desirable biochemical pathways in the body. Because of the minute amounts of physical material of the radionuclide involved, the radioactivity can be simply upscaled from small diagnostic dose to large therapeutic doses while exploiting the same biochemical pathway. This is the basis of routine thyroid cancer imaging using I-131 sodium iodide at small doses (2 mCi) to detect thyroid cancer remnant and then using large dose (100–250 mCi) to ablate confirmed residual thyroid cancer. Isotopes of the same element with different emitted radiations can also be used to attach to the same moiety to produce radiopharmaceuticals with different radiation payloads. The ones with lower radiation absorbed dose (such as 5 mCi of I-123 sodium iodide) can be used for diagnosis, while the ones with higher radiation absorbed dose (I-131) can be used for therapeutic. That is the basis of theranostics for transition between diagnostic use and therapeutic use of radiopharmaceuticals while exploiting the same biochemical pathway. Similarly, the same biochemical mechanism can be investigated with a moiety labeled with radionuclide of lower radiation absorbed dose such as In-111 in Zevalin to detect CD20+ lymphoma. Once CD20 positivity is confirmed, a high radiation load from Y-90 Zevalin can be deployed to ablate systemic lymphomas [22]. In 3/2022, a theranostic agent Lu-177 labeled PSMA [23, 24] received US FDA clearance for treating prostate cancer patients. Multiple radiopharmaceuticals are under industrial pipelines for cancer treatment. Hopefully, some can be developed to treat LM, the deadly cancer complication.

There has been development of a plethora of radiopharmaceuticals (with and without tumor affinities) for clinical applications in oncology. For instance, In-111 DTPA will reveal the spinal fluid flow allowing multiple days of observation. Once it leaves the spinal fluid space to join the general circulation, its whole-body distributions are determined by the DTPA moiety which is secreted by the kidneys into the urinary bladder. As illustrated by I-131 sodium iodide therapy of Grave's disease and thyroid cancer, selected radiopharmaceuticals can be readily upscaled from diagnostic dosage to therapeutic levels to serve as theranostics agent. Current use of diagnostic and therapeutic radiopharmaceuticals in neuro-oncology is reviewed in Chap. 3. Clinical trials involving radiopharmaceuticals to treat LM will be collated according to the mechanism in Chap. 8 to determine the current state of art and to allow design of novel strategies that may be employed to tackle LM. The radiation absorbed doses of intrathecal therapy of LM can be simulated using established models of spinal fluid flow and of human organ distribution. Using a common model, radiation dosimetry to the CSF space and vital organs from different radiopharmaceuticals can be simulated and compared as in Chap. 9. Empirical assessment of radiation dosimetry from image-based dosimetric measurement using established clinical imaging scheme is detailed in Chap. 10.

The use of radiopharmaceuticals is under oversight from the federal levels, state jurisdictions, and local institutional policies. The multiple levels of overseeing entities will be reviewed for practitioners of intrathecal radionuclide therapy in Chap. 11 to provide guidance and considerations for logistics. The last chapter (Chap. 12) is to summarize challenges and opportunities of radiopharmaceuticals therapy schemes to better design LM therapy.

References

1. Siegel RL, et al. Cancer statistics, 2022. CA Cancer J Clin. 2022;72(1):7–33.
2. Enting RH. Leptomeningeal neoplasia: epidemiology, clinical presentation, CSF analysis and diagnostic imaging. Cancer Treat Res. 2005;125:17–30.
3. DeAngelis LM, Boutros D. Leptomeningeal metastasis. Cancer Investig. 2005;23(2):145–54.
4. Herrlinger U, et al. Leptomeningeal metastasis: survival and prognostic factors in 155 patients. J Neurol Sci. 2004;223(2):167–78.
5. O'Meara WP, et al. Leptomeningeal metastasis. Curr Probl Cancer. 2007;31(6):367–424.
6. Wang N, Bertalan MS, Brastianos PK. Leptomeningeal metastasis from systemic cancer: review and update on management. Cancer. 2018;124(1):21–35.
7. Jaeckle KA. Neoplastic meningitis from systemic malignancies: diagnosis, prognosis and treatment. Semin Oncol. 2006;33(3):312–23.
8. Harstad L, Hess KR, Groves MD. Prognostic factors and outcomes in patients with leptomeningeal melanomatosis. Neuro-Oncology. 2008;10(6):1010–8.
9. Niwinska A, et al. Determinants of prolonged survival for breast cancer patient groups with leptomeningeal metastasis (LM). J Neuro-Oncol. 2018;138(1):191–8.
10. Yan W, et al. The clinical characteristic and prognostic factors of leptomeningeal metastasis in patients with non-small-cell lung cancer-a retrospective study from one single cancer institute. Cancer Med. 2019;8(6):2769–76.
11. Kwon JH, et al. Clinical outcome and efficacy of current anti-leukemic therapy for leptomeningeal involvement in acute myeloid leukemia. Int J Hematol. 2016;104(5):574–81.
12. Al Feghali KA, et al. Prognostic value of disease distribution in secondary central nervous system diffuse large B cell lymphoma treated with radiation therapy. Leuk Lymphoma. 2021;62(10):2400–7.
13. Metz O, Stoll W, Plenert W. Meningosis prophylaxis with intrathecal 198Au-colloid and methotrexate in childhood acute lymphocytic leukemia. Cancer. 1982;49(2):224–8.
14. Dichiro G, Reames PM, Matthews WB Jr. Risa-ventriculography and risa-cisternography. Neurology. 1964;14:185–91.
15. Larson SM, et al. The radionuclide ventriculogram. JAMA. 1973;224(6):853–7.
16. Chamberlain MC, Corey-Bloom J. Leptomeningeal metastases: 111indium-DTPA CSF flow studies. Neurology. 1991;41(11):1765–9.
17. Chamberlain MC, Kormanik P, Jaeckle KA. 111Indium-diethylenetriamine pentaacetic acid CSF flow studies predict distribution of intrathecally administered chemotherapy and outcome in patients with leptomeningeal metastases. Neurology. 1999;52(1):216–7.
18. An D, Morgan WH, Yu DY. Glymphatics and lymphatics in the eye and central nervous system. Clin Exp Ophthalmol. 2017;45(5):440–1.

19. Posner JB, Dalmau J. Clinical enigmas of paraneoplastic neurologic disorders. Clin Neurol Neurosurg. 1995;97(1):61–70.
20. Bakshi R, et al. MRI findings in lumbar puncture headache syndrome: abnormal dural-meningeal and dural venous sinus enhancement. Clin Imaging. 1999;23(2):73–6.
21. Chamberlain M, et al. Leptomeningeal metastases: a RANO proposal for response criteria. Neuro-Oncology. 2017;19(4):484–92.
22. Sachpekidis C, Jackson DB, Soldatos TG. Radioimmunotherapy in non-Hodgkin's lymphoma: retrospective adverse event profiling of Zevalin and Bexxar. Pharmaceuticals (Basel). 2019;12(4):141.
23. Tatkovic A, McBean R, Wong D. Lu177-PSMA therapy for men with advanced prostate cancer: 18 months survival analysis in a single Australian tertiary institution. J Med Imaging Radiat Oncol. 2021;65(6):740–7.
24. Schneider CA, et al. Treatment outcome and identification of factors influencing overall survival after Lu-177-PSMA-617 radioligand therapy in metastatic prostate cancer. Nuklearmedizin. 2022;61(1):25–32.

Chapter 2
State of Art of LM Radiographic Diagnosis: Anatomic and Functional Imaging

J. Matthew Debnam and T. Linda Chi

Introduction

Neoplastic leptomeningeal disease (LMD) is a late complication of systemic cancer. LMD causes infiltration of the leptomeninges which consists of the arachnoid, subarachnoid space, and pia mater. LMD occurs in approximately 5% of patients with solid tumors [1, 2]. In autopsy series up to 20% of patients with cancer may have undiagnosed LMD [3–9]. The most common malignancies causing LMD include lymphoma, leukemia, breast cancer, lung cancer, and melanoma [9–11].

Neoplastic cells can disseminate throughout the central nervous system (CNS). A multitude of symptoms and complications may arise from associated compression upon the brain parenchyma or direct invasion, vascular involvement leading to ischemia, disruption of the blood–brain barrier, cranial nerve involvement, and impairment of CSF flow [12]. These symptoms include seizures, headache, nausea and vomiting, somnolence, cranial nerve deficits, visual disturbances including diplopia, hearing loss, back and radicular pain including cauda equina syndrome, and psychiatric disorders [2, 13–15].

The incidence of LMD is increasing and this is likely related to improved diagnostic imaging techniques including MRI and therapies such as anaplastic lymphoma kinase (ALK) inhibitors, epidermal growth factor receptor (EGFR), tyrosine kinase inhibitors, and whole brain radiation [16]. These factors have led to a prolonged survival of patients with cancer and thus a greater opportunity to develop metastases and LMD [17]. The inability of chemotherapy to cross the blood–brain and blood–CSF barriers may also be associated with the increased incidence of LMD [17].

J. M. Debnam (✉) · T. L. Chi
Department of Neuroradiology, The University of Texas M. D. Anderson Cancer Center, Houston, TX, USA
e-mail: matthew.debnam@mdanderson.org; linda.chi@mdanderson.org

F. C. L. Wong (ed.), *Radiopharmaceuticals in the Management of Leptomeningeal Metastasis*, https://doi.org/10.1007/978-3-031-14291-8_2

Unfortunately, LMD is associated with a poor prognosis. Without treatment the median survival is 4–6 weeks. Despite a relative prolonged survival related to recent advances in radiation and chemotherapy, the overall survival after diagnosis has a median survival of 2–6 months [13, 18]. A longer survival may be associated with a younger age at diagnosis, controlled systemic disease, lack of focal neurological deficits or encephalopathy, a Karnofsky Performance Score (KPS) greater than 70, low levels of protein in the cerebrospinal fluid (CSF), and a paucity of extensive disease on imaging [19, 20].

Diagnosis

The initial evaluation of patients suspected of having LMD involves evaluating the CSF including laboratory assessment and cytology and a contrast enhanced MRI of the brain and spine [3, 10, 20]. The National Comprehensive Cancer Network criteria diagnosis of LMD requires one of the following three criteria: (1) cytologic demonstration of malignant cells in the CSF, (2) radiologic findings of LMD, or (3) clinical examination consisting of LMD and CSF laboratory findings including low glucose level and high protein and white blood cell counts in a patient with cancer [21]. An elevated CSF pressure (> 15 cm) may also be a predictor of LMD [16].

At best, CSF cytology is only 80–95% sensitive for diagnosing LMD. The adherence of tumor cells to the leptomeninges has been suggested as the cause of failure to detect LMD [9, 22, 23]. An initially negative CSF evaluation should be followed by at least one additional attempt. False-negative lumbar punctures and repeat attempts may result in a delayed diagnosis [24]. In these instances, suggestive clinical and radiological findings may support the diagnosis [25]. Rarely, leptomeningeal or brain biopsy may be necessary to provide the diagnosis, especially with an unknown primary malignancy [14].

Intrathecal chemotherapy necessitating repeat lumbar punctures may be a component of treatment of LMD. Alternatively, an Ommaya reservoir may be placed directly into the ventricular system [26, 27]. Administration of intrathecal chemotherapy via the Ommaya reservoir is preferred, as it ensures a more homogeneous distribution of chemotherapy over lumbar puncture [7, 28].

MR Imaging

When evaluating a patient for possible LMD, imaging the entire neuraxis, including the brain and spine, needs to be performed [20]. In the imaging assessment of patients with suspected LMD, a contrast enhanced T1-weighted magnetic resonance imaging (MRI) is superior to contrast enhanced CT for the detection of LMD [29, 30]. However, the sensitivity of MRI for detecting LMD is only modest, ranging between 53% and 79% [1, 31–33].

To obtain the MRI sequences, patients are placed in a magnetic field, and a radiofrequency pulse is used to stimulate hydrogen protons and elevate them to a higher energy state. The protons then return to their normal lower resting energy state, releasing electromagnetic energy. A coil receives this electromagnetic energy, and computer manipulation converts it into an image. The time for the hydrogen protons to return to their normal resting state is called the relaxation time. Depending on their chemical composition, tissues have different relaxation times and thus create different signals used for image formation.

Tumor cells can gain access to the CSF in several ways. The most common routes are likely hematogenous, through arachnoid vessels, or direct extension from the brain. Leptomeningeal spread of disease also disseminates from the choroid plexus with metastases spreading into the CSF or from dural-based metastasis [12]. Tumor cells may find sanctuary in the meninges and CSF compartment because many systemic chemotherapeutic agents fail to cross the intact blood–CSF barrier, and tumor cells may proliferate before the instillation of intrathecal chemotherapy.

On MRI, the most common imaging findings of LMD are leptomeningeal enhancement, as thin or thick linear or nodular, diffuse or complex patterns of enhancement with varying sizes. Sites of involvement include the cerebral convexities, basal cisterns, along the tentorium, and/or in the ependymal surfaces of the ventricular system [1, 10, 20, 30, 34, 35] (Fig. 2.1a, b). On imaging, leptomeningeal enhancement has been reported to mainly involve gravity dependent regions, predominately the parietal and occipital lobes and the posterior fossa [11, 36].

Another route of leptomeningeal spread of disease is from the cranial nerves (CN)s into the subarachnoid space (Fig. 2.1c, d) [12]. CN V is the largest of the CNs and expected to be susceptible to leptomeningeal seeding due to a larger surface area. The CN VII/VIII complex has a cisternal component and resides in the bony internal auditory canal. Enzmann et al. [36] reported that CSF within the internal auditory canal pulsates less than CSF within the adjacent cerebellopontine angle. This is suspected to be the cause for more reported leptomeningeal involvement of CN VII/VIII complex than CN V and CN III [11].

Parenchymal brain metastases have also been reported to be associated with LMD in 21–82% of cases of parenchymal metastases [11, 31–33, 37]. In the spine, LMD may also appear as thin or thick linear enhancement, nodular enhancement, or diffuse filling of the spinal canal with enhancing disease (Fig. 2.2) [20].

Enhancement on MRI may not always represent LMD and care should be taken to avoid misdiagnosing LMD. For example, thickened enhancement of the

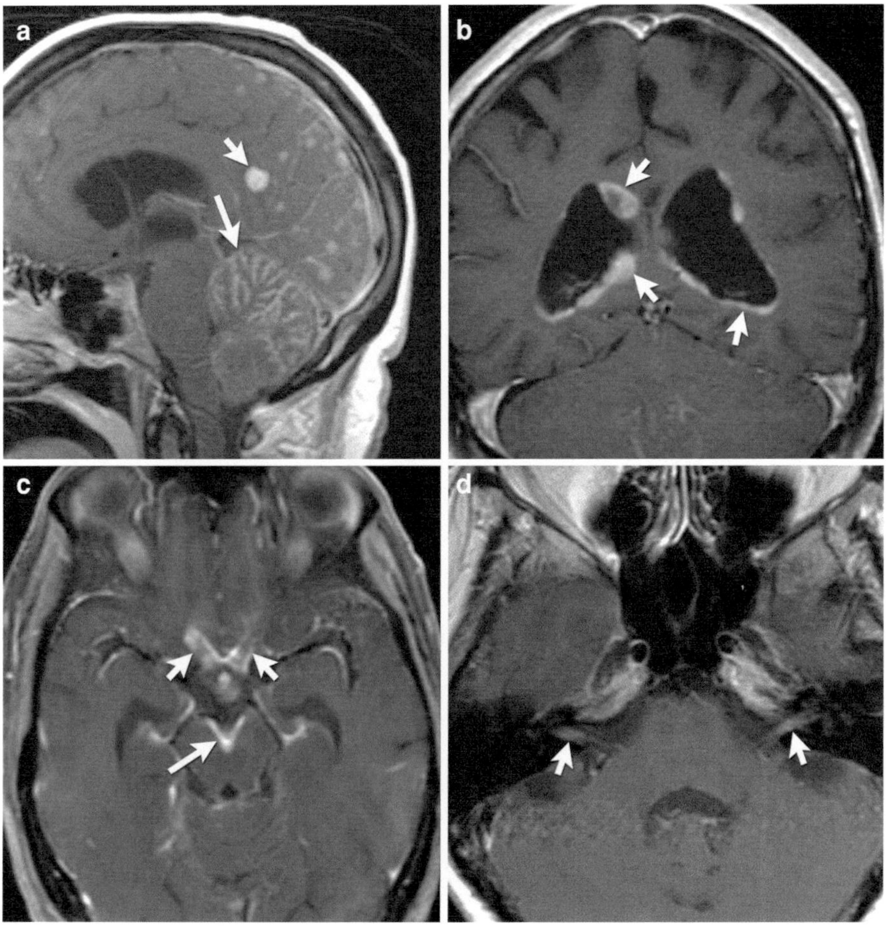

Fig. 2.1 MRI appearance of leptomeningeal disease in the intracranial compartment. (**a**) Sagittal T1 post-contrast, leptomeningeal disease in the cerebellar folia (large arrow) in a patient with parenchymal metastases (small arrow). (**b**) Coronal T1 post-contrast, nodular ependymal enhancement is present in the lateral ventricles (arrows). (**c**) Axial T1 post-contrast, leptomeningeal enhancement is seen in the interpeduncular cistern (large arrow) and lining the pre-chiasmatic optic nerves (small arrows). (**d**) Axial T1 post-contrast, leptomeningeal disease is present in the internal auditory canals involving bilateral 7th/8th cranial nerves (arrows)

meninges may occur after craniotomy [38, 39]. As a lumbar puncture may irritate the meninges and cause pachymeningeal enhancement, the procedure should be performed after the MRI [40]. Similarly, chemotherapy [41, 42] and radiation [43] can alter the pattern of leptomeningeal enhancement leading to imaging findings that appear as LMD or progressive disease.

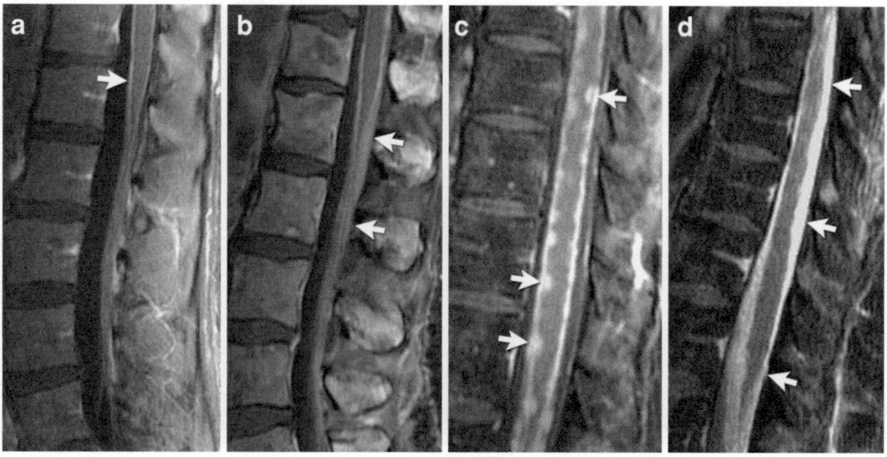

Fig. 2.2 MRI appearance of leptomeningeal disease in the spine. Sagittal T1 post-contrast MRI demonstrates leptomeningeal disease that is either (**a**) thin, (**b**) thick, (**c**) nodular), or (**d**) diffuse filling of the spinal canal (arrows)

CSF Flow Studies

In 30–70% of patients with LMD, obstructed flow of CSF occurs [44]. Failure to diagnose and treat an obstructive lesion is associated with the rapid development of neurological symptoms and death [45]. Prior to initiating intrathecal chemotherapy CSF flow studies can be used to detect regions prone to poor chemotherapy penetration and buildup [16]. Radioisotope cisternography, also referred to as CSF flow studies, is recommended for those patients considered for intra-CSF therapy, as disruption of CSF movement impacts intra-CSF drug delivery [16]. Compared to conventional MRI, CSF flow studies utilizing Indium-111 DTPA or Technetium-99m labeled albumin are more sensitive for detecting the location of obstructed flow (Fig. 2.3). Determining the location of an obstruction allows for palliative treatment with focused radiation therapy [46].

PET/CT

Positron emission tomography/computed tomography (PET/CT) is often used when staging cancer, especially hematologic malignancies, and to exclude osseous spinal metastases. The most common use of PET/CT technique involves the administration of ^{18}F-fluorodeoxyglucose (FDG), a cyclotron-produced radionuclide. FDG is taken up by cells in the same manner as serum glucose. Tumors have a high metabolic demand with increased glucose uptake. When FDG is taken up by tumor cells, the FDG will decay and emit two photons that are detected by a coincidence scanner. The resulting images reflect the concentration of FDG within the tumor. An

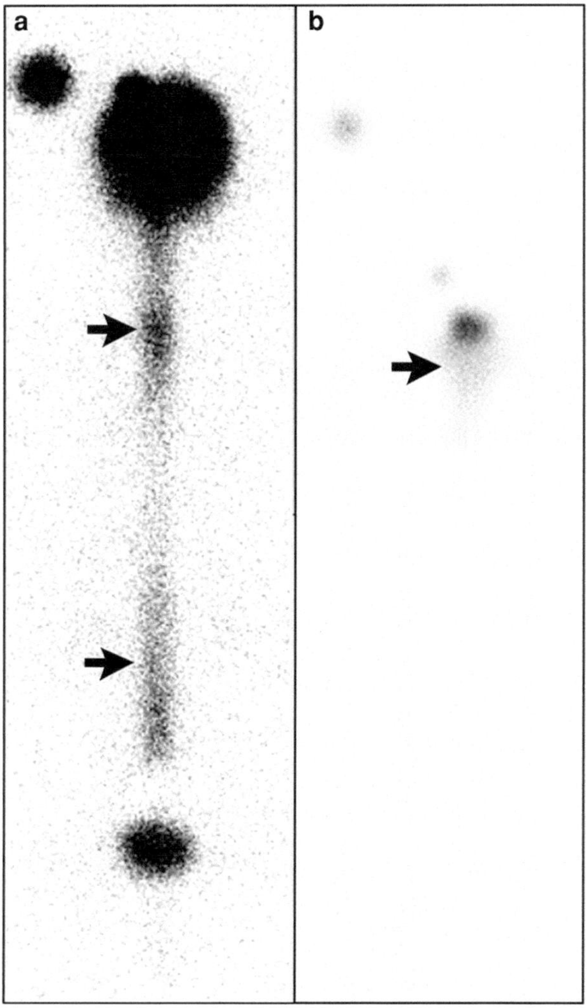

Fig. 2.3 Indium-111 DTPA cisternogram to evaluate patency of the spinal canal before intrathecal chemotherapy. (**a**) Patent cerebrospinal fluid space. Normal activity is demonstrated in the spinal canal at 4 h after injection consistent with patent cerebrospinal fluid flow (arrows). (**b**) Complete block. Lack of activity in the spinal canal beyond the cervical spine at 3 h after injection caused by an obstruction in the cerebrospinal fluid space (arrow)

important clinical use of PET/CT is also the detection of recurrent disease and distant metastasis. It should be noted that tumors of small size, low-grade, or containing significant necrosis may not be FDG-avid.

Several case reports have illustrated that both intracranial and extracranial LMD can be detected on ^{18}F-FDG PET/CT [47–49]. Other authors have suggested that PET may play a supportive role in the diagnosis of intracranial LMD using the radiotracers such as ^{18}F-FDG [50–52] or ^{11}C-methionine [53] if MRI and CSF results are inconclusive [50–52]. However, PET is not specific as inflammatory disorders such as infectious meningitis and neurosarcoidosis may show similar findings.

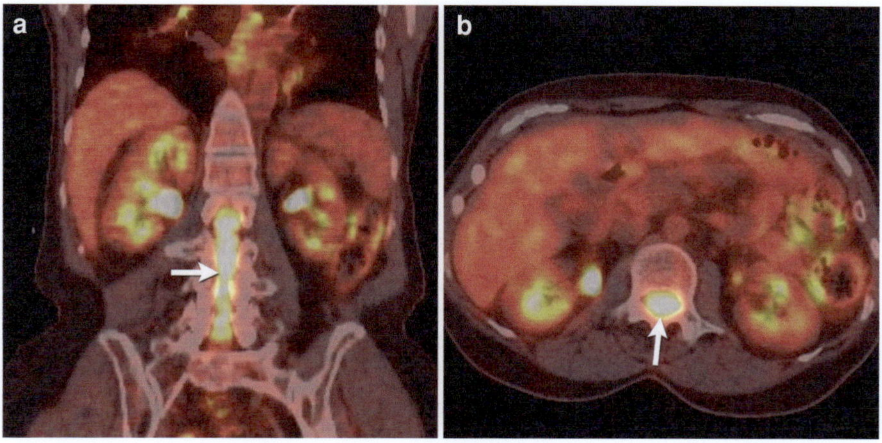

Fig. 2.4 Spinal leptomeningeal disease on an ^{18}FDG PET/CT: (**a**) Coronal and (**b**) axial PET/CT imaging demonstrate activity in the spinal canal in a patient with spinal leptomeningeal tumor spread (arrows)

Patients with the aforementioned hematologic and solid tumors could potentially have spinal LMD. Thus when interpreting PET/CT in these patients the spinal canal needs to be evaluated. The presence of LMD in the spinal canal characterized by ^{18}F-FDG activity (Fig. 2.4) has been described by several authors [24, 54]. When interpreting PET/CT, it should be noted that normal spinal cord ^{18}F-FDG activity decreases in the craniocaudal direction with a nadir near the conus medullaris at approximately the T11/T12 level [55]. No significant ^{18}F-FDG avidity should be present along the nerve roots along the cauda equine. In patients with cancer and FDG activity in the spinal canal, LMD needs to be excluded.

Response Assessment in Neuro-Oncology (RANO) Proposal for Response Criteria

The response to treatment of LMD was without standardized clinical or radiological criteria. Thus, the Response Assessment in Neuro-Oncology (RANO) working group developed a proposal for the initial and follow-up imaging surveillance to assess treatment response to be used in clinical trials across multiple institutions. Three standardized criteria were proposed including (1) the neurological examination, (2) CSF cytology or flow cytometry, and (3) radiological assessment. The clinical assessment and radiological examination should be obtained for the initial diagnosis followed by specified times, for example, after induction therapy is completed. The workgroup's recommendations for a standardized neurological examination and CSF analysis will be discussed in other sections.

Imaging recommendations are that patients be imaged on either a 1.5 or 3T MRI with imaging of both the brain and spine. To avoid difference in the magnetic field between various MRI units, patients should be imaged before treatment (baseline) and throughout surveillance on the same MRI scanner. As a lumbar puncture may lead to false positive intracranial enhancement the lumbar punctures should be performed after MR imaging [34, 40, 56].

The proposed MRI sequences of the brain include "post-contrast volumetric 3D T1 (magnetization-prepared rapid acquisition with gradient echo [MPRAGE] or spoiled gradient [SPGR]) post-contrast images with isotropic 1-mm voxels" that are subsequently reformatted in 3 orthogonal planes (axial, sagittal, and coronal) [20]. For imaging of the spine, "volumetric 3D T1 (MPRAGE or SPGR)" post-contrast imaging in the "sagittal plane with isotropic 1 mm voxels" is acquired and subsequently reformatted in 3 orthogonal planes but at 2–3 mm slice thickness without a gap [20].

As LMD may be seen on imaging as thin or thick linear or nodular, diffuse or complex patterns of enhancement with varying sizes, quantification of disease is often difficult [57–59]. Due to this variation in the presentation of LMD, the RANO workgroup recommends identifying and measuring nodules that are ≥5 × 10 mm in orthogonal diameter at the initial assessment and on serial follow-up while on treatment. Due to differences in MRI slice selection that may exclude a small part of a nodule, and adjacent linear enhancement that may be present, the RANO workgroup recommends excluding nodules that are <5 mm in size.

A scorecard for the radiological assessment has been proposed as outlined in Table 2.1 with five categories in the brain and five in the spine [20]. First, findings in each category are scored as present (1) or absent (0). Second, 5 representative measurable or non-measurable lesions as defined by dimensions of ≥5 × 10 mm in orthogonal diameter are recorded. Third, for follow-up examinations, lesions are recorded as "completely resolved (+3), definitely improved (+2), possibly improved (+1), unchanged (0), possibly worse (−1), definitely worse (−2), or new site of disease (−3)" [20]. For a complete response, the nodules need to completely disappear. Nodules that have decreased in size by >50% as measured by the sum of the product of the orthogonal diameter have "definitely improved," while those with a <50% decrease have "possibly improved." Any nodule with a >25% increase in the sum of the product of the orthogonal diameters is "definitely worse". The score for each category is added together to determine the total score [20].

The RANO workgroup members admit that their proposed criteria will "require prospective validation, is considered a work in progress, and likely will require future revisions as additional knowledge and use are gained." A more complete description of the RANO workgroup is available in the referenced article by Chamberlin et al. [20].

Table 2.1 Scorecard for radiologic assessment in leptomeningeal disease

MRI findings	Present (1) or absent (0) or non-evaluable (NE)	Dimensions of measurable nodules defined as >5 x 10 mm (orthogonal diameters)	Change from previous MRI (−3 to +3)
Brain			
Nodules (subarachnoid or ventricular)			
Leptomeningeal enhancement[a]			
Cranial nerve enhancement			
Hydrocephalus[b]			
Parenchymal (brain metastases)[b]			
Spine			
Nodules (subarachnoid)			
Leptomeningeal enhancement			
Nerve root enhancement			
Parenchymal (intramedullary metastases)[b]			
Epidural metastasis[b]			
Total score			

[b]Leptomeningeal enhancement may include pia, cerebellar folia, ventricular ependyma or cerebral sulci.
[b]Both hydrocephalus and parenchymal metastases, either brain or spine, are noted as present or absent but not used for LM response determination
Column 2: scored as 1 (present) or 0- (absent) or non-evaluable (NE). A maximum of 5 radiographic target lesions are selected from baseline imaging to score on follow-up
Column 3: scores each measurable lesion (at least 5 × 10 mm) excluding parenchymal as I (present with maximum orthogonal diameters) or 0 (absent)
Column 4: change from baseline or prior image scored as same (0), probable improvement (+1), definite improvement (+2), no evidence of disease

References

1. Clarke JL, Perez HR, Jacks LM, Panageas KS, Deangelis LM. Leptomeningeal metastases in the MRI era. Neurology. 2010;74:1449–54.
2. Kaplan JG, DeSouza TG, Farkash A, Shafran B, Pack D, Rehman F, Fuks J, Portenoy R. Leptomeningeal metastases: comparison of clinical features and laboratory data of solid tumors, lymphomas and leukemias. J Neurooncol. 1990;9:225–9.
3. Kesari S, Batchelor TT. Leptomeningeal metastases. Neurol Clin. 2003;21:25–66.
4. Little JR, Dale AJ, Okazaki H. Meningeal carcinomatosis. Clinical manifestations. Arch Neurol. 1974;30:138–43.
5. Olson ME, Chernik NL, Posner JB. Infiltration of the leptomeninges by systemic cancer. A clinical and pathologic study. Arch Neurol. 1974;30:122–37.
6. Posner JB, Chernik NL. Intracranial metastases from systemic cancer. Adv Neurol. 1978;19:579–92.
7. Shapiro WR, Young DF, Mehta BM. Methotrexate: distribution in cerebrospinal fluid after intravenous, ventricular and lumbar injections. N Engl J Med. 1975;293:161–6.
8. Theodore WH, Gendelman S. Meningeal carcinomatosis. Arch Neurol. 1981;38:696–9.

9. Wasserstrom WR, Glass JP, Posner JB. Diagnosis and treatment of leptomeningeal metastases from solid tumors: experience with 90 patients. Cancer. 1982;49:759–72.
10. Gleissner B, Chamberlain MC. Neoplastic meningitis. Lancet Neurol. 2006;5:443–52.
11. Debnam JM, Mayer RR, Chi TL, Ketonen L, Weinberg JS, Wei W, Groves MD, Guha-Thakurta N. Most common sites on MRI of intracranial neoplastic leptomeningeal disease. J Clin Neurosci. 2017;45:252–6.
12. Le Rhun E, Taillibert S, Chamberlain MC. Carcinomatous meningitis: leptomeningeal metastases in solid tumors. Surg Neurol Int. 2013;4:S265–88.
13. Chowdhary S, Chamberlain M. Leptomeningeal metastases: current concepts and management guidelines. J Natl Compr Cancer Netw. 2005;3:693–703.
14. Mack F, Baumert BG, Schafer N, Hattingen E, Scheffler B, Herrlinger U, Glas M. Therapy of leptomeningeal metastasis in solid tumors. Cancer Treat Rev. 2016;43:83–91.
15. Jaeckle KA. Neoplastic meningitis from systemic malignancies: diagnosis, prognosis and treatment. Semin Oncol. 2006;33:312–23.
16. Nayar G, Ejikeme T, Chongsathidkiet P, Elsamadicy AA, Blackwell KL, Clarke JM, Lad SP, Fecci PE. Leptomeningeal disease: current diagnostic and therapeutic strategies. Oncotarget. 2017;8:73312–28.
17. Omar AI, Mason WP. Leptomeningeal metastases. In: Neurologic complications of cancer. 2nd ed. New York: Oxford University Press, Inc; 2009. p. 240–81.
18. Groves MD. Leptomeningeal disease. Neurosurg Clin N Am. 2011;22:67–78.
19. Beauchesne P. Intrathecal chemotherapy for treatment of leptomeningeal dissemination of metastatic tumours. Lancet Oncol. 2010;11:871–9.
20. Chamberlain M, Junck L, Brandsma D, Soffietti R, Ruda R, Raizer J, Boogerd W, Taillibert S, Groves MD, Rhun EL, Walker J, van den Bent M, Wen PY, Jaeckle KA. Leptomeningeal metastases: a RANO proposal for response criteria. Neuro-Oncology. 2017;19:484–92.
21. Brem SS, Bierman PJ, Brem H, Butowski N, Chamberlain MC, Chiocca EA, DeAngelis LM, Fenstermaker RA, Friedman A, Gilbert MR, Hesser D, Junck L, Linette GP, Loeffler JS, Maor MH, Michael M, Moots PL, Morrison T, Mrugala M, Nabors LB, Newton HB, Portnow J, Raizer JJ, Recht L, Shrieve DC, Sills AK Jr, Vrionis FD, Wen PY. National Comprehensive Cancer Network, central nervous system. J Natl Compr Cancer Netw. 2011;9:352–400.
22. Glantz MJ, Cole BF, Glantz LK, Cobb J, Mills P, Lekos A, Walters BC, Recht LD. Cerebrospinal fluid cytology in patients with cancer: minimizing false-negative results. Cancer. 1998;82:733–9.
23. Lossos A, Siegal T. Spinal subarachnoid hemorrhage associated with leptomeningeal metastases. J Neuro-Oncol. 1992;12:167–71.
24. Papasozomenos H, Guha-Thakurta N, Mayer RR, Weinberg JS, Groves MD, Debnam JM. Association between 18F-FDG PET/CT and MRI appearance of spinal leptomeningeal disease before and after treatment at a tertiary referral center. J Solid Tumors. 2016;6:1–8.
25. Klein P, Haley EC, Wooten GF, VandenBerg SR. Focal cerebral infarctions associated with perivascular tumor infiltrates in carcinomatous leptomeningeal metastases. J Neuro-Oncol. 1992;12:167–71.
26. DeAngelis LM. Current diagnosis and treatment of leptomeningeal metastasis. J Neurooncol. 1998;38:245–52.
27. Lin N, Dunn IF, Glantz M, Allison DL, Jensen R, Johnson MD, Friedlander RM, Kesari S. Benefit of ventriculoperitoneal cerebrospinal fluid shunting and intrathecal chemotherapy in neoplastic meningitis: a retrospective, case-controlled study. J Neurosurg. 2011;115:730–6.
28. Dietemann JL, Correia Bernardo R, Bogorin A, Abu Eid M, Koob M, Nogueira T, Vargas MI, Fakhoury W, Zöllner G. Normal and abnormal meningeal enhancement: MRI features. J Radiol. 2005;86:1659–83.
29. Chamberlain MC, Sandy AD, Press GA. Leptomeningeal metastasis: a comparison of gadolinium-enhanced MR and contrast-enhanced CT of the brain. Neurology. 1990;40:435–8.
30. Collie DA, Brush JP, Lammie GA, Grant R, Kunkler I, Leonard R, Gregor A, Sellar RJ. Imaging features of leptomeningeal metastases. Clin Radiol. 1999;54:765–71.

31. Park JH, Kim YJ, Lee JO, Lee KW, Kim JH, Bang SM, Chung JH, Kim JS, Lee JS. Clinical outcomes of leptomeningeal metastasis in patients with non-small cell lung cancer in the modern chemotherapy era. Lung Cancer. 2012;76:387–92.
32. Rudnicka H, Niwińska A, Murawska M. Breast cancer leptomeningeal metastasis: the role of multimodality treatment. J Neuro-Oncol. 2007;84:57–62.
33. Morris PG, Reiner AS, Szenberg OR. Leptomeningeal metastasis from non-small cell lung cancer: survival and the impact of whole brain radiotherapy. J Thorac Oncol. 2012;7:382–5.
34. Pauls S, Fischer AC, Brambs HJ, Fetscher S, Höche W, Bommer M. Use of magnetic resonance imaging to detect neoplastic meningitis: limited use in leukemia and lymphoma but convincing results in solid tumors. Eur J Radiol. 2012;81:974–8.
35. Chamberlain MC. Comprehensive neuraxis imaging in leptomeningeal metastasis: a retrospective case series. CNS Oncol. 2013;2:121–8.
36. Enzmann DR, Rubin JB, DeLaPaz R, Wright A. Cerebrospinal fluid pulsation: benefits and pitfalls in MR imaging. Radiology. 1986;161:773–8.
37. Clatot F, Philippin-Lauridant G, Ouvrier MJ. Clinical improvement and survival in breast cancer leptomeningeal metastasis correlate with the cytologic response to intrathecal chemotherapy. J Neuro-Oncol. 2009;95:421–6.
38. Burke JW, Podrasky AE, Bradley WG Jr. Meninges: benign postoperative enhancement on MR images. Radiology. 1990;174:99–102.
39. Leach JL, Jones BV, Tomsick TA, Stewart CA, Balko MG. Normal appearance of arachnoid granulations on contrast-enhanced CT and MR of the brain: differentiation from dural sinus disease. AJNR Am J Neuroradiol. 1996;17(8):1523–32.
40. Mittl RL Jr, Yousem DM. Frequency of unexplained meningeal enhancement in the brain after lumbar puncture. AJNR Am J Neuroradiol. 1994;15(4):633–8.
41. Weiss HD, Walker MD, Wiernik PH. Neurotoxicity of commonly used antineoplastic drugs. N Engl J Med. 1974;291:75–81.
42. Jacob LA, Sreevatsa A, Chinnagiriyappa LK, Dasappa L, Suresh TM, Babu G. Methotrexate-induced chemical meningitis in patients with acute lymphoblastic leukemia/lymphoma. Ann Indian Acad Neurol. 2015;18:206–9.
43. Muscal JA, Jones JY, Paulino AC, Bertuch AA, Su J, Woo SY, Mahoney DH Jr, Chintagumpala M. Changes mimicking new leptomeningeal disease after intensity-modulated radiotherapy for medulloblastoma. Int J Radiat Oncol Biol Phys. 2009;73:214–21.
44. Chamberlain MC, Kormanik PA. Prognostic significance of 111indium-DTPA CSF flow studies in leptomeningeal metastases. Neurology. 1996;46:1674–7.
45. Chamberlain MC. Radioisotope CSF flow studies in leptomeningeal metastases. J Neurooncol. 1998;38:135–40.
46. Mason WP, Yeh SD, DeAngelis LM. 111Indium-diethylenetriamine pentaacetic acid cerebrospinal fluid flow studies predict distribution of intrathecally administered chemotherapy and outcome in patients with leptomeningeal metastases. Neurology. 1998;50:438–44.
47. Grande ML, Rayo JI, Serrano J, Infante JR, Garcia L, Duran C, Gomez-Caminero F. Leptomeningeal carcinomatosis as only pathological finding at FDG-PET/CT in case of tumor marker elevation in breast cancer. Indian J Nucl Med. 2014;29:53–4.
48. Tripathi M, Jain N, Jaimini A, Garg G, D'souza MM, Sharma R, Grover RK, Mondal A. Demonstration of diffuse leptomeningeal metastasis in a treated case of medulloblastoma with F-18 FDG PET/CT. Clin Nucl Med. 2009;34:530.
49. Intriago B, Danús M, Añaños M, Trampal C, Montero M, Calvo N. 18F-FDG PET detection of spinal leptomeningeal metastases from cerebral glioblastoma multiforme. Eur J Nucl Med Mol Imaging. 2011;38:1392.
50. Short RG, Bal S, German JP, Poelstra RJ, Kardan A. Potential of F-18 PET/CT in the detection of leptomeningeal metastasis. Neuroradiol J. 2014;27:685–9.
51. Carra BJ, Clemenshaw MN. Intracranial leptomeningeal carcinomatosis from breast cancer detected on 18F-FDG PET. J Nucl Med Technol. 2015;43:227–8.

52. Ortapamuk H, Demir MK. Intracranial leptomeningeal carcinomatosis in three cases from breast cancer demonstrated on F-18 fluorodeoxyglucose positron emission tomography/computerized tomography. Indian J Nucl Med. 2017;32:16–8.
53. Padma MV, Jacobs M, Kraus G, Collins M, Dunigan K, Mantil J. 11C-methionine PET imaging of leptomeningeal metastases from primary breast cancer—a case report. J Neuro-Oncol. 2001;55:39–44.
54. Komori T, Delbeke D. Leptomeningeal carcinomatosis and intramedullary spinal cord metastases from lung cancer: detection with FDG positron emission tomography. Clin Nucl Med. 2001;26:905–7.
55. Bhatt G, Li XF, Jain A, Sharma VR, Pan J, Rai A, Rai SN, Civelek AC. The normal variant 18F FDG uptake in the lower thoracic spinal cord segments in cancer patients without CNS malignancy. Am J Nucl Med Mol Imaging. 2013;10:317–25.
56. Chamberlain MC, Kormanik P, Jaeckle KA, Glantz M. 111Indiumdiethylenetriamine pentaacetic acid CSF flow studies predict distribution of intrathecally administered chemotherapy and outcome in patients with leptomeningeal metastases. Neurology. 1999;52:216–7.
57. Quijano S, Lopez A, Manuel SJ, Panizo C, Debén G, Castilla C, Antonio García-Vela J, Salar A, Alonso-Vence N, González-Barca E, Peñalver FJ, Plaza-Villa J, Morado M, García-Marco J, Arias J, Briones J, Ferrer S, Capote J, Nicolás C, Orfao A, Spanish Group for the Study of CNS Disease in NHL. Identification of leptomeningeal disease in aggressive B-cell non-Hodgkin's lymphoma: improved sensitivity of flow cytometry. J Clin Oncol. 2009;27:1462–9.
58. Kraan J, Gratama JW, Haioun C, Orfao A, Plonquet A, Porwit A, Quijano S, Stetler-Stevenson M, Subira D, Wilson W. Flow cytometric immunophenotyping of cerebrospinal fluid. Curr Protoc Cytom. 2008;Chapter 6:Unit 6.25.
59. Nayak L, Fleisher M, Gonzalez-Espinosa R, Lin O, Panageas K, Reiner A, Liu CM, Deangelis LM, Omuro A. Rare cell capture technology for the diagnosis of leptomeningeal metastases in slide tumors. Neurology. 2013;80:1598–605.

Chapter 3
Radionuclides in the Diagnosis and Therapy in Neuro-Oncology

Rodolfo Núñez

Introduction

Brain tumors are considered those that primarily arise from either the brain parenchyma or the ones that are metastatic originating from other organs in the body. Brain metastasis accounts for significantly more than one-half of brain tumors, with up to 30–40% of cancer patients developing brain metastasis at some point during the course of their disease. The most common sites are lung, melanoma, renal, breast, and colorectal cancer. According to the American Cancer Society, in 2021, approximately 24,530 malignant tumors of the brain or spinal cord were diagnosed with 18,600 deaths [1]. Tumors of the brain and the other parts of the nervous system are the leading cause of cancer death among males less than 40 years of age and females aged less than 20 years.

Gliomas, the most fatal type of primary brain tumor, account for roughly 45–50% of all primary brain tumors, followed by meningiomas, which account for nearly 15% of all primary brain neoplasms. The incidence of the other forms of primary brain tumors is lower. Astrocytoma, oligodendroglioma, choroid plexus tumors, ependymal tumors, and embryonal tumors are among the several types of gliomas. Brain tumors are divided into four categories based on histopathologic characteristics, with grade 1 representing benign features and grade 4 indicating the most malignant tumors, according to the WHO Classification of Tumors of the Central Nervous System (CNS) 2016 [2].

Histologic analysis, which requires tissue biopsy of brain neoplasms, is indispensable for tumor grading. The fundamental problems of tumor grading remain the potential complications during and after the surgery, as well as the intrusive nature of tissue sampling. The introduction of novel technologies, such as molecular sequencing, novel tracers, and imaging techniques, has recently opened up the possibility of

R. Núñez (✉)
Tufts Medical Center, Boston, MA, USA
e-mail: rnunez1@tuftsmedicalcenter.org

F. C. L. Wong (ed.), *Radiopharmaceuticals in the Management of Leptomeningeal Metastasis*, https://doi.org/10.1007/978-3-031-14291-8_3

noninvasively identifying the molecular features and grading of neoplastic tissues. Positron emission tomography (PET), is a medical imaging modality that uses a variety of radiotracers, which has the potential to be used as a supplemental imaging technique in clinical practice. Standard therapies include chemotherapy, radiation, surgical resection, and stereotactic radiosurgery (SRS). Prognosis estimation for nervous system neoplasms is a difficult task that remains unsatisfactory, especially for individuals with metastatic tumors. Patients with and without treatment have median survival rates of only 3–21 and 12 months, respectively. Glioblastomas are the most lethal of primary brain tumors. High molecular heterogeneity among glioblastoma phenotypes has been discovered using high throughput molecular and genomic methods, which are the main contributors to treatment failures and poor prognosis in these patients. Given the noninvasive nature of neuroimaging modalities, identifying an imaging prognostic indicator which can be correlated with tumor histopathologic grades, molecular characteristics, or clinical outcome of the disease is critical for disease prognosis and patient care. PET imaging using novel radiotracers has shown promise in tumor grading and molecular characterization.

Several important aspects of brain neoplasms evaluation during the clinical course of the disease rely heavily on neuroimaging. These include precise anatomic localization, tumor grading, delineation of tumor extent and margins for presurgical or radiotherapeutic planning, selection of ideal biopsy site, identification of vital structures involved, early response assessment, differentiation of tumor recurrence from reactive changes after therapy, and prognostication. However, tissue biopsies are still used to get the final diagnosis. In a typical clinical environment, MRI allows for the visualization of anatomic features. Magnetic resonance spectroscopy (MRS) evaluates the concentration of metabolites within tissues, while diffusion tensor imaging (DTI) assesses brain tumors by mapping the white matter. The use of functional MRI (fMRI) with the blood oxygen level dependent (BOLD) approach gives a functional map for each patient, which aids surgical planning and prevents unintended collateral damage to important brain regions during surgery and radiation.

Because of its good soft-tissue contrast, high spatial resolution, and broad availability, contrast-enhanced conventional MRI is the diagnostic method of choice for patients with primary and secondary (metastatic) brain cancers.

Because of its capacity to create surrogate endpoints (e.g., MRI features consistent with tumor development) that can be associated with patient outcomes, MRI is also an important part of many brain tumor therapy trials. However, it has a low specificity for neoplastic tissue, making it difficult to distinguish between cancer and nonneoplastic lesions, delineate tumor extent, particularly non-enhancing tumor sections, and distinguish treatment-related alterations from tumor relapse. PET imaging with multiple radiolabeled molecules has been investigated during the past decades to overcome the limits of conventional MRI, despite a constantly expanding repertoire of advanced MRI techniques. In this regard, the PET task force of the Response Assessment in Neuro-Oncology (RANO) working group, has stressed that the remarkably increased therapeutic value of radiolabeled amino acids (amino acid PET) compared to standard MRI for gliomas justifies its widespread clinical usage [3]. PET imaging has been used to solve a myriad of diagnostic problems in recent years (e.g., noninvasive grading in primary brain tumors, recognition of molecular markers, detection of tumor portions with higher malignant grade, and evaluation of prognosis in newly diagnosed and untreated brain tumors). The following three indications for PET imaging are of particular clinical interest for neuro-oncologists and medical professionals involved in the diagnosis and care of patients with brain tumors: the identification of neoplastic tissue, including the delineation of tumor extent for further diagnostic and therapeutic management, and the differentiation of treatment-related changes from normal changes.

In May 2016, the World Health Organization (WHO) announced a revised classification for CNS malignancies as an update to the 2007 edition, based on advances in diagnostic tools. For the first time, the WHO has used molecular parameters in addition to histology, resulting in the dismissal of a number of entities that are no longer thought to have diagnostic or biological value, as well as the designation of newly recognized neoplasms that should aid in the development of more effective targeted therapies. However, today's diagnostic and treatment techniques have a number of important limitations, some of which are particularly relevant to CNS malignancies. Because the techniques for acquiring biopsy samples or resections are intrusive and come with the danger of injuring healthy (neuronal) structures, the amount of (viable) tumor material for ex vivo analysis is usually restricted. In addition, since MRI is frequently conclusive, not every patient with a newly diagnosed CNS tumor undergoes a biopsy or resection. Moreover, quite frequently just parts of the main tumor are collected, leaving (remote) metastases untreated. Furthermore, tumor material is usually only collected once or twice during the course of the disease, usually at the time of diagnosis and/or disease progression, or in rare cases from post-mortem autopsy. These constraints make it difficult to conduct a complete investigation of both spatial and temporal tumor heterogeneity, as well as treatment effects across time, potentially leading to misclassification and limiting the development of medicines that can circumvent all (adapting) carcinogenic processes. As a result, noninvasive techniques for studying cancer biology in vivo, particularly for CNS malignancies, are greatly needed. Molecular imaging techniques, particularly nuclear techniques like positron emission tomography (PET), have been developed in recent years which combine diagnostic and theranostic applications to directly integrate molecular biology with molecular diagnosis and molecular targeted therapy. This chapter will review some of the major advancements on a number of levels, with a particular focus on the added value in the challenging field of neuro-oncology, where PET imaging cannot only serve as a sensitive diagnostic tool for noninvasive studies of tumor characteristics at multiple sites over time but also as an in vivo theranostic tool for drug development and delivery.

The diagnostic imaging arsenal has vastly improved in recent decades, spanning from computed tomography (CT) and magnetic resonance imaging (MRI) through single-photon emission computerized tomography (SPECT) and PET. Hybrid (i.e., fused) methods, including SPECT-CT, PET-CT, and most recently PET-MR imaging, have been developed during the 1990s and 2000s allowing for combined anatomical and functional studies. Molecular imaging techniques (i.e., SPECT and PET) offer unique opportunities to study the molecular biology of disease

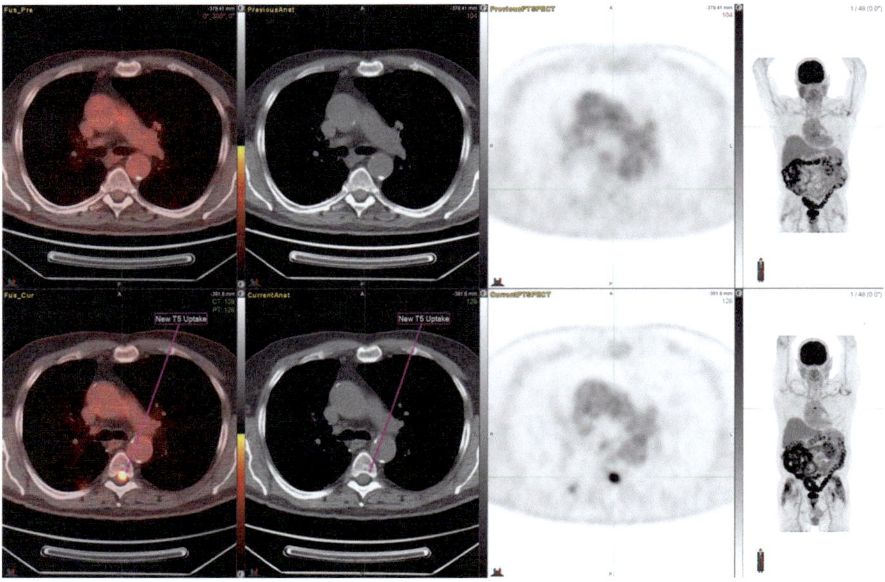

Fig. 3.1 A 72-year-old man with lung cancer. From left to right are the 18F-FDG PET/CT fused, CT, PET, and volume rendered images. Above is the negative 18F-FDG PET/CT scan from October 2020. Below are the images of the 18F-FDG PET/CT scan from January 2021, which shows (arrow) the leptomeningeal site of disease at the level of T5 vertebra. An MRI of the thoracic spine done a few days later was consistent with leptomeningeal disease. (Image courtesy of Dr. F. Wong from MD Anderson Cancer Center, Houston, Texas)

noninvasively by employing radioactive ligands, or tracers, to bind and identify specific targets. SPECT and PET both have the exquisite sensitivity to examine target expression and binding at the picomolar level. In addition, PET imaging has a higher sensitivity, spatial resolution, and quantification capability, Fig. 3.1.

The advent of improved whole-body and more recently digital PET scanners represents a major step forward in this regard, since their broader field of view and digital technology boosts sensitivity, resulting in greater image quality and more accurate assessment of tracer biodistribution at low count rates. Accordingly, PET imaging is gaining favor over SPECT for the reasons stated above. PET tracers can now be utilized in a diagnostic environment to detect the effect of therapy and to do primary staging of CNS malignancies, including assessing how radioactive or non-radioactive targeted medications would behave (i.e., radiopharmaceuticals or pharmaceuticals, respectively) in the treatment of brain tumors.

Small chemical compounds, biologicals such as small peptides, antibodies, antibody fragments, and antibody conjugates, nanoparticles, and effector cells are among the pharmaceuticals utilized for theranostic PET [4]. Targeted medications are initially labeled with a positron-emitting radionuclide for use in a diagnostic role to examine biodistribution and allow dosimetric analysis to estimate radiation exposure to tumors and important normal organs in the case of radiopharmaceuticals. If the results of these tests are positive, the same targeted medication is given, but this time with an alpha or beta particle-emitting radionuclide to induce localized single and/or double-strand DNA breaks and cell death. In comparison to beta-emitting radionuclides, alpha-emitting radionuclides have a much higher relative biological effectiveness. PET tracers used for therapeutic purposes are referred in the literature, with interchangeably terms of "companion diagnostics" or "theranostics," though the term "theranostic" has become increasingly reserved in recent years for cases in which a single molecular entity is used for both diagnostic and therapeutic purposes [5]. To achieve the best possible prediction of theranostic PET tracers, it is critical that the diagnostic and therapeutic compounds behave similarly in vivo (i.e., biodistribution), which necessitates the use of appropriate radionuclides and radiolabeling processes. The development and manufacture of PET tracers is a complex endeavor which necessitates a tailored strategy. First, a target that is known to be particularly overexpressed by the tumor should be chosen. Second, the chosen ligand (i.e., the pharmaceutical of interest) must be selective for the target and bind with sufficient affinity to allow detection in comparison with normal tissue background tracer uptake. Third, the radionuclide's physical half-life should be compatible with the targeted pharmaceutical's biological half-life and pharmacokinetic properties in the body. For instance, amino acids and tyrosine kinase inhibitors (TKIs) are examples of fast kinetic biological or tiny chemical substances that should be conjugated with short half-life radionuclides. By contrast, monoclonal antibodies and other slow-kinetic ligands necessitate the use of longer-lived PET isotopes. The most commonly used PET isotopes have a short half-life (e.g., 2 min for oxygen-15 [15O], 10 min for nitrogen-13 [13N], 20 min for carbon-11 [11C], 68 min for gallium-68 [68Ga], and 110 min for fluorine-18 [18F]), necessitating the use of a local hospital-based cyclotron, as well as quick tracer production and clinical supply. Conversely, PET isotopes with a long half-life (e.g., 12.7 h for copper-64 [64Cu], 78.4 h for zirconium-89 [89Zr], and 4.2 days for iodine-124 [124I]) may not have these logistical problems, but they do come with a greater radiation burden that should be taken into account, Table 3.1. The in vivo performance (i.e., actual binding, accumulation, and retention at the target site) of each newly developed diagnostic or theranostic PET tracer should be thoroughly validated, especially in the field of neuro-oncology, because CNS tumors have high inter- and intratumoral heterogeneity in regard to BBB and blood–tumor barrier permeability. They also have active efflux mechanisms as well as a tumor microenvironment that has been found to reduce the efficacy of therapeutic drugs. Quantification of tracer tissue uptake is critical for arriving at objective performance metrics. Rather than completing genuine quantification based on metabolite analysis and extensive compartmental and kinetic modeling, semi-quantitative parameters are commonly utilized. The ratio of activity per unit volume of a region of interest (ROI) to activity per unit whole-body volume is determined for semi-quantitative analysis, resulting in a standardized uptake value (SUV). The use of SUVs facilitates the comparison of radiopharmaceutical uptake between tumor and healthy tissue, as well as between patients. When compared to healthy tissue SUVs (i.e., background), non-specific tracers have (relatively) low tumor SUVs, resulting in low tumor-to-background ratios (TBRs) and limited

Table 3.1 List of most commonly used imaging radionuclides and their physical characteristics

Radionuclide	Abbreviation	Half-life	Emission	$Energy_{max}$ (KeV)	Method of Production
Indium-111	^{111}In	2.8 days	Auger/gamma	247/173	Cyclotron
Iodine-123	^{123}I	13 h	EC/gamma	159	Cyclotron
Technetium-99m	^{99m}Tc	6 h	IT/gamma	140	Mo^{99} Generator
Fluorine-18	^{18}F	110 min	Beta+ (positron)/EC	511	Cyclotron
Carbon-11	^{11}C	20 min	Beta+(positron)	511	Cyclotron
Gallium-68	^{68}Ga	68 min	Beta+ (positron)/EC	511	Ge^{68} Generator
Copper-62	^{62}Cu	9.7 min	Beta+ (positron)/EC	511	Cyclotron
Copper-64	^{64}Cu	12 h	Beta+ (positron)/EC	511	Cyclotron
Oxigen-15	^{15}O	2 min	Beta+(positron)	511	Cyclotron
Nitrogen-13	^{13}N	10 min	Beta+(positron)	511	Cyclotron
Zirconium-89	^{89}Zr	78.4 h	Beta+(positron)/EC	511	Cyclotron
Iodine-131	^{131}I	8.1 days	Beta−/gamma	364	Fission
Iodine-124	^{124}I	4.2 days	Beta+(positron)	511	Cyclotron

contrast. By contrast, to varying degrees, TBRs are high with tumor selective tracers. The next sections offer a current overview of the most important conventional nuclear medicine, SPECT and PET traces used for diagnostic and theranostic applications in neuro-oncology.

Conventional Nuclear Medicine Studies

CSF is a plasma ultrafiltrate present in the brain's ventricles, as well as the subarachnoid spaces of the cranium and spine. It provides critical functions to the brain such as feeding, waste removal, and protection. Adult CSF is a total volume of 150 mL, including 125 mL in the subarachnoid spaces and 25 mL in the ventricles. The principal source of CSF is the choroid plexus, with other sources playing a less well-defined role. Its secretion varies from person to person in the adult population, but it typically ranges from 400 to 600 mL every day. Continuous CSF secretion allows to complete CSF renewal four to five times every 24-h period. CSF flow studies with radionuclides, also known as radionuclide cisternography, give a safe physiologic assessment of the functional architecture of the CSF spaces. The ventricular system and the subarachnoid area that surrounds the brain and spinal cord both circulate CSF. The CSF is absorbed in the superior sagittal sinus through the Pacchionian granulations of the pia arachnoid villi [6].

Conventional nuclear medicine imaging for the evaluation of cerebrospinal fluid flow, although being a fairly old technique is still being used and has considerable value for the evaluation of leptomeningeal disease, assessment of cerebrospinal shunt patency, and interrogation of the Ommaya reservoir. Injections of radiotracers into the CSF space are only done if they are acceptable for intrathecal administration, aseptic, and pyrogen-free. The carrier molecule diethylenetriamine pentaacetic acid (DTPA) is considered an excellent choice as carrier molecule, since it is not immediately metabolized, tightly binds the radiotracer, is nonlipophilic and it is not readily absorbed from the CSF space until it reaches the arachnoid villi. Compared with Tc-99m, indium-111 (In-111) has poorer imaging characteristics, with two relatively high photopeaks of 245 keV (94% abundance) and 171 keV (90%). Nevertheless, in situations where imaging will be carried out over more than a few hours, indium-111 (In-111) is the more suitable radiolabel because of its 2.8-day half-life. Because of the longer half-life and higher photon energy, the amount of the radiopharmaceutical that can be administered is lower when using In-111 compared with a similar compound labeled with Tc-99m, and this differential can affect sensitivity. However, Tc-99m DTPA is favored for shorter CSF shunt studies, although In-111 DTPA is commonly utilized for cisternography. For instance, a CSF leak will be more easily seen during imaging with Tc-99m DTPA. However, if pledgets are going to be placed in the nose to identify leaks that are not easily visible, it may be preferable to use In-111 to facilitate assessment of the pledgets over longer period of time for evidence of the leak [7].

CSF flow studies allow for the detection of anomalies in the flow of CSF that are often missed by conventional neuroradiographic imaging. The injection of the radiopharmaceuticals is done normally by lumbar puncture or less frequently by intraventricular access. A CSF flow block is defined as the failure of a radionuclide to show in a specific CSF compartment. CSF flow abnormalities are most common at the base of the brain, spinal subarachnoid region, notably at the level of the conus medullaris and cauda equina, or over the cerebral convexities in approximately 50% of patients with leptomeningeal metastases (LM). CSF flow investigations are more sensitive than MR spine, CT myelography, or cranial MR or CT imaging in revealing compartmentalization of CSF channels. The dynamic nature of 111 Indium-DTPA CSF flow investigations, where the radionuclide is passively carried by CSF bulk flow in a physiologic antegrade way, may explain this increased sensitivity. 111 Indium-DTPA CSF flow studies in both adults and children with leptomeningeal metastases, detects CSF compartmentalization, which is a critical issue in intra-CSF medication delivery. Furthermore, 111 indium-DTPA CSF flow investigations visualize intracranial compartmentalization and spinal subarachnoid block better than comparative neuroradiographic studies. However, in radionuclide CSF flow studies (also called radionuclide ventriculography) the information provided is limited to CSF compartmentalization and does not include bulky leptomeningeal disease, which is better addressed by CT Myelography (CY-M) or SpineMR (S-MR). Furthermore, CT-M and S-MR are clearly superior to radionuclide CSF flow studies in identifying epidural spinal cord compression and intraparenchymal spinal cord metastases, two rare consequences of metastatic systemic disease that require emergency treatment, Fig. 3.1 [8]. Despite these limitations, it provides the most accurate radiographic assessment of CSF circulation, being abnormal in 30–40% of individuals with leptomeningeal metastasis. Treatment of CSF flow blocks with involved-field irradiation and subsequent re-establishment of normal CSF flow, as demonstrated by posttreatment 111 indium-DTPA CSF flow tests, ensures both homogeneous chemotherapeutic distribution and treatment of the entire neuraxis. Moreover, CSF compartmentalization appears to be a mechanism of leptomeningeal metastatic relapse, preventing adequate intra-CSF medication distribution [9].

SPECT and PET Radiopharmaceuticals in Neuro-Oncology

SPECT Radiopharmaceuticals

Two main types of SPECT tracers are employed in brain tumor imaging. The first group includes tracers that rely on brain perfusion and BBB disruption (perfusion tracers), whereas the second uses metabolite imaging, Table 3.2. Although there are several options available, 99mTc-based radiotracers are often favored due to their higher photon flux, superior resolution, and lower delivered radioactive doses. However, their sensitivity is reduced because of their removal from tumor cells by p-glycoproteins.

201Tl, 99mTc sestamibi, and 99mTc tetrofosmin are examples of perfusion-based tracers, in which local radiotracer uptake is proportional to local perfusion. When employed to assess radiation necrosis, these tracers rely on higher local perfusion in the tumor. The breakdown of the BBB is required for 99mTc-glucoheptonate uptake. These tracers are less sensitive and specific than metabolite-specific tracers,

Table 3.2 SPECT radiopharmaceuticals in neuro-oncology

Radiopharmaceutical	Target	Mechanism
99mTc-MIBI	Regional blood flow and cellular viability	Mitochondrial uptake and retention
99mTc-Tetrophosmine	Regional blood flow and cellular viability	Mitochondrial uptake and retention
201Tl (chloride)	Regional blood flow and cellular viability	Cell membrane Na/K pump
99mTc-Methionine	Amino acid transport	Amino acid transporter system L
123I-IMT	Amino acid transport	Amino acid transporter system L
123I-VEGF-165	Angiogenesis	Targeting VEGF receptor 1 and VEGF receptor 2
123I-CLINDE	TSPO tracer	Targeting mitochondrial permeability transition pore
131I-TM-601	MMP2 receptor of tumor glioma cells	Targeting chloride channel receptor in glioma cells
123I-L19(scFv)2	Angiogenesis	Antibody mediated imaging

although they perform better with high-grade gliomas than low-grade gliomas. However, their use has all but disappeared with the widespread adoption of MRI. The second group of metabolite-based radiopharmaceuticals is more promising. Only the amino acid based radiotracers have been verified on a wider scale and found usage in routine clinical settings, despite the fact that many experimental radiotracers have been produced. 123I-alpha-methyl tyrosine (IMT) and 99mTc-methionine (MET) are two examples of neutral amino acid transporters that are both carried into cells (expressed in higher concentration in the tumors compared with the inflammatory and reactive processes). Although 123I-IMT and 99mTc-MET can be used to reliably grade tumors and distinguish recurrence from radiation necrosis, their usage in tiny lesions is limited due to low availability and sensitivity. The constraints are more technology-related than tracer-related. The spatial resolution (7 mm), sensitivity, and signal-to-noise ratio of SPECT and SPECT/CT are some of the limitations. In recurrent low grade glyomas (LGGs), these tracers are still superior to 18F-FDG PET/CT and MRI. As a result, they can be used as low-cost PET/CT imaging alternatives [10, 11].

One of the several SPECT radiopharmaceuticals which has been used in smaller clinical trials is [123I]iodo-VEGF-165. Ranier et al. used 123Iodine-labeled recombinant human VEGF165 (rhVEGF165) for brain SPECT scans on 23 patients with histopathologically confirmed primary brain tumors following intravenous injection. Grade IV glioma lesions demonstrated [123I]-VEGF uptake 18 h after the injection, whereas other brain tumors in grades II and III showed negative results. Tumor size did not differ significantly between VEGF positive and VEGF negative tumors. Patients with a T/N ratio of < 1.32 for [123I]-VEGF had significantly longer survival than those with a T/N ratio of ≥ 1.32. They reached the conclusion that [123I]-VEGF scintigraphy could be effective for evaluating tumor angiogenesis. Furthermore, 123I-VEGF scintigraphy may provide useful prognostic information in glioma patients [12].

Jensen et al. compared 123I]-iodo-CLINDE with FET PET in three patients with WHO grade 4 GBM. They concluded that the preliminary findings suggest that translocator protein (TSPO) brain imaging in GBM could be a valuable technique for predicting tumor growth and is less susceptible to changes in blood–brain barrier permeability than 18F-FET. To explore the clinical potential of TSPO imaging in GBM, including presurgical planning and radiotherapy, larger trials are needed [13].

TM-601 is a 36-amino-acid peptide that selectively binds to glioma cells but not normal brain parenchyma. Hockaday et al. published the results of biodistribution and toxicity from a phase I/II clinical trial of intracavitary 131I-TM-601 in adult patients with recurrent high-grade glioma. They evaluated imaging and biodistribution data from this trial to assess whether 131I-TM-601 might be useful in determining tumor extent. They concluded that the primary tumor extent can be accurately estimated using 131I-TM-601. Further customizing this radiopeptide with improved imaging isotopes could give a useful tool for detecting tumor extent and distinguishing between viable and necrotic tumor regions [14, 15].

In a study on 20 patients with different types of tumors including brain cancer, Santimaria et al. evaluated 123I- iodo-L19(scFv)2, which is a radiolabeled antibody fragment against the extra-domain (ED) B of fibronectin. They identified a strong and selective accumulation of 123 I-labeled L19(scFv)2 in a recurrent glioblastoma patient's tumor mass, which grew within the surgical cavity and nearby tissue. In a patient with a benign brain tumor (pilocytic astrocytoma) that could only be partially excised by brain surgery, there was no selective accumulation [16].

PET Radiopharmaceuticals

Most of the new radiopharmaceuticals developed over the last two decades for neuro-oncology have been for PET imaging. This is at least partially explained from the fact that PET imaging is a higher sensitivity imaging modality which facilitates accurate quantification and semi-quantification. In addition, currently, PET/CT can be considered a mainstream imaging modality, widely available, and well established in many countries. Moreover, the more recent introduction of dedicated PET/MRI scanners can be considered an additional incentive for this development of PET radiopharmaceuticals.

PET facilitates in patients with brain tumors to target metabolic and molecular processes that are essential for diagnosis, treatment, and prognosis which cannot be examined with anatomic computed tomography (CT) or magnetic resonance imaging (MRI), Table 3.3. Glucose metabolism, amino acid transport, proliferation, hypoxia, blood flow, and angiogenesis are among these biological processes which

Table 3.3 PET radiopharmaceuticals in neuro-oncology clinically used or as part of clinical research trials

Radiopharmaceutical	Target	Mechanism
18F-FDG	Glucose metabolism	Glucose transporter proteins (GLUT-1 and GLUT-3)
11C-Methionine	Amino acid transport	Amino acid cell membrane transporter proteins
18F-FET	Amino acid transport	Amino acid cell membrane transporter system L
18F-DOPA	Amino acid transport	Amino acid cell membrane transporter system L
18F-FACBC	Amino acid transport	Amino acid cell membrane transporter system L
18F-FGln	Glutamine metabolism	Amino acid transporter ASCT2
11C-AMT	Serotonin synthesis	Substrate of tryptophan hydroxylase
18F-FLT	Cellular proliferation	FLT is a substrate for thymidine kinase I (TK1)
18F-FMISO	Hypoxia imaging	Reductive metabolism followed by glutathione conjugation
62Cu-ATSM	Hypoxia imaging	Selectively reduced in hypoxic cells
15O-H2O	Cerebral flood flow	Free flow through cell membranes
13N-NH3	Cerebral flood flow	Cell membrane diffusion and conversion of ammonia to glutamine, glutamic acid, and carbamyl phosphate

Table 3.3 (continued)

Radiopharmaceutical	Target	Mechanism
89Zr-bevacizumab	Selective binding to VEGF-A	Immuno-imaging of angiogenesis
64Cu-VEGF	Selective binding to VEGFR-2	Angiogenesis
123I-VEGF	Selective binding to VEGFR-2	Angiogenesis
68Ga-DOTATATE	Somatostatin receptor 2	Somatostatin receptor imaging
68Ga-GaPSMA-11	PSMA transmembrane receptor	Small ligand receptor imaging
18F-DCFPyL	PSMA transmembrane receptor	Small ligand receptor imaging
89Zr-IAB2M	PSMA transmembrane receptor	Immuno-imaging of PSMA receptor
68Ga-DOTA-SP	NK-1 receptor	NK-1 receptor imaging
124I-L19SIP	Extracellular domain B of fibronectin	Immuno-imaging of angiogenesis
68Ga-Pentixafor	Chemokine receptor-4 (CXCR4)	Cyclic pentapeptide receptor imaging
11C-erlotinib	EGFR	TKI-mediated imaging
11C-PD153035	EGFR	TKI-mediated imaging
89Zr-DFO-nimotuzumab	EGFR	Immuno-imaging of EGFR
64Cu-DOTA-trastuzumab	HER2	Immuno-imaging of HER2
89Zr-pertuzumab	HER2	Immuno-imaging of HER2
11C-lapatinib	EGFR	TKI-mediated imaging
89Zr-nivolumab	PD-1	Immuno-imaging of PD-1
89Zr-atezolizumab	PD-L1	Immuno-imaging of PD-L1
18F-BMS-986192	PD-L1	Adnectin based imaging
89Zr-IAB22M2C	CD8 receptor	Cell receptor imaging
18F-CFA	Deoxycytidine kinase (dCK)	Targeting the deoxycytidine kinase
18F-FHBG	(HSV1-tk) gene	Imaging of gene transfer therapy
18F-AGI-5198	IDH mutant cells	Imaging of the mutant IDH enzyme
131-81C6	Tenascin	Immuno-imaging of tenascin

can be evaluated by PET tracers that have been studied in patients with gliomas and brain metastases. This section will give an overview of PET tracers used to image brain tumors, especially looking into what can be considered the main indications, namely: noninvasive grading, differential diagnosis, delineation of tumor extent, surgical and radiotherapy treatment planning, posttreatment surveillance, and prognostication.

Glucose Metabolism PET Tracers: FDG

18F-FDG is by far the most popular radiopharmaceutical for PET imaging in oncology. Moreover, some of the first applications of PET imaging started with the use of 18F-FDG in brain tumors, when several decades ago, it was clearly stablished the value of 18F-FDG in brain tumors and the direct relationship between the degree of 18F-FDG uptake and aggressiveness of the tumor [17, 18]. Moreover, although recently other PET radiopharmaceuticals have proven to have better results than 18F-FDG, due to its wider availability and lower price, it is still frequently used in routine clinical practice in neuro-oncology. This use has been further facilitated by the possibility, first, of co-registration of the PET and MRI images, or even sometimes, doing the combined study in a dedicated PET/MRI scanner, allowing a very precise delineation of tumor extension and infiltration on the different set of PET/MRI images. Second, by delayed acquisition of the PET images several hours after the injection of 18F-FDG well beyond the traditional 60 min incubation time, therefore facilitating tracer washout from the normal brain parenchyma and enhancing the relative uptake of 18F-FDG and the contrast of the tumor mass in relation to the lower activity in normal brain parenchyma [19]. 18F-FDG is still being used in routine clinical practice—acknowledging the limitations it has—for tumor delineation, differentiation of low from high-grade tumors, and assessments of response to therapy, Fig. 3.2.

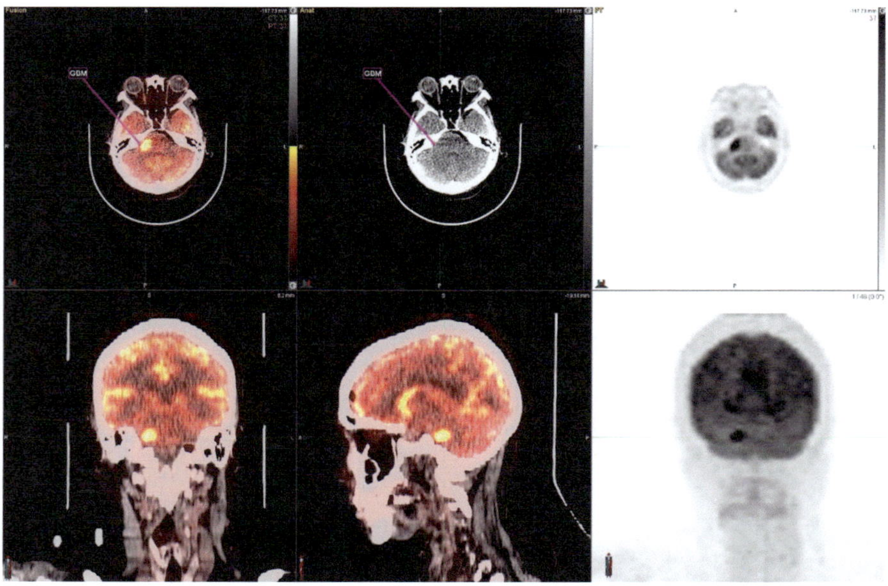

Fig. 3.2 18F-FDG PET/CT images of a 70-year-old woman found to have a 1.3 cm × 1.6 cm hypermetabolic lesion (arrows) with an SUV of 11.5 in the right cerebellopontine angle that was subsequently biopsied and confirmed to be a GBM. (Image courtesy of Dr. F. Wong from MD Anderson Cancer Center, Houston, Texas)

Amino Acid PET Tracers

In most CNS tumor forms, amino acid PET imaging shows enhanced cell metabolism and cell division due to overexpression of amino acid transporters.

The use of amino acid tracers over 18F-FDG is advantageous since amino acid uptake in normal brain tissue is relatively low, resulting in higher lesion contrast, with, for instance, tumor-to-background ratios (TBR) for 18F-DOPA of 2.3 +/ 0.51, compared to 1.03 +/ 0.64 for 18F-FDG [20]. Another advantage of amino acid tracers is that their uptake is independent of BBB permeability because the barrier itself contains amino acid transporters. This allows for the visualization of anaplastic regions even when contrast agents are not used on MRI and the BBB is considered to remain intact [21, 22]. PET imaging of amino acids has demonstrated to be useful for diagnostic purposes as well as planning for biopsy and surgical resection [23–25]. With significantly higher SUVs or TBRs in (recurrent) low-grade gliomas (LGG), high-grade gliomas (HGG), and brain metastases compared to lesions with pseudoprogression, amino acid tracers also perform particularly well in distinguishing early tumor progression from pseudoprogression (i.e., imaging changes that mimic a progressive tumor but are actually due to other causes, most commonly inflammation related to therapy) [26–28]. The capacity to discern pseudoprogression, or treatment-related alterations, is extremely useful in clinical practice since it helps to guide therapeutic decision-making [29].

11C-Methionine (11C-MET) was one of the earliest amino acid tracers employed [30]. The amino acid transporter LAT1 is responsible for 11C-Met absorption, which has been widely used to detect CNS cancers such as glioma, germinoma, CNS lymphoma, CNS metastases, meningioma, mixed neural/glial tumors, and central neurocytoma [31, 32]. Unlike 18F-FDG, 11C-MET can be used to track treatment response over time, as decreased 11C-MET uptake after therapy (i.e., surgery, chemo- or radiation, or a combination of these) has been linked to long-term survival [33], Figs. 3.3 and 3.4.

Next-generation amino acid tracers, including 18F-DOPA, 18F-FET, and 18F-FGln, have been tagged with fluorine-18 to avoid the practical challenges associated with carbon-11's short half-life. 18F-DOPA and18F-FET are also taken up by the tumor via amino acid transporters on the cell surface (i.e., LAT1 and LAT2, respectively), but unlike 11C-MET, they are not integrated into proteins [34, 35]. Both 18F-DOPA and 18F-FET demonstrate selective uptake in tumor cells, yielding similar predictive values for diagnosing CNS malignancies as 11C-MET, Figs. 3.5 and 3.6.

Furthermore, it has been demonstrated that in the vast majority of cases, the metabolically active tumor burden as measured by amino acid PET extends far beyond the volume of MRI contrast enhancement, which is important for treatment planning. For this indication, 11C-MET, 18F-FET, and 18F-FDOPA appear to be equally informative. However, in 20–30% of grade II gliomas there is no amino acid uptake [36–38]. As a result, a negative amino acid PET does not necessarily rule out glioblastoma [21].

Amino acid PET is also useful for distinguishing treatment-related alterations from tumor relapse. The distinction of radiation injury from tumor relapse in glioma

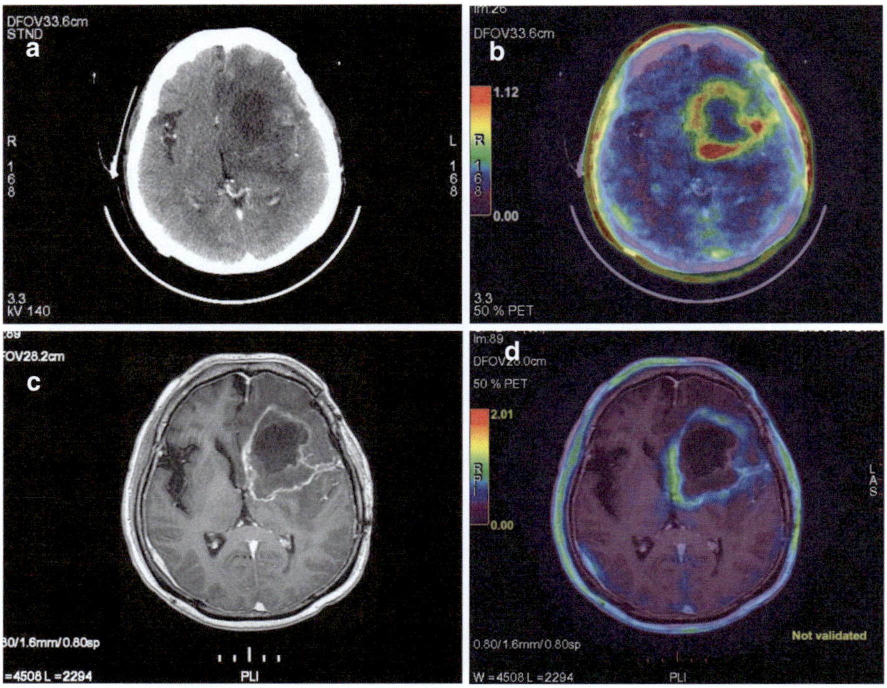

Fig. 3.3 A 35-year-old patient with diagnosis of glioblastoma multiform (GBM). (**a**) Contrast-enhanced TC of the brain, with nodular lesions, perilesional edema, and central necrosis in the left frontal lobe. (**b**) PET/CT of the brain with 11C-MET shows abnormal radiotracer uptake in the left frontoparietal lesion, with a SUVmax of 4.2 and an T/NT ratio of 2.3. (**c**) Contrast-enhanced T1 MRI of the brain shows the left frontal lobe lesion with enhancement and central necrosis. (**d**) Fusion image of the 11C-MET PET and the MRI of the brain. (Image courtesy of Dr. Osvaldo Garcia Perez from the National Cancer Institute, Mexico City, Mexico)

patients, as well as in individuals with brain metastases, can be done with a relatively good diagnostic accuracy of 80–90%, by using18F-FET or 18F-FDOPA PET imaging [39, 40].

Importantly, several parameters generated from dynamic18F-FET PET acquisition may further improve diagnosis accuracy in glioma patients [41, 42]. This has also been reported in patients with brain metastases who had radiosurgery for the treatment of brain metastases. The diagnostic accuracy of 11C-MET PET in this clinical question is slightly lower (around 75%), which is most likely due to 11C-MET's increased affinity for inflammation [43–45]. Preliminary information on the use of 11C-AMT or 18F-FACBC in brain PET imaging suggests that these tracers could be useful in distinguishing between radiation necrosis versus viable glioma.

18F-DOPA has also been demonstrated to aid in the monitoring of treatment response following bevacizumab-based antiangiogenic therapy. The uptake of 18F-FGln is facilitated by a distinct type of amino acid transporter ATB (0), and it

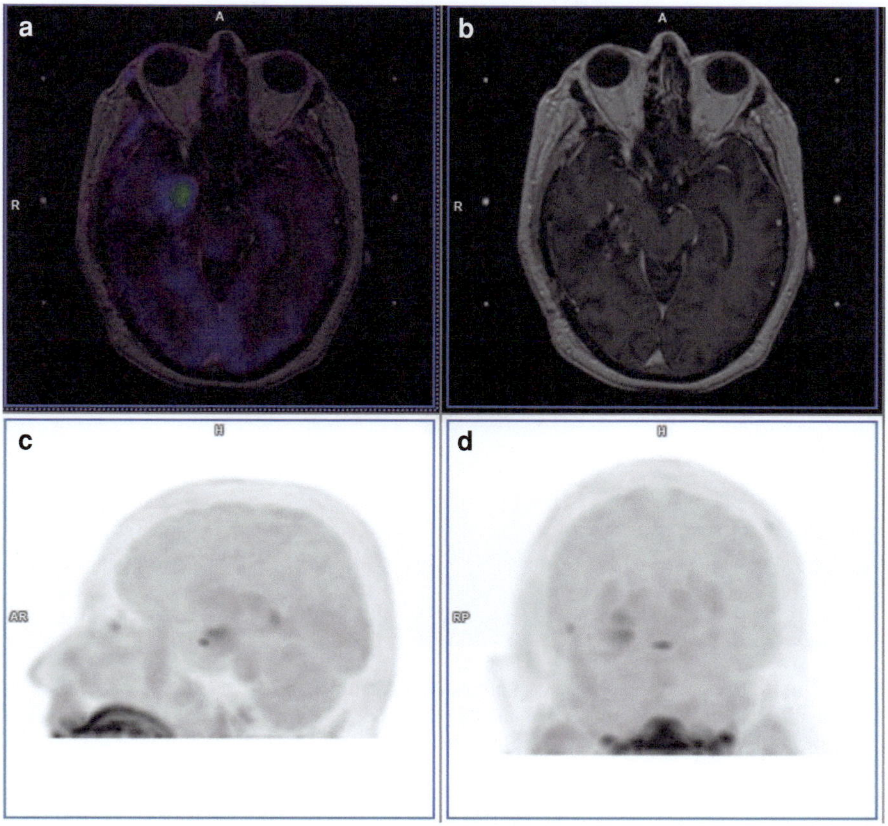

Fig. 3.4 A 51-year-old patient with a diagnosis of glioblastoma multiform (GBM) in the right temporal lobe, treated surgically followed by chemo-RT using temozolomide, is suspected of having tumor recurrence. (**a**) Fusion image of the 11C-MET PET and the contrast-enhanced T1 MRI of the brain show a poorly defined lesion in the mesial gyro of the right temporal lobe, with irregular contrast enhancement and more focal uptake of the radiotracer having an SUVmax of 5.7 and a T/NT ratio of 4.1. (**b**) Contrast-enhanced T1 MRI of the brain. (**c**, **d**). Maximum intensity projection images show in 3D the location of the lesion. (Image courtesy of Dr. Osvaldo Garcia Perez from the National Cancer Institute, Mexico City, Mexico)

is then converted to glutamate, which is utilized for energy production [35].18F-FGln has been proven to be beneficial in glioma patients for distinguishing between progressing and stable disease and for noninvasive tumor delineation [46]. A research study including three patients with brain metastases found that 18F-FGln had a higher detection rate than 18F-FDG (81.6% versus 36.8%, respectively) [47].

For several tracers, PET-based tumor volumes have been demonstrated to extend 2–3.5 cm beyond the contrast-enhancing volume of conventional MRI. Furthermore, delineation of tumor borders by amino acid PET is superior to standard MRI, both in contrast-enhancing and non-contrast-enhancing gliomas.

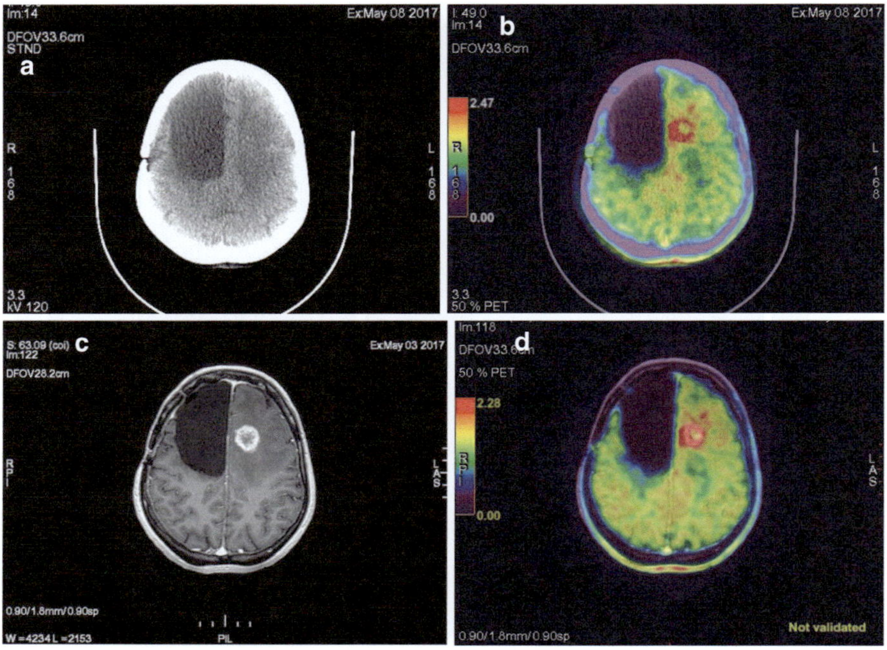

Fig. 3.5 A 43-year-old patient with anatomopathological diagnosis of grade 2 astrocytoma. (**a**) TC scan of the head shows diffuse edema in the left frontal lobe, with no evidence of focal lesion. (**b**) In the 18F-FET PET/CT scan of the head there is abnormal focal uptake of the radiopharmaceutical in the medial aspect of the left frontal lobe with an SUVmax of 2.9 and a T/NT ratio of 1.9. (**c**) Gadolinium enhanced T1 MRI on the brain shows an intraaxial nodular lesion in the left frontal lobe, with enhancement and hyperdense center, suggestive of necrosis and perilesional edema. (**d**) Fusion image of the 18F-FET PET and MRI. (Image courtesy of Dr. Osvaldo Garcia Perez from the National Cancer Institute, Mexico City, Mexico)

The evaluation of a patient's reaction to a certain neurooncological treatment is clinically important since treatment decisions might be influenced by treatment-related changes. Accurate response assessment aids in both terminating an ineffective treatment choice as soon as possible and preventing an effective treatment from being prematurely ended, which could have a negative impact on survival. Furthermore, evaluating response aids in avoiding potential therapy adverse effects, such as bone marrow depression, which translates into maintaining or even improving quality of live. The use of 11C-MET or 18F-FET PET to assess response to alkylating treatment (i.e., temozolomide or lomustine) in glioma patients has been proven to provide useful additional information when compared to contrast-enhanced MRI. Importantly, metabolic PET responders had a considerably longer survival than metabolic non-responders (i.e., patients with a decline in tumor-to-brain ratios or metabolically active tumor volumes at follow-up compared to baseline imaging) [48–50].

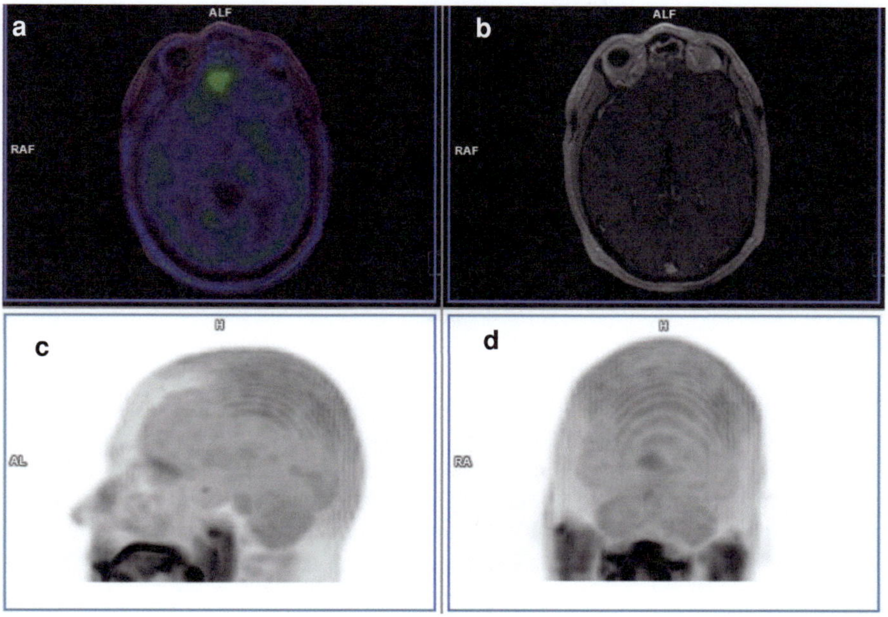

Fig. 3.6 A 43-year-old patient diagnosed with an esthesioneuroblastoma, suspected of having tumor recurrence after being treated with gamma knife. (**a**) Fusion image of the 18F-FET PET and the contrast-enhanced T1MRI of the brain show a hypervascular lesion associated with postsurgical changes in the right olfactory cleft and the right frontal lobe, with intense radiotracer uptake (SUVmax of 5.2) and T/NT ratio of 3.1. (**b**) Contrast-enhanced T1 MRI of the brain shows postsurgical changes with no definitive evidence of tumor recurrence. (**c**, **d**) Maximum intensity projection images show in 3D the location of the lesion. (Image courtesy of Dr. Osvaldo Garcia Perez from the National Cancer Institute, Mexico City, Mexico)

Utilizing reduced contrast enhancement on MRI as a surrogate metric for therapeutic response after antiangiogenic therapy with bevacizumab is not ideal. The term "pseudoresponse" refers to a decline in contrast enhancement caused by antiangiogenic medications that restore the blood–brain barrier quickly, rather than true tumor improvement. Accordingly, it can happen that even in patients who have an excellent radiological response, a clinical benefit is not always present ("pseudoresponse"). The use of 18F-FET and 18F-FDOPA PET in the detection of pseudoresponse may be beneficial. Furthermore, in bevacizumab responders, 18F-FDOPA and 18F-FET PET were able to predict a true good clinical outcome [51–53].

Patients with newly diagnosed glioblastoma can receive tumor-treating fields therapy in addition to adjuvant temozolomide chemotherapy once chemoradiation is completed. Initial research suggests that amino acid PET could be used to detect responding patients having tumor-treating fields therapy, although the response could also be due to concomitant chemotherapy or delayed chemoradiation effects [54].

PET Tracers for Assessment of Tumor Hypoxia

Another type of metabolic PET tracer is for hypoxia imaging, which occurs when quickly expanding tumor cells outgrow their blood supply. Hypoxia has been demonstrated to be a poor prognostic factor for survival because it causes radiation resistance (hypoxia-induced radioresistance) [55]. PET imaging is a noninvasive method for identifying hypoxic areas and mapping oxygenation inside CNS malignancies, and it has the potential to have a significant clinical impact by allowing for treatment customization before and during radiation. 1-(2-Nitro-imidazolyl)-3-[18F] [18F] fluoro-2-propanol (FMISO) is the most commonly researched hypoxia tracer, which is a derivative of nitroimidazole [56]. This nitroimidazole derivative is digested by nitroreductase enzymes at low oxygen levels after diffusion into cells. The tracer is trapped in hypoxic viable cells (not necrotic cells) by binding to these nitroreductase enzymes, which may be seen via PET imaging. 18F-FMISO PET has been shown to identify extra hypoxic tumor subregions outside the contrast-enhancing tumor sections in glioblastoma patients, demonstrating that hypoxia may cause peripheral tumor growth [57]. The metabolically active tumor volume in 11C-MET PET was found to be substantially linked with the hypoxic volume measured by18F-FMISO in a subsequent investigation [58]. Importantly, the tumor size on 11C-MET PET was 20–30% larger than the area of the contrast enhancement on MRI. 18F-MISO PET has recently been utilized to assess the effects of bevacizumab-based antiangiogenic therapy in patients with recurrent malignant glioma [59]. Patients who responded by, both, contrast-enhanced MRI and 18F-FMISO PET, had a considerably longer survival rate than those who just responded just by MRI [60]. A preliminary study of three glioblastoma (GBM) patients found that there was specific uptake of 18F-FMISO in tumor cells but not in healthy brain tissue [61]. 18F-FMISO was similarly useful for distinguishing between LGG and GBM, using lesion to cerebellar uptake ratios of 1.22 and 2.74, respectively [62]. Additional research has revealed a link between the intensity of uptake and volume of the signal with survival after radiation, whereby higher intensity and bigger signal carry a poor prognosis [63, 64]. The lipophilicity of 18F-FMISO is a significant drawback for its clinical application. Although it can pass over an intact BBB, the low clearance from plasma results in a fairly prominent background signal in the brain. Despite this 18F-FMISO has a better sensitivity and specificity than 18F-FDG [62].

Another copper tracer, 62Cu-diacetyl-bis (N4-methylthiosemicarbazone) 62Cu-ATSM has been created as a hypoxia tracer for localizing malignant tumor tissue, but it also showed to be a potential predictor of both PFS and OS in patients with WHO grade II–IV glioma [65]. Because it has shown significant selectivity for hypoxic tumor tissue, 62Cu-ATSM could theoretically be used as a theranostic PET tracer for 67Cu-ATSM radionuclide therapy, but the variable (low) uptake seen in the first human studies necessitates more research into the feasibility of Cu-labeled tracers for targeted therapy in CNS tumors.

PET Tracers for Assessment of Cellular Proliferation

The radiolabeled nucleoside 30-deoxy-30-18F-fluorothymidine (18F-FLT) is a pyrimidine analogue with fast absorption into newly generated DNA, being the most frequently used PET radiopharmaceutical to assess cellular proliferation.

18F-FLT correlates with the activity of thymidine kinase 1 (TK1), a cytosolic enzyme active during the S and G2 phases of the cell cycle [66]. When compared to normal brain tissue, 18F-FLT visualizes increased cell proliferation in cancer cells, providing good contrast and sensitivity for the detection of HGG [67]. Because of its fast absorption into newly generated DNA, it is utilized to assess cellular proliferation. However, because 18F-FLT uptake requires a compromised blood–brain barrier, its diagnostic use may be limited. For example, 18F-FLT PET is less sensitive than 11C-MET PET in detecting WHO grade II gliomas, which normally do not show any contrast enhancement [68]. Furthermore, a meta-analysis of the efficacy of 18F-FLT PET for the diagnosis of glioma recurrence based on a study with 800 patients found that 18F-FLT had no advantage over 18F-FDG (pooled sensitivity, 82%; pooled specificity, 76% versus a pooled sensitivity, 78%; pooled specificity, 77%, respectively) [69]. However, in individuals with recurrent malignant glioma, 18F-FLT PET appears to be useful for assessing response to antiangiogenic therapy with bevacizumab. When compared to metabolic non-responders, 18F-FLT PET was able to detect a reduction in proliferative activity in responding patients with a positive outcome as an indicator for response [70]. 18F-FLT PET has also been employed in patients with brain metastases from malignant melanoma who were receiving targeted therapy or immunotherapy with checkpoint inhibitors [71]. Responding patients have been found to have clearer reduction in proliferative activity as measured by 18F-FLT PET than the decrease in contrast enhancement seen on standard MRI, Fig. 3.7.

The sensitivity of 18F-FLT for tumor detection of all grades is often lower than that of 11C-MET and 18F-FET PET, but it tends to provide superior grading [68, 72]. In most LGGs, there is no increased 18F-FLT uptake. Increased absorption during LGG follow-up, however, was found to be a major negative predictor of overall survival in a study of 41 patients [73]. It is not, however, a predictor of event-free survival because patients may require therapy for symptoms caused by tumors that have grown in size but are still low grade and 18F-FLT negative.

18F-FLT was found to be superior to advanced MRI and MRS for differentiating between tumor grades III and IV in a study of preoperative glioma grading [74]. Obviously, tumor size is a key prognostic factor, and FLT-measured tumor volume is a better predictor of overall survival than uptake intensity [75]. FLT PET detects residual tumor volumes after resection that are similar to CE-MRI but smaller than T2-weighted MR abnormalities [76]. PET utilizing 18F-FLT provides a moderately greater overall accuracy for identifying glioma recurrence than PET using 18F-FDG, according to a meta-analysis of studies with recurring tumors [69]. In individuals with recurrent malignant glioma, the volume and intensity of tracer uptake are both independent predictors of survival [77].

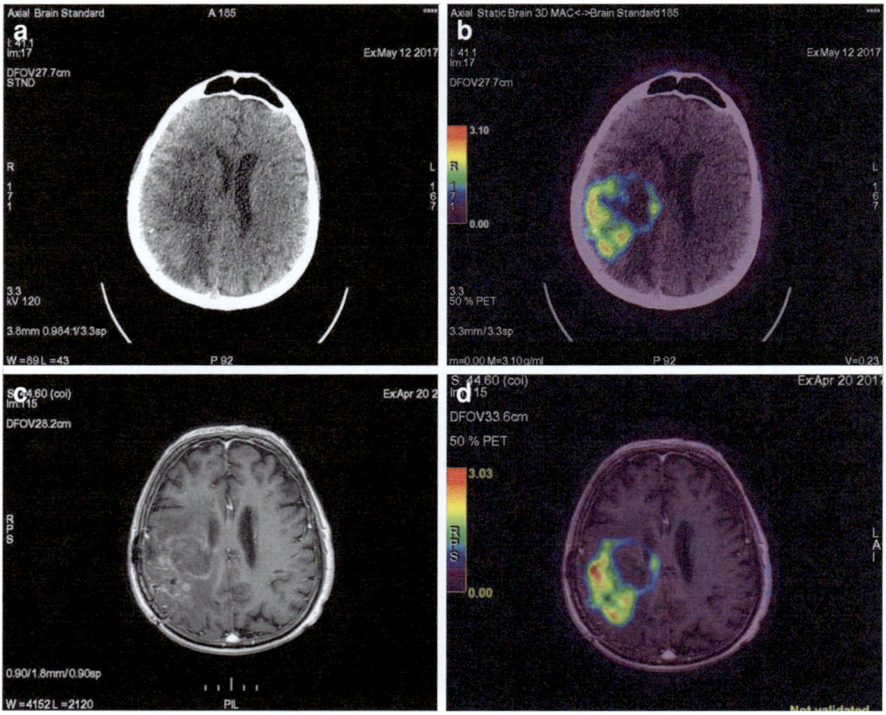

Fig. 3.7 A 70-year-old patient with a gliosarcoma of the right parietal lobe. (**a**) CT scan shows a hyperdense intraaxial lesion of irregular borders and lobulated with associated peritumoral edema. (**b**) PET/CT scan done with 18F-FLT. There is evidence of increased radiotracer uptake by the intraaxial right parietal lesions with central hypodensities compatible with necrosis. The SUVmax is 3.4 and the T/NT ratio is 11.3. (**c**) In the contrast-enhanced axial plane T1 MRI of the brain there is evidence of a diffuse/infiltrative lesion with enhancement in the right parietal lobe and peritumoral edema. (**d**) Fusion image of the 18F-FLT and MRI. (Image courtesy of Dr. Osvaldo Garcia Perez from the National Cancer Institute, Mexico City, Mexico)

PET Tracers for Assessment of Tumor Perfusion

The measurement of regional cerebral blood flow (rCBF) permits identification of brain tumors with high vascularization. PET can be used to measure rCBF using 15O-labeled water. Because of its very short half-life (2 min), 15O-H_2O necessitates the employment of an on-site cyclotron [78]. Since perfusion-weighted CT and MRI imaging are widely available, it has resulted in a large number of studies evaluating brain malignancies, vastly outnumbering 15O-H_2O PET investigations. It has been demonstrated that in direct comparisons, rCBF values vary significantly between CT and MRI-based perfusion measures and 15O-H_2O PET [79].

PET tracers have been utilized to measure the oxygen metabolic rate, cerebral blood flow, and oxygen extraction fraction in malignant gliomas using radiolabeled oxygen, 15O-O_2, water, 15O-H_2O, and carbon monoxide, 15O-CO. Despite having normal blood flow, most investigations have found that oxygen consumption and extraction are lower in brain tumors than in healthy brain cortex. Because energy synthesis by glycolysis, the major energy pathway, occurs without oxygen use, assessing oxygen metabolism with PET is less valuable than 18F-FDG-PET [80].

Another PET radiopharmaceutical that has been used to assess cerebral blood flow is 13N-NH3, which has been used to study cerebral flood flow in patients with glioma, brain metastases, and meningioma [81].

PET Tracers for Assessment of Tumor Angiogenesis

Most cancers, including brain tumors, progress by stimulating the development of new blood vessels, which is predominantly fueled by the overexpression of vascular endothelial growth factor (VEGF) [82]. The resultant vasculature, however, is architecturally and functionally aberrant, contributing to a hostile milieu (low oxygen tension and high interstitial fluid pressure) that favors a more malignant phenotype with higher morbidity and mortality. Anti-VEGF medications may be helpful in glioblastoma, the most common primary brain tumor, and can temporarily normalize tumor vasculature, according to new preclinical and clinical studies. This opens up a window of opportunity for combining chemotherapeutics with radiation in the most effective way possible. In patients with malignant glioma, bevacizumab, a recombinant humanized monoclonal antibody against VEGF, appears to improve progression-free survival and reduce steroid use. 89Zr-labeled bevacizumab PET imaging has been used for tumoral drug accumulation in pediatric patients with diffuse intrinsic pontine glioma (DIPG) based on these features. This investigation revealed a marked inter- and intratumoral heterogeneity in drug accumulation, suggesting considerable variability in tumor delivery of bevacizumab in DIPG patients, possibly related to the heterogeneous expression of VEGF and/or variable integrity of the BBB [83, 84]. Other research in animal models has employed 64Cu-labeled VEGF conjugates with DOTA (1,4,7,10-tetra-azacylododecane N,N0,N00,N000-tetraacetic acid) [85, 86]. Similarly, these methods imply that identifying patients who will benefit from anti-VEGF medication has clinical significance. It has been shown that by utilizing single-photon emission computed tomography (SPECT) imaging, accumulation of 123I-VEGF can be measured in the tumor of adult glioblastoma patients [12]. Moreover, patients with glioblastoma who had a poor clinical prognosis were identified by increased 123I-VEGF uptake.

PET Imaging for Theranostics in Neuro-Oncology

Precision oncology is supported by theranostics, which is a combination of treatments and diagnostics. Peptide receptor radionuclide treatment (PRRT), which uses overexpressed tumor-specific receptors, both, as a diagnostic and therapeutic target, is also a PET-based theranostic technique.

The same PET tracer can be utilized for therapy by replacing the radionuclide used for diagnostic PET, such as 68Ga, with a radiation source, such as ß-emitters like 177Lu or 90Y. Although there are no clinically proven theranostic methods for gliomas or brain metastases at this time, there are several promising possibilities.

Heute et al. published the first study using the so-called peptide receptor radionuclide therapy (PRRT) for the treatment of CNS malignancies in 2010 [87]. The goal of PRRT is to use a therapeutic radionuclide to target upregulated peptide receptors for localized therapy. The expression and accessibility of a target peptide receptor, in this case the somatostatin receptor 2 (SSTR2), were investigated in the first step using an analog of somatostatin, octreotide, labeled with the positron-emitting radionuclide gallium-68 via a so-called DOTA chelator (i.e., 68Ga-Ga-DOTA-TATE) [88]. Patients were judged eligible for targeted therapy utilizing one of the DOTA peptides labeled with a therapeutic beta-particle-emitting radionuclide, either luthetium-177 or yttrium-90, after subsequent PET imaging validated SSTR2 expression and accessibility by exhibiting high tumor uptake [89, 90]. The positron-emitting radionuclide can now be utilized to measure therapy efficacy, as demonstrated in the first study using 90Y-DOTATOC in GBM patients, where post-therapeutic follow-up PET imaging revealed a decreased uptake of 68GaDOTATOC, indicating therapeutic efficacy [87]. Patients with HGG and meningioma were included in subsequent PRRT studies for the treatment of CNS malignancies. The amount of SSTR2 expression, as evaluated by 68Ga-DOTATATE/TOC uptake, has been linked to the therapeutic efficacy of 177Lu-DOTATATE or 90Y-DOTATOC therapy in meningioma [91]. Verburg et al. conducted a PET-guided drug delivery research in four patients with inoperable grade II meningioma in 2019, with the goal of optimizing the impact of PRRT [92]. The tumor absorption of 68Ga-DOTATATE was compared after intra-arterial (IA) and intravenous (IV) injection. When compared to IV administration, IA administration resulted in a 2.7-fold greater tracer absorption. A case report of a grade II meningioma patient treated with 177Lu-DOTATATE showed a 79% decrease in tracer uptake on post-therapeutic 68Ga-DOTATOC imaging, highlighting the potential efficacy of IA PRRT for CNS malignancies [93].

PSMA is expressed in the tumor vasculature of gliomas, breast cancer metastases, schwannomas, and peripheral nerve sheath tumors, according to immunohistochemistry studies of CNS tissues, but not in normal vessels. The first PET experiments using 68Ga-HBED-CC-PSMA also known as 68Ga-PSMA-11 to investigate PSMA expression in CNS malignancies revealed selective target expression and target accessibility in LGG, HGG, and gliosarcoma, with higher expression in HGG than LGG [94–96]. PSMA-PET imaging also exhibited diagnostic value in undefined brain tumors, as lesions with high 68Ga-PSMA-11 uptake were histopathologically proven to be glioma, atypical meningioma, and lymphoma, Figs. 3.8 and 3.9.

Another investigation in three GBM patients verified selective target binding utilizing 2-(3-(1carboxy-5-(6-[18F]fluoro-pyridine-3-carbonyl)-amino]-pentyl)-ureido)-pentanedioic acid (18F-DCFPyL) [97]. Finally, PSMA target expression in patients with HGG and metastatic brain cancers was investigated utilizing the

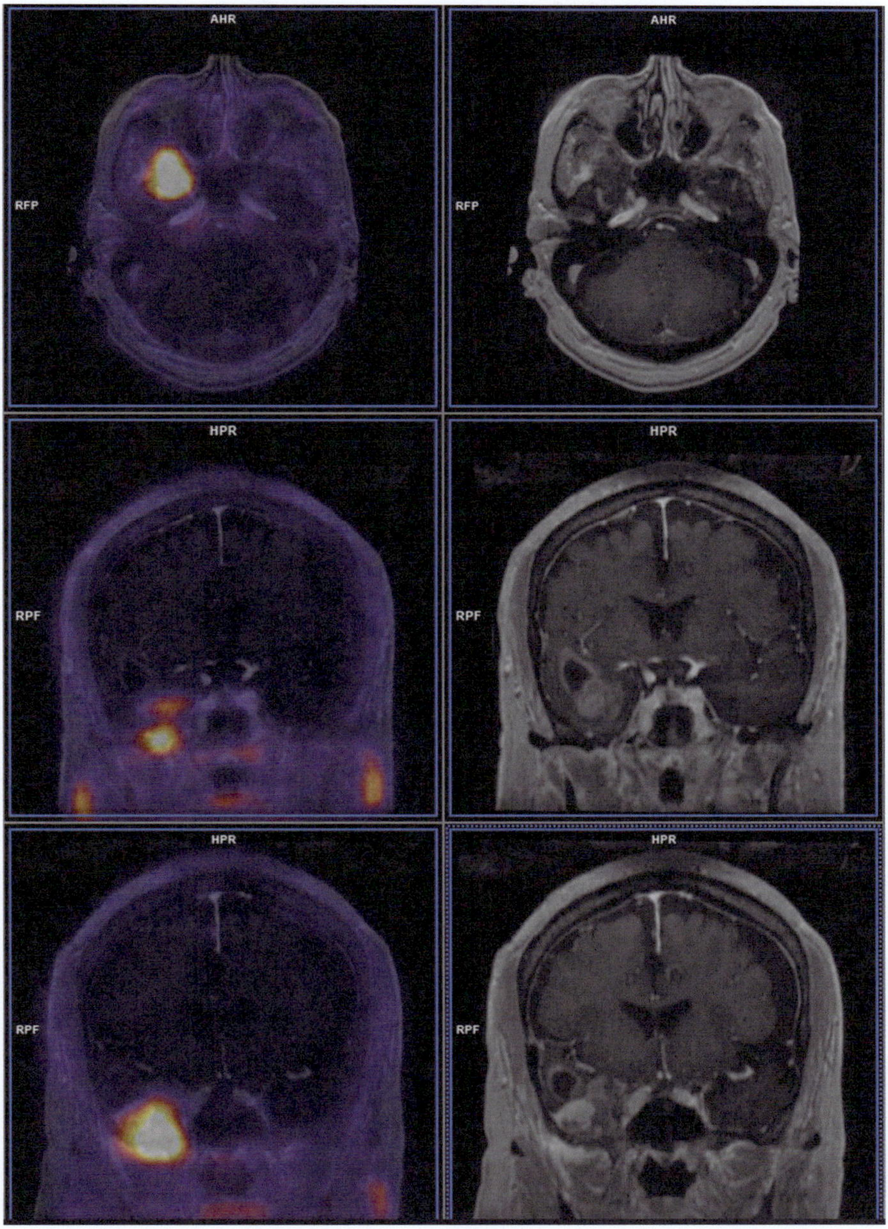

Fig. 3.8 A 68-year-old man with metastatic castrate resistance prostate cancer. Left sided images show the fusion of the 18F-PSMA PET and the contrast-enhanced T1 MRI of the brain, with an extra-axial lesion arising from the meninges in the right temporal lobe, with intense radiotracer uptake and SUVmax of 18.1. Stereotaxic biopsy confirmed the prostatic origin of the lesion. Right sided images correspond to the contrast-enhanced T1 MRI of the brain. (Image courtesy of Dr. Osvaldo Garcia Perez from the National Cancer Institute, Mexico City, Mexico)

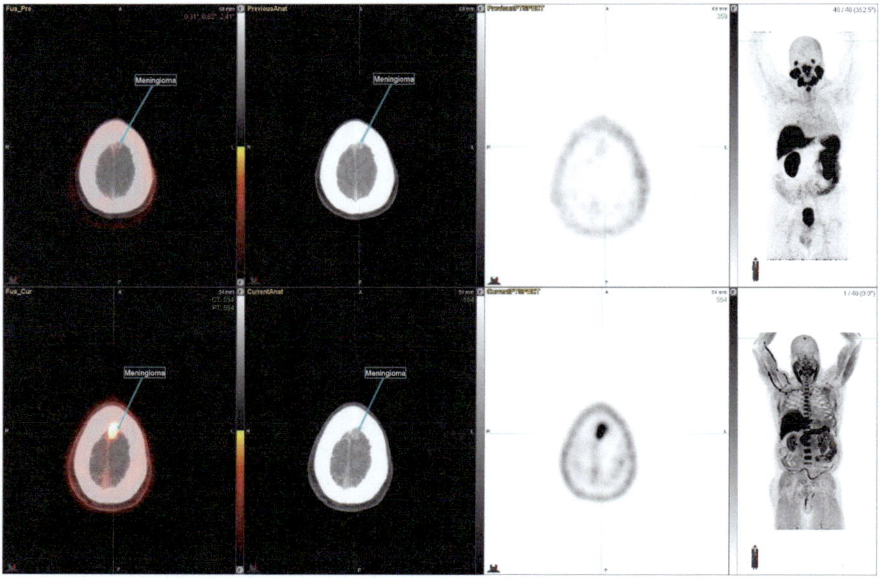

Fig. 3.9 A 57-year-old man with prostate cancer who had surgical resection with no recurrence. As follow-up imaging a 68Ga-PSMA PET/CT scan (images above) was done in December 2020 (from left to right are the 18F-FDG PET/CT fused, CT, PET, and volume rendered images), which was negative. However, a 18F-Fluciclovine PET/CT scan (images below) done in April 2021 shows a lesion in the left dura (arrows) of 1.2 cm × 1.6 cm and SUV of 9.1. This lesion was found to be not prostate cancer, but meningioma. (Image courtesy of Dr. Osvaldo Garcia Perez from the National Cancer Institute, Mexico City, Mexico)

anti-PSMA minibody, IAB2M, tagged with zirconium-89, 89Zr-IAB2M [98]. These results suggest that PSMA has the potential to be a target for the local delivery of therapeutic radionuclides due to its selective target expression and accessibility [99]. This approach's therapeutic efficacy for CNS malignancies has only been demonstrated in individuals who had brain metastases from prostate cancer and were treated with the anti-PSMA-based radiopharmaceuticals 177Lu-PSMA-617 and 225Ac-PSMA-617 [100, 101]. The size of the brain tumors shrank significantly in these investigations. Unfortunately, due to physiologic PSMA expression, 225Ac-PSMA-617 also had considerable toxicity to the salivary glands [100, 102].

Another PRRT target, the transmembrane receptor neurokinin type-1 has been explored since 2018. The neurokinin type 1 receptor (NK-1R) is a 7-transmembrane G protein-coupled receptor that belongs to the tachykinin receptor family in mammals. It works biologically by activating the enzyme phospholipase C, which creates inositol triphosphate. Substance P is NK-1R's biological ligand. On the cell surface and within the neovasculature, brain tumors (of any WHO grade) overexpress NK-1R [103, 104]. As a result, substance P and NK-1R have grown in popularity as a biological target for brain tumor focused therapy. Immunohistochemistry studies have revealed that the neurokinin type-1 receptor is strongly expressed in glioma cells, where it promotes mitogenesis, angiogenesis, cell migration, and metastasis development [105, 106]. 213Bi-DOTA-[Thi8, Met(O_2) [11]-substance P (213Bi-DOTA-SP) is an alpha-particle emitting radionuclide that can be used to target the neurokinin type-1 receptor for theranostic purposes. Two trials exploring the therapeutic use of 213Bi-DOTA-SP in CNS malignancies have been published: one with nine patients and the other with 20 patients with recurrent GBM. Patients in both studies received localized PRRT through an intracavitary injection of 213Bi-DOTA-SP with a co-injection of 68Ga-DOTA-SP to examine pharmacokinetics and biodistribution. Tracer uptake was focused in the target lesions, with limited systemic uptake (less than 5% of total activity) in the kidneys and urine, according to these studies [107, 108].

Fibronectin, which is not strictly a membrane receptor but rather a cell matrix protein involved in cell adhesion and migration, is another target for radionuclide therapy [109]. The expression of fibronectin is downregulated in normal brain cells as they mature. However, expression can be increased in cancer cells in order to promote angiogenesis [110]. In 2013, six patients with inoperable brain and extracranial metastases from NSCLC and breast cancer were enrolled in a PET-guided dose scheduling study. Eligible patients were administered the human small immune protein L19SIP—that targets the ED-B domain of fibronectin—which was labeled with iodine-124, having PET imaging done at 1, 4, 24, 48, and 96 h after injection to assess and predict the optimal protein dose for achieving potentially effective radiation at the target site(s) and to investigate unwanted tracer accumulation at other sites (i.e., bone red marrow and healthy organs) to prevent cancer. Subsequently, patients were given the therapeutic format 131I-L19SIP for treatment purposes after PET-guided drug titration. Despite the fact that the fraction of injected activity in normal organs was equal across patients, antibody absorption in neoplastic lesions differed by up to 60 times. Immuno-PET using 124I-labeled L19SIP was found to have a number of advantages over traditional 131-I imaging, including improved dosimetric accuracy [109].

Overexpressed chemokine receptor-4 (CXCR4), for example, is a potential target in glioblastoma patients and has been linked to a poor clinical outcome [111–113]. Pentixafor is a synthetic, cyclic pentapeptide analog of stromal-cell derived factor-1 (SDF-1 or CXCL12), which is a ligand for chemokine receptor C-X-C chemokine receptor type 4 (CXCR4). CXCR4 expression has been evaluated in glioblastoma patients by PET imaging with CXCR4-directed 68Ga-Pentixafor.

Newer or Potential Tracers for Emerging Cell Targets in Neuro-Oncology PET

There is a growing list of new PET radiopharmaceuticals being explored in neuro-oncology, for the evaluation of never treatment options.

Significant molecular targets have been found as a result of a growing knowledge in cancer biology, leading to the creation of a large spectrum of target therapeutic pharmaceuticals, of which the most rapidly developing are the receptor tyrosine kinase inhibitory drugs. Epidermal growth factor receptor (EGFR), vascular endothelial growth factor receptor (VEGFR), and platelet-derived growth factor receptor (PDGFR) are examples of receptor tyrosine kinases (RTKs).

The epidermal growth factor receptor (EGFR) is a transmembrane cell receptor that is a biological receptor for several epidermal growth factor protein ligands. When a specific ligand attaches to EGFR, it phosphorylates the receptor, which activates intracellular signaling pathways that control cell proliferation, differentiation, and survival. Many malignancies, including brain tumors, overexpress EGFR; for example, GBM overexpresses it in more than 57% of instances. Because EGFR plays such an important role in tumor cell proliferation and survival, it is a promising biological target for targeted therapy. This target has been exploited in radioimmunotherapy clinical studies, in which radiolabeled anti-EGFR mAbs were given to brain tumors with EGFR overexpression validated by immunohistochemistry. The indication with the highest clinical potential for EGFR and HER2 targeted PET is in the evaluation of a response to these targeted therapeutic choices in patients with brain metastases (from melanoma, lung, or breast cancer) as well as in glioma patients. PET imaging agents have included radiolabeled EGFR and HER2 antibodies, as well as tyrosine kinase inhibitors. PET ligands such 11C-erlotinib, 11C-PD153035, and 89Zr-DFO-nimotuzumab have been used to detect EGFR overexpression [114–116]. 64Cu-DOTA-trastuzumab and 89Zr-pertuzumab are the most useful PET tracers for imaging HER2 overexpression. These targets, however, have yet to be investigated in a radiotheranostic context. 11C-lapatinib, another TKI-PET tracer utilized in CNS malignancies, was used to investigate the target expression and accessibility of HER2 in three patients with brain metastases from (HER2-positive) breast cancer. The PET techniques were well tolerated by the patients, and 11C-lapatinib uptake was found in tumor tissue but not in normal brain. Finally, Varrone et al. evaluated the brain accessibility and biodistribution of osimertinib using the TKI-PET tracer 11C-C-osimertinib. Osimertinib, a third-generation tyrosine kinase inhibitor, has been shown to be effective in patients with brain metastases, and it was tested using PET in eight healthy volunteers who had a normal BBB. The findings revealed osimertinib's rapid and high absorption in the brain, underlining the drug's promise and calling for more research in CNS tumor patients.

The use of radiolabeled anti-EGFR mAbs in a radiotheranostic environment has a lot of promise since it can identify patients who have a tumor molecular profile that is most likely to respond to anti-EGFR targeted therapy. While tissue biopsy alone cannot fully reflect the molecular and genetic profile of these heterogeneous malignancies, radiotheranostics can.

In 2010, researchers used the mAb trastuzumab tagged with zirconium-89, 89Zr-trastuzumab, to execute the first PET imaging study for CNS tumor targeting in patients with brain metastases from HER2-positive breast cancer. The researchers discovered an 18-fold higher absorption in tumors in comparison to normal brains, which is intriguing considering that intact antibodies like trastuzumab are thought to be unable to penetrate through the BBB. These findings support the use of trastuzumab therapy in these individuals since they demonstrate local BBB breakdown.

Another study using 64Cu-Cu-DOTA-trastuzumab in breast cancer patients with brain metastases confirmed trastuzumab's transit through the BBB and the ability of PET to noninvasively detect HER2-positive lesions. Finally, the mAb pertuzumab was labeled with zirconium-89 (89Zr-pertuzumab) for use in patients with brain metastases from breast cancer. Similar results were reported with trastuzumab, suggesting that HER2 targeting is safe and effective.

Immunotherapy with antibodies targeting immune checkpoints such as cytotoxic T-lymphocyte antigen-4 (CTLA-4; e.g., ipilimumab), programmed cell death receptor-1 (PD-1; e.g., pembrolizumab, nivolumab), or programmed cell death protein ligand 1 (PD-L1; e.g., atezolizumab) has become increasingly important in clinical oncology. However, the efficacy and responsiveness of these drugs can range significantly between different types of cancer and individuals. Patients can be selected using biomarkers extracted from tumor tissue, such as PD-1 and PD-L1 expression. Nevertheless, these tissue biomarkers are limited, and some patients show no response despite the presence of the target. As a result, PET becomes increasingly important for predicting immunotherapy response and adequate patient selection. Immuno-PET, for example, mixes antibodies or antibody fragments with a radionuclide and takes use of antibodies' specificity and affinity, as well as PET's sensitivity. T-cell markers (e.g., CD4+, CD8+), immunological checkpoints (e.g., CTLA-4, PD-1, PD-L1), and immune response biomarkers (e.g., interferon-, interleukin-2) are all common immuno-PET targets.

Targeting PD-1 with 89Zr-nivolumab or PD-L1 with 89Zr-atezolizumab as imaging biomarkers to noninvasively monitor the expression of these immune checkpoints in patients with extracranial and intracranial cancer has been shown to be feasible in first-in-human studies [117–119]. Engineered target-binding proteins (adnectins) for PD-L1 ligands like 18F-BMS-986192 are currently being tested [120]. Tumor-infiltrating T-cells (such as CD8+) are critical for immune cell activation in response to checkpoint inhibition [121]. A radiolabeled 89Zr-IAB22M2C has recently been proven to have the ability to visualize CD8+ T-cell-enriched tumor tissue [122]. PET has also been used to assess immune cells invading tumors using radiolabeled clofarabine (2-chloro-20-deoxy-20-[18F]fluoro-9-b-D-arabinofranosyl-adenine; 18F-CFA) [123]. The enzyme deoxycytidine kinase, which is overexpressed in immune cells like CD8+ T-cells, uses 18F-CFA as a substrate. In this regard, PET has demonstrated considerable clinical potential in glioblastoma patients treated with dendritic cell immunization paired with immune checkpoint inhibition to pinpoint and quantify immune responses.

Transfection of immune cells with a reporter gene that encodes a protein that can be specifically targeted by a radiolabeled reporter probe is another intriguing technique. Using 9-[4-[18F]fluoro-3 (hydroxymethyl)butyl]guanine, imaging of reporter gene expression in cells transfected with the herpes simplex virus type 1 thymidine kinase reporter gene has been demonstrated by 18F-FHBG PET. Furthermore, using CAR-T cells, this approach offers the potential to assess newly developed cell-based therapeutics [124]. Accordingly, 18F-FHBG can detect by PET/CT imaging, reporter gene expression, in CAR-engineered cytotoxic T-cells.

A new target in brain tumor imaging is the enzyme isocitrate dehydrogenase (IDH). IDH is a Krebs cycle enzyme that catalyzes the conversion of isocitrate to alpha-ketoglutarate through oxidative decarboxylation. Mutations in the IDH1 and IDH2 genes cause a large increase in the oncometabolite 2-hydroxyglutarate, which is commonly found in WHO grade II or III astrocytomas and oligodendrogliomas. The accumulation of 2-hydroxiglutarate (2-HG) in cells with IDH mutant enzymes changes various downstream cellular functions, creating epigenetic instability and, as a result, a stop in cellular development, which leads to oncogenesis. Accordingly, there is interest in the development of inhibitory drugs for the mutant IDH proteins. Selective oral IDH1 inhibitors (ivosidenib, BAY-1436032), pan-IDH1/2 inhibitors (i.e., AG-881), and vaccine techniques targeting the IDH1R132H mutation are now being tested in glioma patients. The preliminary data, mostly from phase 1 studies, are encouraging, indicating that these inhibitors are safe and exhibit anticancer effect. Although immunohistochemistry and genomic sequencing are the preferred approaches for detecting an IDH mutation, both techniques are intrusive and unsuitable for therapy monitoring, which necessitates ongoing evaluation. Furthermore, using magnetic resonance spectroscopy (MRS) to noninvasively test 2-HG is technically demanding, and in 20% of cases, the results may be false-positive. Newer PET probes for imaging mutant IDH expression in gliomas could potentially be a viable option. Triazinediamine or butyl-phenyl sulfonamide analogs labeled with 18F appear to be attractive candidate radiotracers for noninvasive PET imaging of IDH mutations in gliomas, according to recent radiochemical developments. In addition, a 18F-labeled IDH1 inhibitor (AGI-5198) has been studied [125]. Because of the metabolic trapping, 11C-acetate absorption in IDH mutant cells is considerably higher than in IDH wild-type cells. Obviously, further work is needed to transfer these promising techniques for IDH imaging into clinical practice.

Tenascin C (TN-C) is an extracellular matrix (ECM) glycoprotein that is expressed in a variety of physiological and pathologic situations.

For a brief period of time, it is physiologically expressed in the fetus during embryogenesis and organogenesis. Furthermore, it is strongly expressed in a variety of pathological circumstances, including inflammation, wound healing, and tumor formation. TN-C plays a key role in tumor pathogenesis by allowing tumor cells to migrate inside the ECM and to other body regions. Many glioma tumors, such as GBM, overexpress TN-C, although it is expressed to a lesser amount in other healthy tissues. Furthermore, TN-C overexpression is linked to a high rate of proliferation, tumor angiogenesis, and a progressive tumor growth pattern. Because it is overexpressed in gliomas with a critical role in glioma biology and has low expression in normal healthy tissues, TN-C is a potential molecular target. To date, various monoclonal antibodies (mAbs) targeting TN-C have been produced, which are classified as either murine mAbs or chimeric antibodies. ST2146, F16, P12, ST2485, 81C6, BC-2, and BC-4 are anti-TN-C mAbs from mice, while ch81C6 is a chimeric antibody. In a molecular radioimmunotherapy scenario, radiolabeled anti–TN-C mAbs are delivered locoregionally or injected into the systemic circulation to provide targeted therapy. A phase II clinical trial yielded promising results, providing the rationale for the development of a phase III trial [126]. Despite this, anti-TN-C radiopharmaceuticals have yet to be employed in a radiotheranostic setting for the treatment of brain tumors. By including a patient selection phase before the therapy, a radiotheranostic strategy can improve anti-TN-C therapeutic efficacy. This initial step should allow the identification of patients with appropriate target expression.

The low-density lipoprotein receptor (LDLR) expressed at the BBB mediates the transport of endogenous ligands through the BBB, a process referred to as receptor-mediated transcytosis. There is a family of peptide vectors which are being developed to target the LDLR, among others in brain tumors, opening the possibility for brain PET imaging and/or targeted radionuclide therapy with a radiolabeled peptide vector, some of which are under development [127].

Radionuclide Therapy

Introduction

Despite many technological and pharmaceutical advances, the median overall survival of patients with GBM is 15 months. In comparison with other malignancies treatment of brain tumors is especially challenging due to several reasons. The BBB limits the ability of many therapeutic compounds including radionuclide therapy to adequately reach the tumor tissue if injected intravenously, as is not the case in other human organs. Early on, most malignant brain tumors tent to profoundly infiltrate the brain parenchyma over an extend well beyond what it is clearly visibly by MRI. Moreover, small clusters of tumor cells can frequently be present at 4–7 cm from the original tumor site. In addition, even if localized, the position of the tumor mass in relationship to vital neurological structures limits the capacity for adequate treatment, since it can have significant neurological implications. To further compound the challenge, many brain tumors are extremely heterogeneous even between the core of the tumor, with areas of necrosis and hypoxia. Tumor cells, at the genetic level, can have multiple deletions, point mutations, or amplifications that trigger signal transduction pathways for several tyrosine kinase receptors, such as epidermal growth factor receptor and platelet-derived growth factor receptor. Cell cycle arrest pathways are also disrupted by these mutations. In conclusion, malignant brain tumors are exceptionally proliferative and invasive, have significantly abnormal vascularization, and are resistant to standard radio- and chemotherapeutic treatments.

Radionuclide therapy is an appealing technique for individuals with brain tumors because it has the ability to more selectively irradiate tumor cells, benefiting from the selective targeting of many different tumor receptors that have been identified over the last few decades. Furthermore, the localized radiation not only will spare the normal brain tissue but at the same time, depending on the specific type of radionuclide used, benefit from the "cross fire effect" radiating immediately adjacent tumor cells, in addition to the ones the radiopharmaceutical has specifically targeted, Table 3.4.

Table 3.4 List of most commonly used therapeutic radionuclides in neuro-oncology and their physical characteristics

Radionuclide	Abbreviation	Half-life	Emission	$Energy_{max}$ (KeV)	Method of production
Bismuth-213	^{213}Bi	45.6 min	Beta-/alpha	1423/5981	^{225}Ac generator
Actinium-225	^{225}Ac	9.9 days	Alpha	5800	Nuclear reactor
Iodine-131	^{131}I	8 days	Beta-/gamma	606/364	Nuclear reactor
Astatin-211	^{211}At	7.2 h	Alpha/EC	5900/7450	Cyclotron
Iodine-125	^{125}I	59.5 days	EC	35	Nuclear reactor
Rhenium-188	^{188}Re	17 h	Beta-	2100	W-188/Re-188 generator
Yttrium-90	^{90}Y	2.6 days	Beta-	2280	Nuclear reactor
Lutetium-177	^{177}Lu	7 days	Beta-/gamma	498/208	Nuclear reactor

Table 3.5 Therapeutic radiopharmaceuticals in neuro-oncology used in clinical studies

Radiopharmaceutical	Target	Mechanism
213Bi-DOTA-SP	Neurokinin type 1 receptor (NK-1R)	Small peptide tachykinin receptor therapy
225Ac-DOTAGA-SP	Neurokinin type 1 receptor (NK-1R)	Small peptide tachykinin receptor therapy
131I- 81C6	Tenascin C (TN-C)	Monoclonal antibody
211At-labeled 81C6	Tenascin C (TN-C)	Monoclonal antibody
131I-L19SIP	Fibronectin monoclonal	Monoclonal antibody
125I-mAb 425	EGFR	Monoclonal antibody
188Re-Nimotuzumab	EGFR	Monoclonal antibody
131I-chTNT-1/B	Histone H1 complexed into DNA	Monoclonal antibody
90Y-DOTATOC	Somatostatin receptor 2	Somatostatin receptor therapy
177Lu-PSMA	PSMA transmembrane receptor	Small ligand receptor therapy
131I-IPA	LAT 1	Amino acid cell membrane transporter system L
131I-TM-601	Phosphatidyl inositide	Binding to phosphorylated lipid on tumor cell lamellipodia

There are several biological targets that have been identified in brain tissues for which a whole range of different targeted radiopharmaceuticals have been developed over the last few decades. However, all of them are still considered investigational agents. I will review the main ones, according to the specific receptor targeted, Table 3.5.

Neurokinin Type-1 Receptor

The neurokinin type 1 receptor (NK-1R) is one of the three types of mammalian tachykinin receptors in the 7 transmembrane G-protein coupled receptor family. Its effects are mediated through the activation of phospholipase C, which produces inositol triphosphate. Substance P belongs to the neurokinins (NKs) family of small peptides found throughout the central nervous system (CNS) and peripheral nervous system (PNS). Substance P's biological effects in the CNS, such as control of emotional behavior and emesis in the brain and nociception in the spinal cord, are mediated via the NK1 receptor. The most thoroughly researched NK route is the substance P-NK1(SP-NK1) receptor system. NK-1R-targeted therapies for the treatment of glioma tumors have been developed in response to the overexpression of NK1-R found in glioma tumors. The two most frequently used radiopharmaceuticals in small clinical trials are 213Bi-DOTA-SP and 225Ac-DOTAGA-SP.

In one study including 20 patients with recurrent glia tumor grade IV, were treated with 1–7 cycles of 213Bi-DOTA-SP, with mean doses for one course of 1.8 GBq in 2-month intervals. The median progression-free survival was 2.7 months. The median overall survival from the first diagnosis was 23.6 months and median survival after recurrence was 10.9 months. The median survival time from the start of 213Bi-DOTA-SP was 7.5 months [108]. In another study, 9 patients with recurrence of secondary GBM were treated with 1–6 cycles of 213Bi-DOTA-SP in 2 months intervals, with a median total injected activity of 5.8 GBq. The median OS from the time of diagnosis was 52.3 months, the OS time from the time of conversion was 18.6 months. From the initiation of treatment with the 213Bi-DOTA-SP analogue, the median PFS was 5.8 months and the median OS was 16.4 months [107]. However, it is the opinion of some investigators that the relatively short half-life of 213Bi can limit the optimal biodistribution of the radiopharmaceuticals in larger tumors. Accordingly, an isotope with a longer half-life may be preferable in these cases. To this end, 225Ac- with a half-life of 9.9 days has been applied.

In one study 225 Ac-DOTA-SP treatment was performed as salvage therapy in 21 patients with recurrence glioblastoma WHO grade IV, primary and secondary. The treatment was well tolerated, with the majority of moderate transient side effects (edema, epileptic seizures, aphasia, and hemiparesis) occurring mostly in the group of patients given 30 MBq of 225Ac-DOTA-SP. Only one patient who received 30 MBq developed grade 3 thrombopenia. In all groups, there was no other grade 3 or 4 toxicity due to 225Ac-DOTA therapy. The median overall survival time (OS-d) from the main diagnosis was 35.0 months, and the median overall survival time (OS-r/c) from the diagnosis of the recurrence/conversion was 13.2 months. The median PFS was 2.4 months and the OS-t was 9.0 months after starting therapy with 225Ac-DOTA-SP. There were no statistically significant changes between the dose escalation groups that were evaluated [128, 129].

Tenascin C

Tenascin C (TN-C) is a glycoprotein encoded by the TNC gene in humans. During development, disease, and injury, it is found in the extracellular matrix (ECM) of many tissues, as well as in restricted neurogenic areas of the central nervous system. Tenascin C is the first member of the tenascin protein family to be discovered. It is produced by migrating cells such as the neural crest in the embryo, and it is abundant in growing tendons, bone, and cartilage.

Furthermore, it is strongly expressed in a variety of pathological circumstances, including inflammation, wound healing, and tumor formation. TN-C plays a key role in tumor pathogenesis by allowing tumor cells to migrate inside the ECM and to other body regions. Many glioma tumors, such as GBM, overexpress TN-C, although it is expressed to a lesser degree in other healthy tissues. Furthermore, TN-C overexpression is linked to a high rate of proliferation, tumor angiogenesis, and a progressive tumor growth pattern. Because it is extensively expressed in gliomas, plays a critical role in glioma biology, and has low expression in normal healthy tissues, TN-C is a potential molecular target. To date, various monoclonal antibodies (mAbs) targeting TN-C have been developed, which are classified as murine mAbs and chimeric antibodies. ST2146, F16, P12, ST2485, 81C6, BC-2, and BC-4 are anti–TN-C mAbs from mice, while ch81C6 is a chimeric antibody. The radiolabeled antitenascin murine monoclonal antibody 81C6 was used in five phase I/II clinical trials at Duke Comprehensive Cancer Center. Many patients have had promising results, with median survival times of up to 22 months in GBM patients treated with 131I- and 211At-labeled 81C6 compared to about 11 months for traditional therapies [130].

Riva et al. explored the use of radiolabeled antitenascin mAbs BC-2 and BC-4 in the treatment of anaplastic astrocytomas and glioblastoma. In a phase II research, 91 patients (74 with glioblastoma, 9 with anaplastic astrocytoma, 7 with anaplastic oligodendroglioma, and 1 with oligodendroglioma) were treated with 131I-labeled antitenascin mAbs. The mean radiation dose administered to the walls of the surgically formed resection cavity was 150 Gy, and the median effective half-life of 131I in the tumor was 57.1 h. Patients with glioblastoma, anaplastic astrocytoma, and anaplastic oligodendroglioma had median survival times of 19, 46, and 23 months, respectively [131].

In a molecular radioimmunotherapy scenario, radiolabeled anti-TN-C mAbs are delivered locoregionally or injected into systemic circulation to provide targeted therapy. A phase II clinical trial yielded promising results, concluding that a phase III trial is required [132]. Despite this, anti-TN-C radiopharmaceuticals have yet to be employed in a radiotheranostic setting for the treatment of brain tumors. By including a patient selection phase before the therapy, a radiotheranostic strategy can improve anti-TN-C therapeutic efficacy. This stage facilitates patients with appropriate target expression to be identified.

In 18 patients with recurring malignant brain tumors, Zalutsky et al. investigated the feasibility, safety, and efficacy of injecting chimeric antitenascin monoclonal antibody (mAb) 81C6 (ch81C6) labeled with 211At-ch81C6 into the surgically formed resection cavity. IgG2b was the monoclonal antibody used (ch81C6). The reservoir was injected with 10 mg of ch81C6 tagged with 71-347 MBq of 211At before being treated with salvage chemotherapy. Those patients with glioblastoma multiforme, anaplastic astrocytoma, or oligodendroglioma had median survival periods of 54, 52, and 116 weeks, respectively. They found that regional delivery of 211-At-ch81C6 in patients with malignant central nervous system tumors is practical, safe, and associated with a beneficial anticancer effect [133].

Fibronectin

Fibronectin is a high-molecular-weight extracellular matrix glycoprotein that interacts with integrins which are membrane-spanning receptor proteins. Other extracellular matrix proteins that fibronectin binds to include collagen, fibrin, and heparan sulfate proteoglycans. It plays a key role in cell adhesion, migration, development, and differentiation by mediating a wide range of cellular interactions with the extracellular matrix (ECM).

Fibronectin can be expressed in a variety of ways based on alternative splicing, with three isoforms detected in tumor tissue: IIICS, extra-domain (ED) A, and ED-B. An 80 kDa construct was created using a human antibody targeting the ED-B, named "L19" which consisted of two single-chain variable segments linked by a CH4 domain of the human IgE [134]. After intravenous injection, this construct, L19SIP, was radioiodinated using a modified chloramine-T technique and clinically studied in numerous solid tumor types, including metastatic solid brain tumors [135]. Poli et al. employed 124I-labeled L19SIP in immune-PET imaging to estimate the administered dose to metastatic lesions and healthy organs in patients with solid tumor brain metastases. The administered dose to the bone red marrow, which is the principal dose-limiting organ for this form of therapy, was found to be 2 Gy. Depending on the extent of the lesion, intracranial lesions received 0.73–8.15 Gy. These values are close to those observed in extracranial metastatic lesions. Patients who met the criteria for RIT (target/background ratio of brain metastases >4 and bone marrow dose 2 Gy) were given 131I-L19SIP treatment at a dose of 4.107 GBq/m^2. Preliminary findings reveal that intracranial and extracranial lesions showed reduced 18F-FDG uptake throughout the 6-month follow-up in three out of four individuals. The reduction in glucose metabolism in the lesions suggests that 131I-L19SIP-mediated RIT may be clinically effective [109].

Epidermal Growth Factor Receptor

The epidermal growth factor receptor (EGFR) is a transmembrane cell receptor that is a biological receptor for epidermal growth factor family of protein ligands. When a specific ligand attaches to EGFR, it phosphorylates the receptor, which activates intracellular signaling pathways that control cell proliferation, differentiation, and survival. Many malignancies, including brain tumors, overexpress EGFR. For instance, GBM overexpresses it in more than 57% of cases [136]. Because EGFR plays such an important role in tumor cell proliferation and survival, it is a promising biological target for targeted therapy. This target has been exploited in radioimmunotherapy clinical studies, in which radiolabeled anti-EGFR mAbs were given to brain tumors with EGFR overexpression validated by immunohistochemistry.

The use of the murine anti-EGFR mAb 425 antibody, radiolabeled with 125I by the Iodogen method, has been reported in several clinical trials. Because EGFR is an internalizing receptor, an Auger-emitter, like 125I, will ensure that routinely used radionuclides have the most specific targeting potential. Intravenous delivery of

125I-mAb 425, either alone or in combination with standard of care treatment, enhanced median survival considerably. The combination of 125I-mAb 425 plus TMZ produced the greatest survival advantage in the largest phase II trial to date, with a median survival of 20.4 months, compared to therapy with 125I-mAb 425 alone, which was 14.5 months [137]. In contrast to most clinical trials involving TRNT in the brain, 125I-mAb 425 was delivered via intravenous injection rather than local injection into the resection cavity. Given the radiopharmaceutical's systemic distribution, it emphasizes the treatment's efficacy. Aside from skin discomfort at the injection site, the intravenous injection was found to have no significant side effects. The 188Re-labeled Nimotuzumab, a humanized anti-EGFR antibody, was used in a small-scale phase I single-dose clinical trial. 188Re is a beta-emitting radionuclide with a short half-life that can be directly bound to antibodies as a glucoheptonate complex. 188Re can be generated quickly using an in-house 188W/188Re generator, which is identical to the 99Mo/99mTc generator, making it ideal for clinical applications. Three patients with anaplastic astrocytoma (AA) and eight patients with GBM received 188Re-labeled Nimotuzumab into the resection cavity after surgery. One GBM patient died from progression 6 months after TRNT, while one GBM and one Anaplastic Astrocitoma patient had stable disease for 3 months. After 3 years of treatment, one GBM patient had a partial response for more than a year, while two patients (1 GBM and 1 AA) were asymptomatic and in total response. In two of the individuals who were given the drug, dose-dependent neurotoxicity was seen [138].

The use of radiolabeled anti-EGFR mAbs in a radiotheranostic environment has a lot of promise since it can identify patients who have a tumor molecular profile that is most likely to benefit from anti-EGFR targeted therapy. As a result, whereas tissue biopsies cannot fully reflect the molecular and genetic characteristics of these heterogeneous malignancies, radiotheranostics may do it.

DNA–Histone H1 Complex

131I-chTNT-1/B MoAb is a 131I-labeled chimeric monoclonal antibody that targets a universal intracellular antigen, namely histone H1 complexed to DNA. This protein is found in high concentrations within the necrotic core of patients with high-grade glioma and GBM. Healthy cells with an intact cell membrane are not penetrated by this MoAb. This abundant, non-diffusible protein, however, offers an anchor in the necrotic portions of malignant solid tumors, where it delivers a lethal dose of 131I radiation to the neighboring viable tumor cells. 131I-chTNT-1/B MoAb can be delivered via convection-enhanced delivery system to irradiate not only the bulk of the tumor but also the invasive glial cells dispersed throughout normal brain tissue. In 51 individuals with high-grade glioma who have been treated in phase I/II clinical trials, treatment-related side effects included cerebral edema (16%), hemiparesis (14%), and headache (14%), all of which were reversible with corticosteroids. Despite the fact that the phase II trial showed therapeutic efficacy, there were insufficient patients for therapy with a constant dose [139, 140]. Therapeutic efficacy was not formally studied in phase I and II trials because of the small number of patients treated at a constant dose, albeit trends were detected in a subset of patients who received total activity between 1.25 and 2.5 mCi/cm^3. These delivered activity cutoffs were chosen based on findings that below 1.25 mCi/cm^3, progression occurred at 8 weeks, and over 2.5 mCi/cm^3, there was increased toxicity. The median survival time in this subset was 41 weeks.

Somatostatin Receptors

Somatostatin receptor (SSTR) is a transmembrane receptor that belongs to a family of G protein-coupled 7-transmembrane receptors. There are five different SSTR subtypes (SSTR1-5). Somatostatin (SST), the SSTR ligand, is a neuropeptide generated by immunological, inflammatory, and neuroendocrine cells that is involved in neuromodulation (sensory, motor, and cognition) and cell growth inhibition via autocrine and paracrine routes. Gliomas and meningiomas, medulloblastomas, pituitary adenomas, and primitive neuroendocrine cancers are all known to overexpress SSTR and have been effectively targeted using SST agonists and antagonists. According to Dutour and colleagues, glioma and meningioma, the most common primary brain tumors, overexpress various subtypes of SSTRs [141]. They also discovered that, although having diverse profiles of SSTR overexpression, all brain tumors expressed at least one form of SSTR [141]. Furthermore, they discovered distinct SSTR expression profiles in low-grade and high-grade gliomas. Until yet, four kinds of 1,4,7,10-tetraazacyclododecane have been identified. DOTATATE, DOTANOC, DOTAGA, and DOTATOC stand for tetraacetic acid-d-Phe1-Tyr3-octreotide. These peptides have been radionuclide-labeled with beta- and alpha-emitter radionuclides and are now being used in a growing number of clinical trials [103].

In one small study, three grade IV recurrent GBM patients were treated with 90Y-DOTATOC. 68Ga-DOTATOC PET was performed to evaluate the expression of somatostatin receptor 2 prior to the administration of the therapeutic drug. A subcutaneous reservoir system placed into the resection cavity was used to supply the radiopharmaceutical locally. With only modest side effects, MRI and PET confirmed complete remission in one patient and partial remission in the other. Patients also reported a significant increase in their quality of life. Tumor cells got a two-fold higher dose from a single cycle of locally delivered 90Y-DOTATOC than from normal whole-brain irradiation, whereas surrounding brain tissue was spared, according to whole-body dosimetry [87].

Ten glioma patients (WHO grades II and III; 5 progressing gliomas, 5 extensively debulked) underwent local administration of different fractions of 90Y-DOTATOC, either in the bulk tumor or into the resection cavity, in an extended pilot trial by Schumacher et al. PRRT was the sole treatment option for the five patients with glioma whose tumors were progressing. All five patients had tumor progression arrested for 13–45 months, and even one solid, mostly inoperable anaplastic astrocytoma slowly shrinked into a resectable multicystic lesion 2 years after PRRT. PRRT was well tolerated and had no intermediate or long-term side effects. There are currently one phase I and two phase II clinical trials investigating 90Y-DOTATOC's safety, side effects, maximum tolerated dose, and efficacy [142].

Prostate Membrane Antigen

PSMA is a type II transmembrane glycoprotein that normally resides in the cytoplasm of normal prostate cells; however, in prostate carcinoma, it binds to the cancer cell membrane, resulting in a membrane-bound protein. PSMA expression has also been found in the brain, kidneys, salivary glands, and intestine, indicating that it is not confined to the prostate. Furthermore, the endothelium of the neovasculature of many forms of solid tumors, including brain tumors, overexpresses PSMA, but in the normal endothelium does not. Because of their significant neovascularization, vasculature-targeted therapy has a lot of promise in the context of targeted therapies for brain tumors. Verma and colleagues used 68Ga-PSMA 11 PET/CT imaging and histopathologic analysis to assess the degree of PSMA expression in high-grade gliomas versus low-grade gliomas [94]. They discovered that PSMA 11 uptake on PET/CT was much higher in high-grade gliomas than in low-grade gliomas and that the PSMA 11 uptake on PET/CT was associated with the histologic proliferation index in both tumor types. There are a few reports on the beneficial results of 177Lu-PSMA combined with external beam radiation therapy for metastatic brain lesions in patients with prostate cancer [143]. The noninvasive PSMA-based theranostic platform may open up a new frontier in the treatment of these highly diverse and aggressive brain tumors.

Amino Acid Metabolism

In gliomas, the membrane-bound L-amino acid transporter 1 (LAT1) is overexpressed, and the level of expression is related to histological tumor grade [144]. As a result, LAT1 is a promising target for molecular treatment. Indeed, radiolabeled amino acid derivatives that are substrates for the LAT1 transporter, such as 11C-labeled methionine (11C-MET), 123I-methyltyrosine (123I-IMT), and 18F-fluoroethyltyrosine (18F-FET) have been used in clinical PET and single-photon emission computed tomography (SPECT) imaging of gliomas. While they are effective in targeting glioma cells in vivo, they cannot be employed as scaffolds for therapeutic iodine-131 labeling because they are retained in tumor tissue for less than 90 min or have a chemical structure that is unsuitable for radiohalogenation. 4-123I-Iodo-L-phenylalanine (123I-IPA) is a new SPECT tracer that was recently described in a validation study in 35 patients with histologically confirmed glioma

(WHO grade I–IV, primary tumors as well as recurrences) and demonstrated retention in glioma tissue for up to 24 h, high metabolic stability, and uptake by >85% of gliomas WHO grade I–IV [145]. These properties encouraged the testing of 131I-IPA, a 131I-labeled analogue, as a therapeutic agent for glioma endoradiotherapy. Baum et al. reported on two patients with heavily pretreated and progressing gliomas, who were treated with 2 and 4 GBq of 131I-IPA. The treatment was well tolerated by both patients. There was no evidence of immediate or delayed organ toxicity. PET revealed steadily decreasing maximum standardized uptake values (SUVmax) in one patient over a 10-month period, indicating metabolic response, which was accompanied by decreased contrast enhancement and tumor volume on MRI. After 18 months of therapy, the patient progressed. No response was detected when the treatment was repeated with 6.6 GBq of 131I-IPA. The second patient was observed for 3 months following treatment and MRI and PET scans revealed stable illness [146]. In another study by Verburg et al. 5 patients with GBM were treated with 131I-iodo-L-phenylalanine (131-IPA) combined with hypo-fractionated external beam radiation therapy. The patients received a single intravenous infusion of 2–7 GBq of 131IPA according to their individual dosimetry, resulting in radiation absorbed doses to the blood of 0.80–1.47 Gy. The treatment was well tolerated, with the first two patients reporting just moderate nausea and vomiting that responded to ondansetron and pantoprazole. The final three patients had no problems during therapy after receiving prophylactic medicine. There was no evidence of a drop in leukocyte or thrombocyte counts below the baseline level or the lower normal limit in any of the individuals. The tumor doses from 131IPA were minimal (less than 1 Gy), and all of the patients died 3–8 months (median 5.5) after treatment [147]. There is new phase 1/2 clinical trial (IPAX-1) which hopefully will provide additional information after the intended enrolment of 44 GBM patients, on the tolerability and clinical benefits of combined 131IPA with external bean radiation therapy.

Matrix Metalloproteinase

TM-601 is a synthetic version of a peptide (chlorotoxin) identified in the venom of the Leiurus quinquestriatus, a giant yellow Israeli scorpion. This 36-amino-acid peptide has been studied as a potential glioma target. TM-601 binds to a phosphatidyl inositide, a phosphorylated lipid on tumor cell lamellipodia, and penetrates blood–brain and tissue barriers. Radioiodinated TM-601 was found to be stable, safe, effective, and immunogenic in preclinical trials. Mamelak et al. conducted a phase I research in adult patients with recurrent high-grade glioma to assess the safety, biodistribution, and dosimetry of intracavitary iodine-131 (131I)-TM-601. The study included eighteen adult patients with histologically confirmed recurrent glioblastoma and a Karnofsky performance status of 60% who were candidates for cytoreductive craniotomy. Patients were given a single dosage of 131I-TM-601 (0.25, 0.50, or 1.0 mg of TM-601) from one of three dosing panels, each labeled with 10 mCi of 131I. There were no dose-limiting effects detected after intracavitary delivery. 131I-TM-601 adhered to the tumor perimeter and remained there for a long time, with negligible uptake in other organ systems. Four patients had radiographic stable illness on day 180, while one had a partial response. Two of these patients continued to improve and were in disease-free progression for more than 30 months [15].

Radiopharmaceuticals Used in Preclinical Studies

There is a long list of different radiopharmaceuticals that have been used in preclinical studies, including, but not limited to, 177Lu-6A10Fab targeting Carbonic anhydrase XII, 225Ac-E4G10 targeting Cadherin, 64Cu/177Lu-IIIA4 targeting the Ephin receptor A3, 131-I-PARPi targeting the poly(AND-ribose) polymerase, 131-I-hyaluronectin glycoprotein, 177Lu-CXCR4-L targeting the chemokine receptor, 225Ac-Pep-1L targeting the interleukin-13 receptor, and 125-I- 2′deoxy-uridine 9UdR targeting DNA synthesis. One receptor with great potential is the low-density lipoprotein receptor (LDLR), expressed at the BBB since it mediates the transport of endogenous ligands through the BBB. A family of peptide vectors has been identified and chemically optimized targeting both the human and murine LDLR, with the ability to cross the BBB and accordingly target tumors such as glioblastoma that express high levels of the LDLR. Nevertheless, the two preclinical radiopharmaceuticals with the largest number of publications are one which is targeting the integrin receptors and the second which is targeting the human epidermal growth factor 2 (HER2).

Human epidermal growth factor 2 (HER2) is a member of the human growth factor receptor family that is overexpressed in about 30% of breast cancers. It is involved in tumor cell proliferation, cell survival, and angiogenesis. Moreover, it is considered an independent factor for metastatic disease. HER2-positive breast cancers are more likely to metastasize to the brain in up to 37% of cases. Targeted therapy for breast cancer using trastuzumab, a monoclonal antibody targeting HER2 receptors, is a well-stablished treatment strategy. However, breast cancer metastasis to the brain significantly accelerates progression to death for patients who have otherwise treatable primary tumors. Therefore, there is still a need for effective treatment strategies to treat brain metastasis of HER2-positive breast cancer. Puttemans and colleagues studied the therapeutic efficacy of 2Rs15d, a novel anti-HER2 Camelid single-domain antibody fragment, for treating intracranial metastases of breast cancer in a theranostic setting in mice. The results were promising and radiolabeled 2Rs15d was able to increase the survival in trastuzumab-resistant tumors [148]. These results warrant future translational studies to assess the therapeutic effect of 2Rs15d in vivo.

$\alpha_v\beta_3$ is a cell adhesion molecule found in glioblastoma multiforme tumor cells and actively angiogenic endothelium. Integrin $\alpha_v\beta_3$ controls extracellular matrix adherence to facilitate the recruitment of endothelial progenitor cells during angiogenesis. Furthermore, malignant gliomas have been demonstrated to exhibit a high density of $\alpha_v\beta_3$ on their cell surface. As a result of its significant connection with tumor invasiveness, metastasis, and poor clinical prognosis, integrin $\alpha_v\beta_3$ is a reliable diagnostic target to identify malignant from benign cancer phenotype. In a study by Veeravagu et al., they used Abegrin with is a monoclonal antibody against the integrin $\alpha_v\beta_3$ cell adhesion molecule. MTD and dose response analysis revealed 200 μCi per mouse as appropriate treatment dose with hepatic clearance and no organ toxicity. 90Y-Abegrin treated U87MG tumor mice showed partial regression of tumor volume, in comparison to increased tumor volumes in 90Y-IgG, Abegrin, and saline groups. 18F-FDG imaging revealed a reduction of cell proliferation and metabolic activity, whereas 18F-FLT PET showed decreased DNA synthesis in the 90Y-Abegrin group [149]. Another study by Jian Lei et al. used cystine knot peptides (knottins) labeled with 177Lu to form 177Lu-DOTA-2.5D and 177Lu-DOTA-2.5F, to target integrins receptors with high affinity. They found that Knottin 2.5F labeled with 177Lu exhibits favorable distribution in murine U87MG xenograft model; thus, it is a promising agent for radionuclide therapy of integrin positive tumors [150]. In their work, Shi J et al. proceeded to investigate and optimize the integrin αvβ3 mediated therapeutic effect of 177Lu-3PRGD2 (a dimeric RGD peptide with 3 PEG4 linkers) in the animal model. The targeted radiotherapy (TRT) with a single dose and repeated doses, as well as the combined therapy of TRT and the antiangiogenic therapy (AAT) with Endostar were conducted in U87MG tumor models. They found that tumor growth was significantly delayed by 177Lu-3PRGD2 TRT. Significantly increased anti-tumor effects were observed in the two doses or combined (combined with the antiangiogenic therapy with Endostar) treatment groups [151].

Conclusions

The number of radiopharmaceuticals available for the diagnosis and therapy in neuro-oncology has increased considerably over the last few decades. This growth has been mainly driven by, the superior knowledge on cancer cell biology which the recognition of a myriad of cell receptors adequate for targeting to facilitate molecular imaging and radionuclide therapy, the advances in technology such as hybrid PET/CT and PET/MRI scanners, and the improvements in radiochemistry including an easier access to previously less frequently used isotopes such as alpha-particle emitters. Unfortunately, most of these new radiopharmaceuticals are not commercially available and are being used only for research.

Although MRI of the brain currently constitutes the standard of care for imaging of tumors on the brain and the spinal cord, there is an increasing recognition of the unique and complementary information that can be obtained from PET imaging. Moreover, there are current recommendations from professional societies on the use of PET such as the 2018 Joint EANM/EANO/RANO practice guidelines/SNMMI procedure standards for imaging of gliomas using PET with radiolabeled amino acids and18F-FDG that unequivocally recommend the use of amino acid PET brain imaging [152]. In addition to FDG, FDOPA and F-18 Fluciclovine are commercially available in the USA. Nevertheless, there is an increased awareness on the potential of molecular PET brain imaging due to the unique ability to provide non-invasive exquisitely sensitive information on multiple different aspects of tumor cell biology that are critical for the adequate clinical management of such a complex malignancy as are brain tumors.

The use of radionuclide therapy in brain tumors has been mostly limited to small phase 1 and 2 clinical studies. However, recognizing the limitations of the currently available standard of care treatments, especially for high-grade malignant brain tumors, there is an increased recognition of the potential of radionuclide therapy. There are unique challenges for the treatment of brain tumors, such as the BBB, that also need to be overcome by radionuclide therapy. However, development of dedicated catheters systems or new radiopharmaceuticals targeting low-density lipoprotein receptor (LDLR), expressed at the BBB which mediates the transport of endogenous ligands through the BBB, can overcome some of these challenges. Futures studies should focus on sequential treatments using different peptides and isotopes, or even dual targeting of different receptors of the same tumor cells, taking advantage of the theranostics potential of PET imaging, guiding drug development and drug delivery studies and facilitating a multidisciplinary integrated system for the treatment of patients with brain tumors.

References

1. Siegel RL, Miller KD, Fuchs HE, Jemal A. Cancer statistics, 2021. CA Cancer J Clin. 2021;71(1):7–33. https://doi.org/10.3322/caac.21654.
2. Wesseling P, Capper D. WHO 2016 classification of gliomas. Neuropathol Appl Neurobiol. 2018;44(2):139–50. https://doi.org/10.1111/nan.12432.
3. Albert NL, Weller M, Suchorska B, Galldiks N, Soffietti R, Kim MM, et al. Response Assessment in Neuro-Oncology working group and European Association for Neuro-Oncology recommendations for the clinical use of PET imaging in gliomas. Neuro Oncol. 2016;18(9):1199–208. https://doi.org/10.1093/neuonc/now058.
4. Bolcaen J, Kleynhans J, Nair S, Verhoeven J, Goethals I, Sathekge M, et al. A perspective on the radiopharmaceutical requirements for imaging and therapy of glioblastoma. Theranostics. 2021;11(16):7911–47. https://doi.org/10.7150/thno.56639.
5. Shooli H, Nemati R, Ahmadzadehfar H, Aboian M, Jafari E, Jokar N, et al. Theranostics in brain tumors. PET Clin. 2021;16(3):397–418. https://doi.org/10.1016/j.cpet.2021.03.005.
6. Chamberlain MC. Leptomeningeal metastases: a review of evaluation and treatment. J Neurooncol. 1998;37(3):271–84. https://doi.org/10.1023/a:1005976926058.
7. Chamberlain MC. Leptomeningeal metastasis. Curr Opin Oncol. 2010;22(6):627–35. https://doi.org/10.1097/CCO.0b013e32833de986.
8. Chamberlain MC. Spinal 111Indium-DTPA CSF flow studies in leptomeningeal metastasis. J Neurooncol. 1995;25(2):135–41. https://doi.org/10.1007/bf01057757.
9. Chamberlain MC. Neoplastic meningitis. Oncologist. 2008;13(9):967–77. https://doi.org/10.1634/theoncologist.2008-0138.
10. Weber W, Bartenstein P, Gross MW, Kinzel D, Daschner H, Feldmann HJ, et al. Fluorine-18-FDG PET and iodine-123-IMT SPECT in the evaluation of brain tumors. J Nucl Med. 1997;38(5):802–8.

11. Rani N, Singh B, Kumar N, Singh P, Hazari PP, Jaswal A, et al. The diagnostic performance of 99mTc-methionine single-photon emission tomography in grading glioma preoperatively: a comparison with histopathology and Ki-67 indices. Nucl Med Commun. 2020;41(9):848–57. https://doi.org/10.1097/mnm.0000000000001230.
12. Rainer E, Wang H, Traub-Weidinger T, Widhalm G, Fueger B, Chang J, et al. The prognostic value of [(123)I]-vascular endothelial growth factor ([(123)I]-VEGF) in glioma. Eur J Nucl Med Mol Imaging. 2018;45(13):2396–403. https://doi.org/10.1007/s00259-018-4088-y.
13. Jensen P, Feng L, Law I, Svarer C, Knudsen GM, Mikkelsen JD, et al. TSPO imaging in glioblastoma multiforme: a direct comparison between 123I-CLINDE SPECT, 18F-FET PET, and gadolinium-enhanced MR imaging. J Nucl Med. 2015;56(9):1386–90. https://doi.org/10.2967/jnumed.115.158998.
14. Hockaday DC, Shen S, Fiveash J, Raubitschek A, Colcher D, Liu A, et al. Imaging glioma extent with 131I-TM-601. J Nucl Med. 2005;46(4):580–6.
15. Mamelak AN, Rosenfeld S, Bucholz R, Raubitschek A, Nabors LB, Fiveash JB, et al. Phase I single-dose study of intracavitary-administered iodine-131-TM-601 in adults with recurrent high-grade glioma. J Clin Oncol. 2006;24(22):3644–50. https://doi.org/10.1200/jco.2005.05.4569.
16. Santimaria M, Moscatelli G, Viale GL, Giovannoni L, Neri G, Viti F, et al. Immunoscintigraphic detection of the ED-B domain of fibronectin, a marker of angiogenesis, in patients with cancer. Clin Cancer Res. 2003;9(2):571–9.
17. Di Chiro G, DeLaPaz RL, Brooks RA, Sokoloff L, Kornblith PL, Smith BH, et al. Glucose utilization of cerebral gliomas measured by [18F] fluorodeoxyglucose and positron emission tomography. Neurology. 1982;32(12):1323–9. https://doi.org/10.1212/wnl.32.12.1323.
18. Patronas NJ, Di Chiro G, Kufta C, Bairamian D, Kornblith PL, Simon R, et al. Prediction of survival in glioma patients by means of positron emission tomography. J Neurosurg. 1985;62(6):816–22. https://doi.org/10.3171/jns.1985.62.6.0816.
19. Özütemiz C, Neil EC, Tanwar M, Rubin NT, Ozturk K, Cayci Z. The role of dual-phase FDG PET/CT in the diagnosis and follow-up of brain tumors. AJR Am J Roentgenol. 2020;215(4):985–96. https://doi.org/10.2214/ajr.19.22571.
20. Tripathi M, Sharma R, D'Souza M, Jaimini A, Panwar P, Varshney R, et al. Comparative evaluation of F-18 FDOPA, F-18 FDG, and F-18 FLT-PET/CT for metabolic imaging of low grade gliomas. Clin Nucl Med. 2009;34(12):878–83. https://doi.org/10.1097/RLU.0b013e3181becfe0.
21. Galldiks N, Lohmann P, Albert NL, Tonn JC, Langen KJ. Current status of PET imaging in neuro-oncology. Neurooncol Adv. 2019;1(1):vdz010. https://doi.org/10.1093/noajnl/vdz010.
22. Filss CP, Cicone F, Shah NJ, Galldiks N, Langen KJ. Amino acid PET and MR perfusion imaging in brain tumours. Clin Transl Imaging. 2017;5(3):209–23. https://doi.org/10.1007/s40336-017-0225-z.
23. Misch M, Guggemos A, Driever PH, Koch A, Grosse F, Steffen IG, et al. (18)F-FET-PET guided surgical biopsy and resection in children and adolescence with brain tumors. Childs Nerv Syst. 2015;31(2):261–7. https://doi.org/10.1007/s00381-014-2552-y.
24. Rosenfeld A, Etzl M, Bandy D, Carpenteri D, Gieseking A, Dvorchik I, et al. Use of positron emission tomography in the evaluation of diffuse intrinsic brainstem gliomas in children. J Pediatr Hematol Oncol. 2011;33(5):369–73. https://doi.org/10.1097/MPH.0b013e31820ad915.
25. Pafundi DH, Laack NN, Youland RS, Parney IF, Lowe VJ, Giannini C, et al. Biopsy validation of 18F-DOPA PET and biodistribution in gliomas for neurosurgical planning and radiotherapy target delineation: results of a prospective pilot study. Neuro Oncol. 2013;15(8):1058–67. https://doi.org/10.1093/neuonc/not002.
26. Grosu AL, Astner ST, Riedel E, Nieder C, Wiedenmann N, Heinemann F, et al. An interindividual comparison of O-(2-[18F]fluoroethyl)-L-tyrosine (FET)- and L-[methyl-11C]methionine (MET)-PET in patients with brain gliomas and metastases. Int J Radiat Oncol Biol Phys. 2011;81(4):1049–58. https://doi.org/10.1016/j.ijrobp.2010.07.002.

27. Kebir S, Fimmers R, Galldiks N, Schäfer N, Mack F, Schaub C, et al. Late pseudoprogression in glioblastoma: diagnostic value of dynamic O-(2-[18F]fluoroethyl)-L-tyrosine PET. Clin Cancer Res. 2016;22(9):2190–6. https://doi.org/10.1158/1078-0432.Ccr-15-1334.
28. Zikou A, Sioka C, Alexiou GA, Fotopoulos A, Voulgaris S, Argyropoulou MI. Radiation necrosis, pseudoprogression, pseudoresponse, and tumor recurrence: imaging challenges for the evaluation of treated gliomas. Contrast Media Mol Imaging. 2018;2018:6828396. https://doi.org/10.1155/2018/6828396.
29. Tsiouris S, Bougias C, Fotopoulos A. Principles and current trends in the correlative evaluation of glioma with advanced MRI techniques and PET. Hell J Nucl Med. 2019;22(3):206–19.
30. Långström B, Antoni G, Gullberg P, Halldin C, Malmborg P, Någren K, et al. Synthesis of L- and D-[methyl-11C]methionine. J Nucl Med. 1987;28(6):1037–40.
31. Glaudemans AW, Enting RH, Heesters MA, Dierckx RA, van Rheenen RW, Walenkamp AM, et al. Value of 11C-methionine PET in imaging brain tumours and metastases. Eur J Nucl Med Mol Imaging. 2013;40(4):615–35. https://doi.org/10.1007/s00259-012-2295-5.
32. Okochi Y, Nihashi T, Fujii M, Kato K, Okada Y, Ando Y, et al. Clinical use of (11) C-methionine and (18)F-FDG-PET for germinoma in central nervous system. Ann Nucl Med. 2014;28(2):94–102. https://doi.org/10.1007/s12149-013-0787-4.
33. Van Laere K, Ceyssens S, Van Calenbergh F, de Groot T, Menten J, Flamen P, et al. Direct comparison of 18F-FDG and 11C-methionine PET in suspected recurrence of glioma: sensitivity, inter-observer variability and prognostic value. Eur J Nucl Med Mol Imaging. 2005;32(1):39–51. https://doi.org/10.1007/s00259-004-1564-3.
34. Mansoor NM, Thust S, Militano V, Fraioli F. PET imaging in glioma: techniques and current evidence. Nucl Med Commun. 2018;39(12):1064–80. https://doi.org/10.1097/mnm.0000000000000914.
35. Kim MM, Parolia A, Dunphy MP, Venneti S. Non-invasive metabolic imaging of brain tumours in the era of precision medicine. Nat Rev Clin Oncol. 2016;13(12):725–39. https://doi.org/10.1038/nrclinonc.2016.108.
36. Hutterer M, Nowosielski M, Putzer D, Jansen NL, Seiz M, Schocke M, et al. [18F]-fluoro-ethyl-L-tyrosine PET: a valuable diagnostic tool in neuro-oncology, but not all that glitters is glioma. Neuro Oncol. 2013;15(3):341–51. https://doi.org/10.1093/neuonc/nos300.
37. Jansen NL, Graute V, Armbruster L, Suchorska B, Lutz J, Eigenbrod S, et al. MRI-suspected low-grade glioma: is there a need to perform dynamic FET PET? Eur J Nucl Med Mol Imaging. 2012;39(6):1021–9. https://doi.org/10.1007/s00259-012-2109-9.
38. Pichler R, Dunzinger A, Wurm G, Pichler J, Weis S, Nussbaumer K, et al. Is there a place for FET PET in the initial evaluation of brain lesions with unknown significance? Eur J Nucl Med Mol Imaging. 2010;37(8):1521–8. https://doi.org/10.1007/s00259-010-1457-6.
39. Mehrkens JH, Pöpperl G, Rachinger W, Herms J, Seelos K, Tatsch K, et al. The positive predictive value of O-(2-[18F]fluoroethyl)-L-tyrosine (FET) PET in the diagnosis of a glioma recurrence after multimodal treatment. J Neurooncol. 2008;88(1):27–35. https://doi.org/10.1007/s11060-008-9526-4.
40. Lizarraga KJ, Allen-Auerbach M, Czernin J, DeSalles AA, Yong WH, Phelps ME, et al. (18) F-FDOPA PET for differentiating recurrent or progressive brain metastatic tumors from late or delayed radiation injury after radiation treatment. J Nucl Med. 2014;55(1):30–6. https://doi.org/10.2967/jnumed.113.121418.
41. Galldiks N, Stoffels G, Filss C, Rapp M, Blau T, Tscherpel C, et al. The use of dynamic O-(2-18F-fluoroethyl)-l-tyrosine PET in the diagnosis of patients with progressive and recurrent glioma. Neuro Oncol. 2015;17(9):1293–300. https://doi.org/10.1093/neuonc/nov088.
42. Ceccon G, Lohmann P, Stoffels G, Judov N, Filss CP, Rapp M, et al. Dynamic O-(2-18F-fluoroethyl)-L-tyrosine positron emission tomography differentiates brain metastasis recurrence from radiation injury after radiotherapy. Neuro Oncol. 2017;19(2):281–8. https://doi.org/10.1093/neuonc/now149.
43. Nihashi T, Dahabreh IJ, Terasawa T. Diagnostic accuracy of PET for recurrent glioma diagnosis: a meta-analysis. AJNR Am J Neuroradiol. 2013;34(5):944–50., s1-11. https://doi.org/10.3174/ajnr.A3324.

44. Minamimoto R, Saginoya T, Kondo C, Tomura N, Ito K, Matsuo Y, et al. Differentiation of brain tumor recurrence from post-radiotherapy necrosis with 11C-methionine PET: visual assessment versus quantitative assessment. PLoS One. 2015;10(7):e0132515. https://doi.org/10.1371/journal.pone.0132515.
45. Salber D, Stoffels G, Pauleit D, Oros-Peusquens AM, Shah NJ, Klauth P, et al. Differential uptake of O-(2-18F-fluoroethyl)-L-tyrosine, L-3H-methionine, and 3H-deoxyglucose in brain abscesses. J Nucl Med. 2007;48(12):2056–62. https://doi.org/10.2967/jnumed.107.046615.
46. Venneti S, Dunphy MP, Zhang H, Pitter KL, Zanzonico P, Campos C, et al. Glutamine-based PET imaging facilitates enhanced metabolic evaluation of gliomas in vivo. Sci Transl Med. 2015;7(274):274ra17. https://doi.org/10.1126/scitranslmed.aaa1009.
47. Xu X, Zhu H, Liu F, Zhang Y, Yang J, Zhang L, et al. Imaging brain metastasis patients with 18F-(2S,4R)-4-fluoroglutamine. Clin Nucl Med. 2018;43(11):e392–e9. https://doi.org/10.1097/rlu.0000000000002257.
48. Galldiks N, Kracht LW, Burghaus L, Thomas A, Jacobs AH, Heiss WD, et al. Use of 11C-methionine PET to monitor the effects of temozolomide chemotherapy in malignant gliomas. Eur J Nucl Med Mol Imaging. 2006;33(5):516–24. https://doi.org/10.1007/s00259-005-0002-5.
49. Herholz K, Kracht LW, Heiss WD. Monitoring the effect of chemotherapy in a mixed glioma by C-11-methionine PET. J Neuroimaging. 2003;13(3):269–71.
50. Roelcke U, Wyss MT, Nowosielski M, Rudà R, Roth P, Hofer S, et al. Amino acid positron emission tomography to monitor chemotherapy response and predict seizure control and progression-free survival in WHO grade II gliomas. Neuro Oncol. 2016;18(5):744–51. https://doi.org/10.1093/neuonc/nov282.
51. Hutterer M, Nowosielski M, Putzer D, Waitz D, Tinkhauser G, Kostron H, et al. O-(2-18F-fluoroethyl)-L-tyrosine PET predicts failure of antiangiogenic treatment in patients with recurrent high-grade glioma. J Nucl Med. 2011;52(6):856–64. https://doi.org/10.2967/jnumed.110.086645.
52. Galldiks N, Rapp M, Stoffels G, Fink GR, Shah NJ, Coenen HH, et al. Response assessment of bevacizumab in patients with recurrent malignant glioma using [18F]Fluoroethyl-L-tyrosine PET in comparison to MRI. Eur J Nucl Med Mol Imaging. 2013;40(1):22–33. https://doi.org/10.1007/s00259-012-2251-4.
53. Schwarzenberg J, Czernin J, Cloughesy TF, Ellingson BM, Pope WB, Grogan T, et al. Treatment response evaluation using 18F-FDOPA PET in patients with recurrent malignant glioma on bevacizumab therapy. Clin Cancer Res. 2014;20(13):3550–9. https://doi.org/10.1158/1078-0432.Ccr-13-1440.
54. Ceccon G, Lazaridis L, Stoffels G, Rapp M, Weber M, Blau T, et al. Use of FET PET in glioblastoma patients undergoing neurooncological treatment including tumour-treating fields: initial experience. Eur J Nucl Med Mol Imaging. 2018;45(9):1626–35. https://doi.org/10.1007/s00259-018-3992-5.
55. Gérard M, Corroyer-Dulmont A, Lesueur P, Collet S, Chérel M, Bourgeois M, et al. Hypoxia imaging and adaptive radiotherapy: a state-of-the-art approach in the management of glioma. Front Med (Lausanne). 2019;6:117. https://doi.org/10.3389/fmed.2019.00117.
56. Lee ST, Scott AM. Hypoxia positron emission tomography imaging with 18f-fluoromisonidazole. Semin Nucl Med. 2007;37(6):451–61. https://doi.org/10.1053/j.semnuclmed.2007.07.001.
57. Swanson KR, Chakraborty G, Wang CH, Rockne R, Harpold HL, Muzi M, et al. Complementary but distinct roles for MRI and 18F-fluoromisonidazole PET in the assessment of human glioblastomas. J Nucl Med. 2009;50(1):36–44. https://doi.org/10.2967/jnumed.108.055467.
58. Kawai N, Maeda Y, Kudomi N, Miyake K, Okada M, Yamamoto Y, et al. Correlation of biological aggressiveness assessed by 11C-methionine PET and hypoxic burden assessed by 18F-fluoromisonidazole PET in newly diagnosed glioblastoma. Eur J Nucl Med Mol Imaging. 2011;38(3):441–50. https://doi.org/10.1007/s00259-010-1645-4.

59. Barajas RF, Krohn KA, Link JM, Hawkins RA, Clarke JL, Pampaloni MH, et al. Glioma FMISO PET/MR imaging concurrent with antiangiogenic therapy: molecular imaging as a clinical tool in the burgeoning era of personalized medicine. Biomedicines. 2016;4(4). https://doi.org/10.3390/biomedicines4040024.
60. Yamaguchi S, Hirata K, Toyonaga T, Kobayashi K, Ishi Y, Motegi H, et al. Change in 18F-fluoromisonidazole PET is an early predictor of the prognosis in the patients with recurrent high-grade glioma receiving bevacizumab treatment. PLoS One. 2016;11(12):e0167917. https://doi.org/10.1371/journal.pone.0167917.
61. Valk PE, Mathis CA, Prados MD, Gilbert JC, Budinger TF. Hypoxia in human gliomas: demonstration by PET with fluorine-18-fluoromisonidazole. J Nucl Med. 1992;33(12):2133–7.
62. Hirata K, Terasaka S, Shiga T, Hattori N, Magota K, Kobayashi H, et al. ^{18}F-Fluoromisonidazole positron emission tomography may differentiate glioblastoma multiforme from less malignant gliomas. Eur J Nucl Med Mol Imaging. 2012;39(5):760–70. https://doi.org/10.1007/s00259-011-2037-0.
63. Spence AM, Muzi M, Swanson KR, O'Sullivan F, Rockhill JK, Rajendran JG, et al. Regional hypoxia in glioblastoma multiforme quantified with [18F]fluoromisonidazole positron emission tomography before radiotherapy: correlation with time to progression and survival. Clin Cancer Res. 2008;14(9):2623–30. https://doi.org/10.1158/1078-0432.Ccr-07-4995.
64. Gerstner ER, Zhang Z, Fink JR, Muzi M, Hanna L, Greco E, et al. ACRIN 6684: assessment of tumor hypoxia in newly diagnosed glioblastoma using 18F-FMISO PET and MRI. Clin Cancer Res. 2016;22(20):5079–86. https://doi.org/10.1158/1078-0432.Ccr-15-2529.
65. Toriihara A, Ohtake M, Tateishi K, Hino-Shishikura A, Yoneyama T, Kitazume Y, et al. Prognostic implications of (62)Cu-diacetyl-bis (N(4)-methylthiosemicarbazone) PET/CT in patients with glioma. Ann Nucl Med. 2018;32(4):264–71. https://doi.org/10.1007/s12149-018-1241-4.
66. Lopci E, Franzese C, Grimaldi M, Zucali PA, Navarria P, Simonelli M, et al. Imaging biomarkers in primary brain tumours. Eur J Nucl Med Mol Imaging. 2015;42(4):597–612. https://doi.org/10.1007/s00259-014-2971-8.
67. Chen W, Cloughesy T, Kamdar N, Satyamurthy N, Bergsneider M, Liau L, et al. Imaging proliferation in brain tumors with 18F-FLT PET: comparison with 18F-FDG. J Nucl Med. 2005;46(6):945–52.
68. Jacobs AH, Thomas A, Kracht LW, Li H, Dittmar C, Garlip G, et al. 18F-fluoro-L-thymidine and 11C-methylmethionine as markers of increased transport and proliferation in brain tumors. J Nucl Med. 2005;46(12):1948–58.
69. Li Z, Yu Y, Zhang H, Xu G, Chen L. A meta-analysis comparing 18F-FLT PET with 18F-FDG PET for assessment of brain tumor recurrence. Nucl Med Commun. 2015;36(7):695–701. https://doi.org/10.1097/mnm.0000000000000302.
70. Chen W, Delaloye S, Silverman DH, Geist C, Czernin J, Sayre J, et al. Predicting treatment response of malignant gliomas to bevacizumab and irinotecan by imaging proliferation with [18F] fluorothymidine positron emission tomography: a pilot study. J Clin Oncol. 2007;25(30):4714–21. https://doi.org/10.1200/jco.2006.10.5825.
71. Nguyen NC, Yee MK, Tuchayi AM, Kirkwood JM, Tawbi H, Mountz JM. Targeted therapy and immunotherapy response assessment with F-18 fluorothymidine positron-emission tomography/magnetic resonance imaging in melanoma brain metastasis: a pilot study. Front Oncol. 2018;8:18. https://doi.org/10.3389/fonc.2018.00018.
72. Ferdová E, Ferda J, Baxa J, Tupý R, Mraček J, Topolčan O, et al. Assessment of grading in newly-diagnosed glioma using 18F-fluorothymidine PET/CT. Anticancer Res. 2015;35(2):955–9.
73. Belohlavek O, Fencl P, Majovsky M, Jaruskova M, Benes V. FLT-PET in previously untreated patients with low-grade glioma can predict their overall survival. Nucl Med Rev Cent East Eur. 2014;17(1):7–12. https://doi.org/10.5603/nmr.2014.0003.
74. Collet S, Valable S, Constans JM, Lechapt-Zalcman E, Roussel S, Delcroix N, et al. [(18) F]-fluoro-L-thymidine PET and advanced MRI for preoperative grading of gliomas. Neuroimage Clin. 2015;8:448–54. https://doi.org/10.1016/j.nicl.2015.05.012.

75. Idema AJ, Hoffmann AL, Boogaarts HD, Troost EG, Wesseling P, Heerschap A, et al. 3'-Deoxy-3'-18F-fluorothymidine PET-derived proliferative volume predicts overall survival in high-grade glioma patients. J Nucl Med. 2012;53(12):1904–10. https://doi.org/10.2967/jnumed.112.105544.
76. Zhao F, Li M, Wang Z, Fu Z, Cui Y, Chen Z, et al. (18)F-Fluorothymidine PET-CT for resected malignant gliomas before radiotherapy: tumor extent according to proliferative activity compared with MRI. PLoS One. 2015;10(3):e0118769. https://doi.org/10.1371/journal.pone.0118769.
77. Zhao F, Cui Y, Li M, Fu Z, Chen Z, Kong L, et al. Prognostic value of 3'-deoxy-3'-18F-fluorothymidine ([(18)F] FLT PET) in patients with recurrent malignant gliomas. Nucl Med Biol. 2014;41(8):710–5. https://doi.org/10.1016/j.nucmedbio.2014.04.134.
78. Ter-Pogossian MM, Eichling JO, Davis DO, Welch MJ. The measure in vivo of regional cerebral oxygen utilization by means of oxyhemoglobin labeled with radioactive oxygen-15. J Clin Invest. 1970;49(2):381–91. https://doi.org/10.1172/jci106247.
79. Lüdemann L, Warmuth C, Plotkin M, Förschler A, Gutberlet M, Wust P, et al. Brain tumor perfusion: comparison of dynamic contrast-enhanced magnetic resonance imaging using T1, T2, and T2* contrast, pulsed arterial spin labeling, and H2(15)O positron emission tomography. Eur J Radiol. 2009;70(3):465–74. https://doi.org/10.1016/j.ejrad.2008.02.012.
80. Spence AM, Mankoff DA, Muzi M. Positron emission tomography imaging of brain tumors. Neuroimaging Clin N Am. 2003;13(4):717–39. https://doi.org/10.1016/s1052-5149(03)00097-2.
81. Yi C, Shi X, Yu D, Luo G, Zhang B, He Q, et al. The combination of 13N-ammonia and 18F-FDG PET/CT in the identification of metabolic phenotype of primary human brain tumors. Nuklearmedizin. 2019;58(3):272–8. https://doi.org/10.1055/a-0835-5746.
82. Jain RK, di Tomaso E, Duda DG, Loeffler JS, Sorensen AG, Batchelor TT. Angiogenesis in brain tumours. Nat Rev Neurosci. 2007;8(8):610–22. https://doi.org/10.1038/nrn2175.
83. Jansen MH, Veldhuijzen van Zanten SEM, van Vuurden DG, Huisman MC, Vugts DJ, Hoekstra OS, et al. Molecular drug imaging: (89)Zr-bevacizumab PET in children with diffuse intrinsic pontine glioma. J Nucl Med. 2017;58(5):711–6. https://doi.org/10.2967/jnumed.116.180216.
84. Veldhuijzen van Zanten SEM, Sewing ACP, van Lingen A, Hoekstra OS, Wesseling P, Meel MH, et al. Multiregional tumor drug-uptake imaging by PET and microvascular morphology in end-stage diffuse intrinsic pontine glioma. J Nucl Med. 2018;59(4):612–5. https://doi.org/10.2967/jnumed.117.197897.
85. Chen K, Cai W, Li ZB, Wang H, Chen X. Quantitative PET imaging of VEGF receptor expression. Mol Imaging Biol. 2009;11(1):15–22. https://doi.org/10.1007/s11307-008-0172-1.
86. Cai W, Chen K, Mohamedali KA, Cao Q, Gambhir SS, Rosenblum MG, et al. PET of vascular endothelial growth factor receptor expression. J Nucl Med. 2006;47(12):2048–56.
87. Heute D, Kostron H, von Guggenberg E, Ingorokva S, Gabriel M, Dobrozemsky G, et al. Response of recurrent high-grade glioma to treatment with (90)Y-DOTATOC. J Nucl Med. 2010;51(3):397–400. https://doi.org/10.2967/jnumed.109.072819.
88. Breeman WA, de Blois E, Sze Chan H, Konijnenberg M, Kwekkeboom DJ, Krenning EP. (68) Ga-labeled DOTA-peptides and (68)Ga-labeled radiopharmaceuticals for positron emission tomography: current status of research, clinical applications, and future perspectives. Semin Nucl Med. 2011;41(4):314–21. https://doi.org/10.1053/j.semnuclmed.2011.02.001.
89. Collamati F, Pepe A, Bellini F, Bocci V, Chiodi G, Cremonesi M, et al. Toward radioguided surgery with β- decays: uptake of a somatostatin analogue, DOTATOC, in meningioma and high-grade glioma. J Nucl Med. 2015;56(1):3–8. https://doi.org/10.2967/jnumed.114.145995.
90. Seystahl K, Stoecklein V, Schüller U, Rushing E, Nicolas G, Schäfer N, et al. Somatostatin receptor-targeted radionuclide therapy for progressive meningioma: benefit linked to 68Ga-DOTATATE/-TOC uptake. Neuro Oncol. 2016;18(11):1538–47. https://doi.org/10.1093/neuonc/now060.
91. Parghane RV, Talole S, Basu S. Prevalence of hitherto unknown brain meningioma detected on (68)Ga-DOTATATE positron-emission tomography/computed tomography in patients

with metastatic neuroendocrine tumor and exploring potential of (177)Lu-DOTATATE peptide receptor radionuclide therapy as single-shot treatment approach targeting both tumors. World J Nucl Med. 2019;18(2):160–70. https://doi.org/10.4103/wjnm.WJNM_39_18.
92. Verburg FA, Wiessmann M, Neuloh G, Mottaghy FM, Brockmann MA. Intraindividual comparison of selective intraarterial versus systemic intravenous 68Ga-DOTATATE PET/CT in patients with inoperable meningioma. Nuklearmedizin. 2019;58(1):23–7. https://doi.org/10.1055/a-0802-5039.
93. Braat A, Snijders TJ, Seute T, Vonken EPA. Will (177)Lu-DOTATATE treatment become more effective in salvage meningioma patients, when boosting somatostatin receptor saturation? A promising case on intra-arterial administration. Cardiovasc Intervent Radiol. 2019;42(11):1649–52. https://doi.org/10.1007/s00270-019-02262-1.
94. Verma P, Malhotra G, Goel A, Rakshit S, Chandak A, Chedda R, et al. Differential uptake of 68Ga-PSMA-HBED-CC (PSMA-11) in low-grade versus high-grade gliomas in treatment-naive patients. Clin Nucl Med. 2019;44(5):e318–22. https://doi.org/10.1097/rlu.0000000000002520.
95. Sasikumar A, Joy A, Pillai MR, Nanabala R, Anees KM, Jayaprakash PG, et al. Diagnostic value of 68Ga PSMA-11 PET/CT imaging of brain tumors-preliminary analysis. Clin Nucl Med. 2017;42(1):e41–e8. https://doi.org/10.1097/rlu.0000000000001451.
96. Unterrainer M, Niyazi M, Ruf V, Bartenstein P, Albert NL. The endothelial prostate-specific membrane antigen is highly expressed in gliosarcoma and visualized by [68Ga]-PSMA-11 PET: a theranostic outlook for brain tumor patients? Neuro Oncol. 2017;19(12):1698–9. https://doi.org/10.1093/neuonc/nox172.
97. Salas Fragomeni RA, Menke JR, Holdhoff M, Ferrigno C, Laterra JJ, Solnes LB, et al. Prostate-specific membrane antigen-targeted imaging with [18F]DCFPyL in high-grade gliomas. Clin Nucl Med. 2017;42(10):e433–5. https://doi.org/10.1097/rlu.0000000000001769.
98. Matsuda M, Ishikawa E, Yamamoto T, Hatano K, Joraku A, Iizumi Y, et al. Potential use of prostate specific membrane antigen (PSMA) for detecting the tumor neovasculature of brain tumors by PET imaging with (89)Zr-Df-IAB2M anti-PSMA minibody. J Neurooncol. 2018;138(3):581–9. https://doi.org/10.1007/s11060-018-2825-5.
99. Van de Wiele C, Sathekge M, de Spiegeleer B, de Jonghe PJ, Beels L, Maes A. PSMA-targeting positron emission agents for imaging solid tumors other than non-prostate carcinoma: a systematic review. Int J Mol Sci. 2019;20(19). https://doi.org/10.3390/ijms20194886.
100. Kratochwil C, Bruchertseifer F, Rathke H, Hohenfellner M, Giesel FL, Haberkorn U, et al. Targeted α-therapy of metastatic castration-resistant prostate cancer with (225) Ac-PSMA-617: swimmer-plot analysis suggests efficacy regarding duration of tumor control. J Nucl Med. 2018;59(5):795–802. https://doi.org/10.2967/jnumed.117.203539.
101. Wen PY, Chang SM, Van den Bent MJ, Vogelbaum MA, Macdonald DR, Lee EQ. Response assessment in neuro-oncology clinical trials. J Clin Oncol. 2017;35(21):2439–49. https://doi.org/10.1200/jco.2017.72.7511.
102. Sathekge M, Bruchertseifer F, Knoesen O, Reyneke F, Lawal I, Lengana T, et al. (225) Ac-PSMA-617 in chemotherapy-naive patients with advanced prostate cancer: a pilot study. Eur J Nucl Med Mol Imaging. 2019;46(1):129–38. https://doi.org/10.1007/s00259-018-4167-0.
103. Kneifel S, Cordier D, Good S, Ionescu MC, Ghaffari A, Hofer S, et al. Local targeting of malignant gliomas by the diffusible peptidic vector 1,4,7,10-tetraazacyclododecane-1-glutaric acid-4,7,10-triacetic acid-substance p. Clin Cancer Res. 2006;12(12):3843–50. https://doi.org/10.1158/1078-0432.Ccr-05-2820.
104. Cordier D, Forrer F, Bruchertseifer F, Morgenstern A, Apostolidis C, Good S, et al. Targeted alpha-radionuclide therapy of functionally critically located gliomas with 213Bi-DOTA-[Thi8,Met(O2)11]-substance P: a pilot trial. Eur J Nucl Med Mol Imaging. 2010;37(7):1335–44. https://doi.org/10.1007/s00259-010-1385-5.
105. Schulz S, Stumm R, Röcken C, Mawrin C, Schulz S. Immunolocalization of full-length NK1 tachykinin receptors in human tumors. J Histochem Cytochem. 2006;54(9):1015–20. https://doi.org/10.1369/jhc.6A6966.2006.

106. Rosso M, Muñoz M, Berger M. The role of neurokinin-1 receptor in the microenvironment of inflammation and cancer. ScientificWorldJournal. 2012;2012:381434. https://doi.org/10.1100/2012/381434.
107. Krolicki L, Bruchertseifer F, Kunikowska J, Koziara H, Królicki B, Jakuciński M, et al. Prolonged survival in secondary glioblastoma following local injection of targeted alpha therapy with (213)Bi-substance P analogue. Eur J Nucl Med Mol Imaging. 2018;45(9):1636–44. https://doi.org/10.1007/s00259-018-4015-2.
108. Królicki L, Bruchertseifer F, Kunikowska J, Koziara H, Królicki B, Jakuciński M, et al. Safety and efficacy of targeted alpha therapy with (213)Bi-DOTA-substance P in recurrent glioblastoma. Eur J Nucl Med Mol Imaging. 2019;46(3):614–22. https://doi.org/10.1007/s00259-018-4225-7.
109. Poli GL, Bianchi C, Virotta G, Bettini A, Moretti R, Trachsel E, et al. Radretumab radioimmunotherapy in patients with brain metastasis: a 124I-L19SIP dosimetric PET study. Cancer Immunol Res. 2013;1(2):134–43. https://doi.org/10.1158/2326-6066.Cir-13-0007.
110. Zamecnik J. The extracellular space and matrix of gliomas. Acta Neuropathol. 2005;110(5):435–42. https://doi.org/10.1007/s00401-005-1078-5.
111. Bailly C, Vidal A, Bonnemaire C, Kraeber-Bodéré F, Chérel M, Pallardy A, et al. Potential for nuclear medicine therapy for glioblastoma treatment. Front Pharmacol. 2019;10:772. https://doi.org/10.3389/fphar.2019.00772.
112. Burger JA, Kipps TJ. CXCR4: a key receptor in the crosstalk between tumor cells and their microenvironment. Blood. 2006;107(5):1761–7. https://doi.org/10.1182/blood-2005-08-3182.
113. Bian XW, Yang SX, Chen JH, Ping YF, Zhou XD, Wang QL, et al. Preferential expression of chemokine receptor CXCR4 by highly malignant human gliomas and its association with poor patient survival. Neurosurgery. 2007;61(3):570–8; discussion 8–9. https://doi.org/10.1227/01.Neu.0000290905.53685.A2.
114. Sun J, Cai L, Zhang K, Zhang A, Pu P, Yang W, et al. A pilot study on EGFR-targeted molecular imaging of PET/CT With 11C-PD153035 in human gliomas. Clin Nucl Med. 2014;39(1):e20–6. https://doi.org/10.1097/RLU.0b013e3182a23b73.
115. Weber B, Winterdahl M, Memon A, Sorensen BS, Keiding S, Sorensen L, et al. Erlotinib accumulation in brain metastases from non-small cell lung cancer: visualization by positron emission tomography in a patient harboring a mutation in the epidermal growth factor receptor. J Thorac Oncol. 2011;6(7):1287–9. https://doi.org/10.1097/JTO.0b013e318219ab87.
116. Tang Y, Hu Y, Liu W, Chen L, Zhao Y, Ma H, et al. A radiopharmaceutical [(89)Zr]Zr-DFO-nimotuzumab for immunoPET with epidermal growth factor receptor expression in vivo. Nucl Med Biol. 2019;70:23–31. https://doi.org/10.1016/j.nucmedbio.2019.01.007.
117. Cole EL, Kim J, Donnelly DJ, Smith RA, Cohen D, Lafont V, et al. Radiosynthesis and preclinical PET evaluation of (89)Zr-nivolumab (BMS-936558) in healthy non-human primates. Bioorg Med Chem. 2017;25(20):5407–14. https://doi.org/10.1016/j.bmc.2017.07.066.
118. Bensch F, van der Veen EL, Lub-de Hooge MN, Jorritsma-Smit A, Boellaard R, Kok IC, et al. (89)Zr-atezolizumab imaging as a non-invasive approach to assess clinical response to PD-L1 blockade in cancer. Nat Med. 2018;24(12):1852–8. https://doi.org/10.1038/s41591-018-0255-8.
119. Niemeijer AN, Leung D, Huisman MC, Bahce I, Hoekstra OS, van Dongen G, et al. Whole body PD-1 and PD-L1 positron emission tomography in patients with non-small-cell lung cancer. Nat Commun. 2018;9(1):4664. https://doi.org/10.1038/s41467-018-07131-y.
120. Donnelly DJ, Smith RA, Morin P, Lipovšek D, Gokemeijer J, Cohen D, et al. Synthesis and biologic evaluation of a novel (18)F-labeled adnectin as a PET radioligand for imaging PD-L1 expression. J Nucl Med. 2018;59(3):529–35. https://doi.org/10.2967/jnumed.117.199596.
121. Tumeh PC, Harview CL, Yearley JH, Shintaku IP, Taylor EJ, Robert L, et al. PD-1 blockade induces responses by inhibiting adaptive immune resistance. Nature. 2014;515(7528):568–71. https://doi.org/10.1038/nature13954.
122. Pandit-Taskar N, Postow MA, Hellmann MD, Harding JJ, Barker CA, O'Donoghue JA, et al. First-in-humans imaging with (89)Zr-Df-IAB22M2C anti-CD8 minibody in patients with

solid malignancies: preliminary pharmacokinetics, biodistribution, and lesion targeting. J Nucl Med. 2020;61(4):512–9. https://doi.org/10.2967/jnumed.119.229781.
123. Antonios JP, Soto H, Everson RG, Moughon DL, Wang AC, Orpilla J, et al. Detection of immune responses after immunotherapy in glioblastoma using PET and MRI. Proc Natl Acad Sci U S A. 2017;114(38):10220–5. https://doi.org/10.1073/pnas.1706689114.
124. Wei W, Jiang D, Ehlerding EB, Luo Q, Cai W. Noninvasive PET Imaging of T cells. Trends Cancer. 2018;4(5):359–73. https://doi.org/10.1016/j.trecan.2018.03.009.
125. Chitneni SK, Yan H, Zalutsky MR. Synthesis and evaluation of a (18)F-labeled triazinediamine analogue for imaging mutant IDH1 expression in gliomas by PET. ACS Med Chem Lett. 2018;9(7):606–11. https://doi.org/10.1021/acsmedchemlett.7b00478.
126. Reardon DA, Akabani G, Coleman RE, Friedman AH, Friedman HS, Herndon JE II, et al. Phase II trial of murine (131)I-labeled antitenascin monoclonal antibody 81C6 administered into surgically created resection cavities of patients with newly diagnosed malignant gliomas. J Clin Oncol. 2002;20(5):1389–97. https://doi.org/10.1200/jco.2002.20.5.1389.
127. David M, Lécorché P, Masse M, Faucon A, Abouzid K, Gaudin N, et al. Identification and characterization of highly versatile peptide-vectors that bind non-competitively to the low-density lipoprotein receptor for in vivo targeting and delivery of small molecules and protein cargos. PLoS One. 2018;13(2):e0191052. https://doi.org/10.1371/journal.pone.0191052.
128. Królicki L, Kunikowska J, Bruchertseifer F, Koziara H, Królicki B, Jakuciński M, et al. (225)Ac- and (213)Bi-substance P analogues for glioma therapy. Semin Nucl Med. 2020;50(2):141–51. https://doi.org/10.1053/j.semnuclmed.2019.11.004.
129. Królicki L, Bruchertseifer F, Kunikowska J, Koziara H, Pawlak D, Kuliński R, et al. Dose escalation study of targeted alpha therapy with [225Ac]Ac-DOTA-substance P in recurrence glioblastoma—safety and efficacy. Eur J Nucl Med Mol Imaging. 2021;48(11):3595–605. https://doi.org/10.1007/s00259-021-05350-y.
130. Zalutsky MR. Current status of therapy of solid tumors: brain tumor therapy. J Nucl Med. 2005;46 Suppl 1:151s–6s.
131. Riva P, Franceschi G, Riva N, Casi M, Santimaria M, Adamo M. Role of nuclear medicine in the treatment of malignant gliomas: the locoregional radioimmunotherapy approach. Eur J Nucl Med. 2000;27(5):601–9. https://doi.org/10.1007/s002590050549.
132. Akabani G, Reardon DA, Coleman RE, Wong TZ, Metzler SD, Bowsher JE, et al. Dosimetry and radiographic analysis of 131I-labeled anti-tenascin 81C6 murine monoclonal antibody in newly diagnosed patients with malignant gliomas: a phase II study. J Nucl Med. 2005;46(6):1042–51.
133. Zalutsky MR, Reardon DA, Akabani G, Coleman RE, Friedman AH, Friedman HS, et al. Clinical experience with alpha-particle emitting 211At: treatment of recurrent brain tumor patients with 211At-labeled chimeric antitenascin monoclonal antibody 81C6. J Nucl Med. 2008;49(1):30–8. https://doi.org/10.2967/jnumed.107.046938.
134. Borsi L, Balza E, Bestagno M, Castellani P, Carnemolla B, Biro A, et al. Selective targeting of tumoral vasculature: comparison of different formats of an antibody (L19) to the ED-B domain of fibronectin. Int J Cancer. 2002;102(1):75–85. https://doi.org/10.1002/ijc.10662.
135. Sauer S, Erba PA, Petrini M, Menrad A, Giovannoni L, Grana C, et al. Expression of the oncofetal ED-B-containing fibronectin isoform in hematologic tumors enables ED-B-targeted 131I-L19SIP radioimmunotherapy in Hodgkin lymphoma patients. Blood. 2009;113(10):2265–74. https://doi.org/10.1182/blood-2008-06-160416.
136. Brennan CW, Verhaak RG, McKenna A, Campos B, Noushmehr H, Salama SR, et al. The somatic genomic landscape of glioblastoma. Cell. 2013;155(2):462–77. https://doi.org/10.1016/j.cell.2013.09.034.
137. Li L, Quang TS, Gracely EJ, Kim JH, Emrich JG, Yaeger TE, et al. A phase II study of anti-epidermal growth factor receptor radioimmunotherapy in the treatment of glioblastoma multiforme. J Neurosurg. 2010;113(2):192–8. https://doi.org/10.3171/2010.2.Jns091211.
138. Casacó A, López G, García I, Rodríguez JA, Fernández R, Figueredo J, et al. Phase I single-dose study of intracavitary-administered nimotuzumab labeled with 188 Re in adult recurrent high-grade glioma. Cancer Biol Ther. 2008;7(3):333–9. https://doi.org/10.4161/cbt.7.3.5414.

139. Hdeib A, Sloan A. Targeted radioimmunotherapy: the role of ^{131}I-chTNT-1/B mAb (Cotara) for treatment of high-grade gliomas. Future Oncol. 2012;8(6):659–69. https://doi.org/10.2217/fon.12.58.
140. Shapiro WR, Carpenter SP, Roberts K, Shan JS. (131)I-chTNT-1/B mAb: tumour necrosis therapy for malignant astrocytic glioma. Expert Opin Biol Ther. 2006;6(5):539–45. https://doi.org/10.1517/14712598.6.5.539.
141. Dutour A, Kumar U, Panetta R, Ouafik L, Fina F, Sasi R, et al. Expression of somatostatin receptor subtypes in human brain tumors. Int J Cancer. 1998;76(5):620–7. https://doi.org/10.1002/(sici)1097-0215(19980529)76:5<620::aid-ijc2>3.0.co;2-s.
142. Schumacher T, Hofer S, Eichhorn K, Wasner M, Zimmerer S, Freitag P, et al. Local injection of the 90Y-labelled peptidic vector DOTATOC to control gliomas of WHO grades II and III: an extended pilot study. Eur J Nucl Med Mol Imaging. 2002;29(4):486–93. https://doi.org/10.1007/s00259-001-0717-x.
143. Wei X, Schlenkhoff C, Schwarz B, Essler M, Ahmadzadehfar H. Combination of 177Lu-PSMA-617 and external radiotherapy for the treatment of cerebral metastases in patients with castration-resistant metastatic prostate cancer. Clin Nucl Med. 2017;42(9):704–6. https://doi.org/10.1097/rlu.0000000000001763.
144. Nawashiro H, Otani N, Shinomiya N, Fukui S, Ooigawa H, Shima K, et al. L-type amino acid transporter 1 as a potential molecular target in human astrocytic tumors. Int J Cancer. 2006;119(3):484–92. https://doi.org/10.1002/ijc.21866.
145. Hellwig D, Ketter R, Romeike BF, Sell N, Schaefer A, Moringlane JR, et al. Validation of brain tumour imaging with p-[123I]iodo-L-phenylalanine and SPECT. Eur J Nucl Med Mol Imaging. 2005;32(9):1041–9. https://doi.org/10.1007/s00259-005-1807-y.
146. Baum RP, Kluge A, Gildehaus FJ, Bronzel M, Schmidt K, Schuchardt C, et al. Systemic endoradiotherapy with carrier-added 4-[(131)I]Iodo-L-phenylalanine: clinical proof-of-principle in refractory glioma. Nucl Med Mol Imaging. 2011;45(4):299–307. https://doi.org/10.1007/s13139-011-0116-6.
147. Verburg FA, Sweeney R, Hänscheid H, Dießl S, Israel I, Löhr M, et al. Patients with recurrent glioblastoma multiforme. Initial experience with p-[(131)I]iodo-L-phenylalanine and external beam radiation therapy. Nuklearmedizin. 2013;52(1):36–42. https://doi.org/10.3413/Nukmed-0510-12-06.
148. Puttemans J, Dekempeneer Y, Eersels JL, Hanssens H, Debie P, Keyaerts M, et al. Preclinical targeted α- and β(-)-radionuclide therapy in HER2-positive brain metastasis using camelid single-domain antibodies. Cancers (Basel). 2020;12(4). https://doi.org/10.3390/cancers12041017.
149. Veeravagu A, Liu Z, Niu G, Chen K, Jia B, Cai W, et al. Integrin alphavbeta3-targeted radioimmunotherapy of glioblastoma multiforme. Clin Cancer Res. 2008;14(22):7330–9. https://doi.org/10.1158/1078-0432.Ccr-08-0797.
150. Jiang L, Miao Z, Kimura RH, Liu H, Cochran JR, Culter CS, et al. Preliminary evaluation of (177)Lu-labeled knottin peptides for integrin receptor-targeted radionuclide therapy. Eur J Nucl Med Mol Imaging. 2011;38(4):613–22. https://doi.org/10.1007/s00259-010-1684-x.
151. Shi J, Fan D, Dong C, Liu H, Jia B, Zhao H, et al. Anti-tumor effect of integrin targeted (177) Lu-3PRGD2 and combined therapy with Endostar. Theranostics. 2014;4(3):256–66. https://doi.org/10.7150/thno.7781.
152. Law I, Albert NL, Arbizu J, Boellaard R, Drzezga A, Galldiks N, et al. Joint EANM/EANO/RANO practice guidelines/SNMMI procedure standards for imaging of gliomas using PET with radiolabelled amino acids and [(18)F]FDG: version 1.0. Eur J Nucl Med Mol Imaging. 2019;46(3):540–57. https://doi.org/10.1007/s00259-018-4207-9.

Chapter 4
Scintigraphy of Human CSF Flow in Patients with Leptomeningeal Metastasis

Franklin C. L. Wong and Ian E. McCutcheon

Introduction: Imaging of Human CSF Flow

Human cerebrospinal fluid is produced from the choroid plexus in the roof of lateral ventricles [1]. It passes through the third ventricle to reach the fourth ventricle and then further down the spinal cord, then back over the cerebral convexity to return to the systemic circulation through the cristae villi along the parasagittal sinuses and likely through one-way-valves [2]. The flow of CSF in the cervical spinal canal consists of bulk flow which is likely propelled by respiration [3] and also occurs through pulsatile flow driven by vascular pulsation during the cardiac cycle [4]. The combination of respiratory and vascular pulsation results in opposite CSF flows in the anterior (cephalic) versus the posterior (caudal) spinal subarachnoid space across the dentate ligament partition [5]. CSF in the cephalad flow joins the rest of the CSF distributed to the cerebral convexity to be returned to the general circulation. Small amounts of CSF also directly return to the general circulation from each compartment.

Leptomeningeal metastasis (LM) is a unique disease process predominantly involving tumor deposits in the arachnoid [6]. It is a high-risk area for clinical care and for research because of the surrounding eloquent brain and spinal cord as well as the high mortality and treatment resistance as stated in Chap. 1. Nevertheless, LM has remained an unmet need in the care of cancer patients. It is also a potentially high-reward area because any gain can be measured in weeks and months of

F. C. L. Wong (✉)
Department of Nuclear Medicine, University of Texas M. D. Anderson Cancer Center, Houston, TX, USA
e-mail: fwong@mdanderson.org

I. E. McCutcheon
Neurosurgery, The University of Texas M. D. Anderson Cancer Center, Houston, Texas, USA
e-mail: imccutch@mdanderson.org

F. C. L. Wong (ed.), *Radiopharmaceuticals in the Management of Leptomeningeal Metastasis*, https://doi.org/10.1007/978-3-031-14291-8_4

survival and tumor-free periods. It has been referred to as a test tube for cancer treatment [7]. The intrathecal space has become a delight for LM researchers and clinicians because with intrathecal access, many biological barriers are overcome to allow direct diagnostic and therapeutic interventions within tumor proximity. The main challenge has remained heterogeneous flow distribution over tumors and leptomeninges spreading over convoluted areas [8] within intracranial subarachnoid spaces [9] and spinal subarachnoid spaces [10]. One estimate of human subarachnoid space area reports a total of 3130 cm^2 (cerebral surface 1660 cm^2, free cerebral surface 458 cm^2, cerebellar surface 843 cm^2, and free cerebellar surface 163 cm^2) [9]. Imaging of the CSF space and intrathecal intervention has been a challenge as well as a focus of interest for scientists and physicians and requires multidisciplinary collaborations.

Iodine-based contrast agents (such as metrizamide [11]) have been used in gram quantities to evaluate CSF flow in myelography, with radiograms and/or CT. They are less often used today because of tedious procedures and potential adverse effects including arachnoiditis. Current spiral CT scanners can image the anatomic structures of the entire neural axis in seconds but repetitive serial imaging to determine CSF flow over time may result in unacceptably high radiation exposure risk.

MRI of spinal fluid compartments has superior spatial resolution of anatomic details. Qualitative evaluation of the CSF space by MRI has become the dominant imaging modality, with or without contrast. However, MRI has relatively low temporal resolution for directly monitoring CSF flow from one compartment to another. With cardiac gating or respiratory gating, CSF flow within regular cardiac cycles or respiratory cycles can be, respectively, assessed by accumulating the signals over many cycles. When MRI images were acquired over multiple cardiac cycles or respiratory cycles, spinal fluid motions and directional flow have demonstrated details of CSF flow superior to those acquired from scintigraphy. Under research settings, CSF flow could be quantified from MRI after the nonlinear signals were calibrated and normalized. Because of the high signal-to-noise ratios in CSF scintigraphy, CSF flow could be quantified with less rigor than with MRI.

Current scanners of MRI, PET, and SPECT are limited by an axial field of view of up to about 20 cm. Therefore, serial scanning sessions of imaging along the neural axis take at least 20 min, resulting in lower temporal resolution. Advances in whole-body PET-CT and MRI scanners with field of views up to 1.2 m [12–18] have remarkably shortened temporal resolution to perform whole-body PET scanning in research settings and may soon benefit clinical studies.

Scintigraphic images have lower spatial resolution because of the requirement of the "as low as reasonably achievable" (ALARA) principle for the use of radioactive material resulting in lower radioactivity counts to form high resolution images. Conversely, scintigraphic studies have critical advantages over MRI and CT with the use of radionuclides that have longer half-lives and enable serial imaging over days. Furthermore, the physical amounts of radiopharmaceuticals used are typically in the nanogram to microgram range resulting in minimal perturbation of physiologic processes. This advantage is in contrast to the multi-gram range of contrast agents for CT and MRI that may cause perturbation of meninges resulting in adverse effects including arachnoiditis. The use of hybrid imaging of SPECT-CT or PET-CT also allows evaluation of sub-centimeter volume-of-interest below resolution of the nuclear imaging modality. Therefore, scintigraphy has remained a crucial imaging modality of human CSF flow.

Intrathecal Radiopharmaceuticals Used in Humans (Table 4.1)

Although there have been innovative initiatives involving the use of intrathecal radiopharmaceuticals in nonspecific solutions and colloidal forms as well as labeled monoclonal antibodies against tumor antigens (Table 4.1), only a single intrathecal radiopharmaceutical has gained US FDA approval. Indium-111 diethylenetriamine pentaacetic acid (In-111 DTPA) obtained FDA approval in 1982 for diagnostic evaluation of intrathecal CSF flow with an expiration date in December 2021 by which time its manufacturer was expected to request continuation. This radiopharmaceutical has remained on the FDA-approved drug database in February 2022, indicating that it has gained continuation. The lack of additional approved intrathecal radiopharmaceuticals is the result of heightened regulatory scrutiny of radioactive material (RAM) use, good manufacturing practice (GMP), current good clinical practice (cGCP), and intrathecal medication's benefits to patients and returns to commercial investment.

In this chapter, discussion of intrathecal radiopharmaceuticals focuses mostly on diagnostic use. Intrathecal radiopharmaceuticals could be in particulate versus soluble forms. The latter can be macromolecules (MW > 2000 Da) versus small

Table 4.1 Intrathecal radiopharmaceuticals used in clinical studies

Intrathecal radiopharmaceutical	Radionuclide	Tp1/2 (h)	Molecular class	Radiation emission(s)	Detection	Source
Nonspecific solution:						
In-111 DTPA **(FDA approval)**	In-111	67.2	Chelate	Electrons, photons	Gamma camera/SPECT	Grossman [19]
In-111 EDTA	In-111	67.2	Chelate	Electrons, photons	Gamma camera	Goodwin [20]
In-111 transferrin	In-111	67.2	Protein	Electrons, photons	Gamma camera	Goodwin [20]
Tc99m DTPA	Tc99m	6.0	Chelate	Photons	Gamma camera	Larson SM 1973
Tc99m pertechnetate	Tc99m	6.0	Anion	Photons	Gamma camera	Lette [25]
Yb-169 DTPA	Yb-169	768.6	Chelate	Photons	Gamma camera	Hosain [24]
I-125 iododeoxyuridine (IUDR)	I-125	1425.6	Nucleoside	Electrons		Rebischung [28]
I-131 Sodium iodide (NaI)	I-131	193.7	Anion	Electrons, photons	Radioactivity count	Rougemont [26]
I-131 Sodium iodide (NaI)	I-131	193.7	Anion	Electrons, photons	Gamma camera	Wong [27]
I-131 Human serum albumin	I-131	193.7	Protein	Electrons, photons	Gamma camera	Di Chiro [22]
Ga-67 citrate	Ga-67	78.3	Cation	Electrons, photons	Gamma camera	Wong (2022) (this chapter)
Ga-68 EDTA	Ga-68	1.1	Chelate	Positron, photons	PET	Bergstran [29]
Co-55 DTPA	Co-55	17.5	Chelate	Positron, photons	PET	Maziere [30]
Cu-64 DOTA	Cu-64	12.7	Chelate	Positron, photons	PET	Freesmeyer [31]
Nonspecific colloids:						
P-32 chromic phosphate	P-32	343.2	Microparticles	Electrons	Gamma camera	Muriel [32]
Au-198 colloid	Au-198	64.8	Microparticles	Electrons		Doge [9]
Target-specific antibodies:						
I-131 HMFG1	I-131	193.7	Protein	Electrons, photons	Gamma camera	Moseley [33]
I-131 HMFG2 UJ181.4 4C6 FD32	I-131	193.7	Protein	Electrons, photons	Gamma camera	Lashford [34]
I-131 3F8	I-131	193.7	Protein	Electrons, photons	Gamma camera	Kramer K 2007
I-131 Mel 14	I-131	193.7	Protein	Electrons, photons	Gamma camera	Moseley [37]
I-131 81C6	I-131	193.7	Protein	Electrons, photons	Gamma camera	Moseley [37]
I-131 Omburtamab	I-131	193.7	Protein	Electrons, photons	Gamma camera	Pandit-Taska [36]
I-124 Omburtamab	I-124	100.8	Protein	Positron, photons	PET	Pandit-Taska [36]
Lu-177 Omburtamab	Lu-177	159.6	Protein	Electrons, photons	Gamma camera/SPECT	Wong (2022) (Chap. 8)

molecules that include anions, cations, and adducts of radionuclide as in Table 4.1. Intrathecal radiopharmaceuticals in colloid forms (P-32 and Au-198), nucleoside (I-125 IUDR), and tumor-targeting antibody forms have been used for LM therapy and will be discussed in Chap. 8.

The small molecules In-111 DTPA [19, 20] and In-111 EDTA [20] are radiolabeled chelates with similar imaging characteristics, but In-111 DTPA has been favored for quality control reasons and it developed further after 1973 to gain FDA approval in 1982. The biological half-life of DTPA is 10–12 h [21, 22]. Since the tracer pharmacodynamics mostly depend on the biochemical properties of the labeled moiety, In-111 DTPA and Tc99m DTPA [23] share similar biologic behavior. However, with a shorter physical half-life for Tc99m, the effective half-life of Tc99m DTPA is 3.75 h (harmonic mean of the physical half-life and biologic half-life of 6 and 10 h, respectively) in the CSF space and is less likely to yield important diagnostic information at 24 h.

Macromolecules In-111 transferrin [20], Tc99m albumin, and I-131 HSA [22] were reported to have longer biologic half-lives in the CSF (30 h) and in the body (315 h) resulting in higher radiation exposure [20]. They were also reported to have higher rates of febrile reactions (up to 38%) after intrathecal injection. Yb-192 DTPA [21, 24] has not been further pursued, likely related to the low availability of the radionuclide and its long physical half-life (of 32 days) resulting in higher radiation absorbed dose to the body and longer periods of radiation safety precautions. Intrathecal injection of Tc-99m pertechnetate (an anion) for imaging of CSF has been reported [25] and is subject to limits of short effective half-life and perhaps of choroidal uptake. Intrathecal injection of the anion I-131 (as sodium iodide) in microcurie activity with subsequent radioactivity counting was reported in an earlier French study [26]. Intraventricular and intralumbar injection of larger activities of the anion I-131 sodium iodide with imaging were reported in two US trials [27]. I-125 labeled iododeoxyuridine (IUDR) has been injected intrathecally along with methotrexate to treat LM and to inhibit IUDR degradation [28]. Additional small molecule radiopharmaceuticals (shown in Table 4.1) have been reported with Ga-67 citrate (Fig. 4.10), Ga-68 EDTA [29], Co-55 DTPA, Cu-64 DTPA [30], and Cu-64 DOTA [31]. Radiolabeled colloids (P-32 chromic phosphate [32] and Au-198 colloids [9]), radioiodide-labeled monoclonal antibodies (HNFG1, HMFG2, Mel 14, 81C6, and Omburtamab [33–37]), and Lu-177 labeled Omburtamab will be discussed in detail including therapeutic trials (Chap. 8).

A cisternogram is typically performed after intralumbar injections of indium-111 DTPA followed by serial imaging of the neural axis. Historically, cisternograms have been used to confirm and study different types of hydrocephalus which now are typically evaluated by MRI because of better spatial resolution. Cisternography has remained a useful diagnostic tool for patients with LM for detection of spinal fluid leakage and confirmation of CSF flow patency. The standard of care for patients with LM includes neuroaxis radiation therapy and intrathecal therapy. The latter has better outcomes after intraventricular injection than with intralumbar injection, as illustrated by an Italian study of patients with acute lymphoblastic leukemia who showed an 88% versus 33% rate of response, respectively [38]. The reason for this difference is that intraventricular injection provides more drug exposure within CSF spaces (including the cerebral ventricles) that are less likely to be reached by retrograde CSF flow from the lumbar spine. Intraventricular injection is often accomplished via an Ommaya reservoir [39] surgically implanted beneath the scalp. Evaluation of CSF flow patency from Ommaya reservoir injection has thus become an important task to assure tracer transit between CSF compartments before initiation of intrathecal therapy. Access to the CSF via the Ommaya reservoir also provides an invaluable route to studying the pharmacokinetics and pharmacodynamics of LM treatment.

Imaging: Multiple Planar Scans of Multiple Time Points

Because of the limited field of view of an Anger gamma camera of less than 20 cm, earlier cisternogram studies prior to the 1970s were performed with multiple 15-min sessions of the head, thoracic spine, and lumbar spine in the anterior and posterior positions (totaling over 100 min) at each time point. Between 3 and 4 such imaging sessions were carried out for up to 48 h in order to visualize and determine the arrival and clearance of tracer in the head, thorax, and abdomen in a qualitative manner [20, 21, 23]. Quantification was difficult, although possible, with multiple standards within the field of view to account for the decay and difference in body thickness and considerations of uneven attenuation. Multiregional kinetic modeling could still be accomplished but was subject to a low temporal resolution [40].

Qualitative evaluation could be accomplished by counting the time of tracer arrival to each CSF compartment and has been correlated with LM prognosis [41, 42]. It is technically possible but tedious and subject to observer bias and arbitrary intensity windowing. With advances in gamma cameras having larger field of view and dual-headed gamma camera in the 1990s, imaging durations for each session have been halved and last about 1 h for each time point. Newer gamma cameras also allow simultaneous acquisition of multiple photo peaks to account for scattering to enhance count statistics and imaging quality. Although imaging duration has been reduced, serial imaging sessions at multiple time points are still needed to observe physiology and pathologies.

CSF Flow Abnormalities in LM

Cisternograms via lumbar injection were used extensively to identify hydrocephalus and monitor normal pressure hydrocephalus by revealing persistent abnormal retention of tracer in the ventricles [43–46]. Qualitative evaluation of hydrocephalus and normal pressure hydrocephalus using cisternograms would typically take up to 3 days for comprehensive assessment of tracer appearance and clearance from each CSF compartment. The 3-day half-life of In111- aptly allows prolonged periods of observation. Typical findings in normal pressure hydrocephalus can only be made by qualitative terms and include delayed clearance of tracer from the CSF compartments and retrograde flow to the ventricles. These findings have been correlated with the clinical triad of headache, ataxia, and dementia. However, reviews of the use of spinal fluid flow scintigraphy [47–53] have suggested that the cardinal imaging signs of ventriculomegaly as well as parenchymal flow and other neurologic structural anomalies in NPH are better evaluated by MRI which has provided more detailed imaging of anatomic features than has spinal fluid flow scintigraphy. For similar reasons, cisternograms are rarely required to evaluate hydrocephalus in the clinical setting nowadays.

Radiotracer appearance outside of the CSF compartments is the key finding in patients with CSF leakage that could be iatrogenic (for instance, after transsphenoidal resection of pituitary tumors), occur after trauma, or arise spontaneously (spontaneous intracranial hypotension). Identification of abnormal extra-thecal tracer activities has been enhanced by SPECT-CT resulting in prompt 3D localization and co-registration with CT of diagnostic quality.

The typical findings for confirming CSF leakage as a cause for rhinorrhea by nuclear studies are:

1. Abnormal tracer collection outside of CSF on scintigrams [54] or SPECT [55] in head or spine. Abnormal tracer collection in the stomach or bowel is also an indirect finding of CSF leak [56];
2. Elevated nasal pledget radioactivity counts over 1000 cpm [57] and radioactivity counting ratio (compared to 0.5 mL serum for a threshold ratio of 1.3 [58] or 2 mL of serum for threshold ratio of 2.0 [59]); and
3. Abnormally fast clearance from CSF space (Te <10 h) [60].

Confirmation and localization of CSF leakage will provide valuable guidance for surgical intervention for alleviating rhinorrhea.

For the care of patients with LM, cisternograms are most useful in detecting CSF flow abnormalities (mostly blockades from LM) and abnormalities in preparation for intrathecal therapy. There have been efforts to correlate cisternogram findings with LM prognosis [41, 61]. Spinal fluid flow blockade has been reported to correlate with improvement and progression of LM [42, 62]. Successful subsequent LM treatment with radiation therapy has been correlated with improvement of CSF flow abnormalities that were assessed in qualitative terms. These earlier studies were based on qualitative evaluation of serial multi-planar images and indeed have shed light in predicting LM prognosis from CSF flow study. Their findings need to be independently confirmed in other institutions.

Additional uses of cisternography in LM patients focus on confirmation of the patency of CSF flow from Ommaya reservoir injection. Assessment of Ommaya reservoir patency is typically carried out in LM patients requiring intrathecal therapy to assure tracer and chemotherapeutics distribution to CSF compartments without significant blockade of CSF flow [63]. Such studies typically occur over 24–48 h. It has been demonstrated from a retrospective study of 31 patients with LM requiring intrathecal therapy that patients having a CSF flow study confirming CSF flow patency have less toxicity and better outcome than do those without such a study [64].

Evaluation of ventriculoperitoneal or ventriculoatrial shunt patency allowing CSF to reach the peritoneal cavity (or atrium) take less time (0.5–1 h) as long as there is prompt visualization of tracer transit from the shunt with no significant blockade. This is often done in a qualitative manner. One study of pediatric CSF shunts reports four patterns of findings denoting normal patency of flow (clearance half-life less than 5 min), distal obstruction, proximal obstruction with reflux to the ventricle, and rapid clearance of tracer [65]. A retrospective analysis of 49 ventriculoatrial shunt studies in 41 patients reported a normal clearance half-time of 3.9–8.0 min [66] and correlation with over drainage for clearance below 3.9 min, and with obstruction for a clearance half-time above 8.0 min. Compared with ventriculoatrial shunts, ventriculoperitoneal shunts have longer tubing and a slower clearance of tracer from peritoneal cavity (because of the faster blood flow in the atrium). Clearance of tracer from the VP shunt is expected to be longer, up to 4 h as shown in Fig. 4.12b below. More meticulous efforts with shorter scanning time will be required than the current duration of 20 min to estimate the half-time of VP shunt clearance and to establish a threshold to determine VP shunt blockade. Without established standards, the current state of the art for determination of VP shunt blockade by scintigraphy is at best qualitative, as illustrated in 3-s static images in Fig. 4.11b. For evaluation of continuous or intermittent CSF drainage through VP shunts, detection and quantification of the small amounts of tracer in the short and long segments of the shunt tubing are indeed limited by the spatial and temporal resolution of current gamma scintigraphy.

Intrathecal In-111 DTPA and Pharmacokinetics in LM

From serial CSF sampling, intrathecal pharmacokinetics of methotrexate have been noted to be altered by severe leptomeningeal metastasis in three patients [67]. It is desirable to noninvasively interrogate the intrathecal pharmacokinetics of therapeutics to predict toxicity and efficacy. Soluble radiopharmaceuticals with lower molecular weights including In-111 DTPA (MW 545.3) and methotrexate (MW 454.44) are cleared from the CSF pathways predominantly by bulk flow. The intrathecal radioactivity counts of In-111 DTPA from CSF sampling were compared with the intrathecal concentration of methotrexate and revealed a high degree of correlation. Therefore, the intrathecal pharmacokinetics and biodistribution of methotrexate can be predicted by the pharmacokinetics of In111- DTPA [68]. It was concluded that In-111 DTPA radioactivities can predict intrathecal methotrexate distribution and the outcome of treatment. A subsequent critique cautioned about the futility of treating bulky LM, but emphasized that an In-111 DTPA CSF flow study should be done on all patients being considered for intrathecal therapy [69].

Since In-111 DTPA reveals the bulk flow of CSF which is the pathway for most low molecular weight soluble pharmaceuticals, both potential toxicity and efficacy of low molecular weight therapeutics may thus be predicted by the pharmacokinetic of radioactivity of In-111 DTPA, measured from CSF sampling and scintigraphy. In pharmacokinetic terms, the total exposure to a pharmaceutical can be measured by the area under curve on a time–activity curve. Therefore, the intrathecal exposure (potential efficacy and toxicity) of small molecule soluble therapeutics may be estimated from the time-activity curve of In-111 DTPA.

Whole-Body Scan Can Derive Effective Half-Life (Te) in CSF

Since the 1990s, advances in instrumentation have allowed gamma cameras to acquire images while moving from the head down to the pelvis in less than 20 min to present digital data as a whole-body scan. Through coupling between a gamma camera in the anterior position and another gamma camera in the conjugate posterior position, whole-body scans can be acquired. The conjugated (simultaneously obtained) anterior and posterior images also allow determination of the depth of tracer uptake and enable normalization of body depth to determine radioactivity within the body by taking into account the uneven attenuation of photons at different body depths. Selected cases of whole-body cisternograms have been reported as allowing prompt assessment of tracer in the CSF space [60].

Serial whole-body scintigraphic images in the anterior and posterior projections can be acquired by a dual-headed gamma scanner to allow visual qualitative evaluation of the tracer distribution over time after intralumbar injection of In-111 DTPA (Fig. 4.1a). Similarly, In-111 DTPA biodistribution over time can be assessed after intraventricular injection, most frequently done via an Ommaya reservoir in preparation of LM intrathecal therapy (Fig. 4.1b). Geographic-mean images of each pixel of the conjugated anterior and posterior images in combination with an external standard of In-111 DTPA in the field of view allow quantification of In-111 in each pixel and hence dynamic analysis. The tracer effective half-life (Te) is the harmonic mean of the physical half-life (Tp) and biologic half-life (Tb). Based on monoexponential decay over time, the correct expression for effective half-life (Te) is that the reciprocal of Te is the sum of reciprocals of Tb and Tb ($1/Te = 1/Tp + 1/Tb$). When the irregular depth of CSF in the body is accounted for by geometric-mean (GM) images, Te can be estimated by serial measurement of radioactivity in the region-of-interest (ROI) over time.

An IRB-approved retrospective review (DR10-0344) of 498 consecutive cisternograms or Ommayagrams of 241 unique subjects (0.5 mCi of intrathecal tracer) between 1996 and 2006 was conducted to evaluate the usefulness of whole-body cisternograms done to assess human CSF flow for the management of patients with LM. The hypothesis was that whole-body cisternograms can provide reliable measures to correlate with CSF block, CSF leak, and CSF pathway patency.

Whole-body scans using a dual-headed gamma camera were obtained at the following time points (0.5–2 h), (3–6 h), (18–22 h), and (23–28 h) with optional additional time points, static images, nasal pledget radioactivity counts (against 0.5 whole-blood), and SPECT or SPECT-CT. Typically, an external standard of 0.01 mCi was placed by the right side of the skull. In addition to routine qualitative evaluations of static images, whole-body images in anterior and posterior views were generated, as were geometric-mean images of conjugated anterior and posterior images. This methodology allows measurement of radioactivity independent of body depth so as to construct time–activity curves of regions of interest. The effective half-life of tracer in the CSF pathways was calculated for each study, which typically lasted over 24 h. Examples of normal and abnormal spinal fluid flow patterns are illustrated

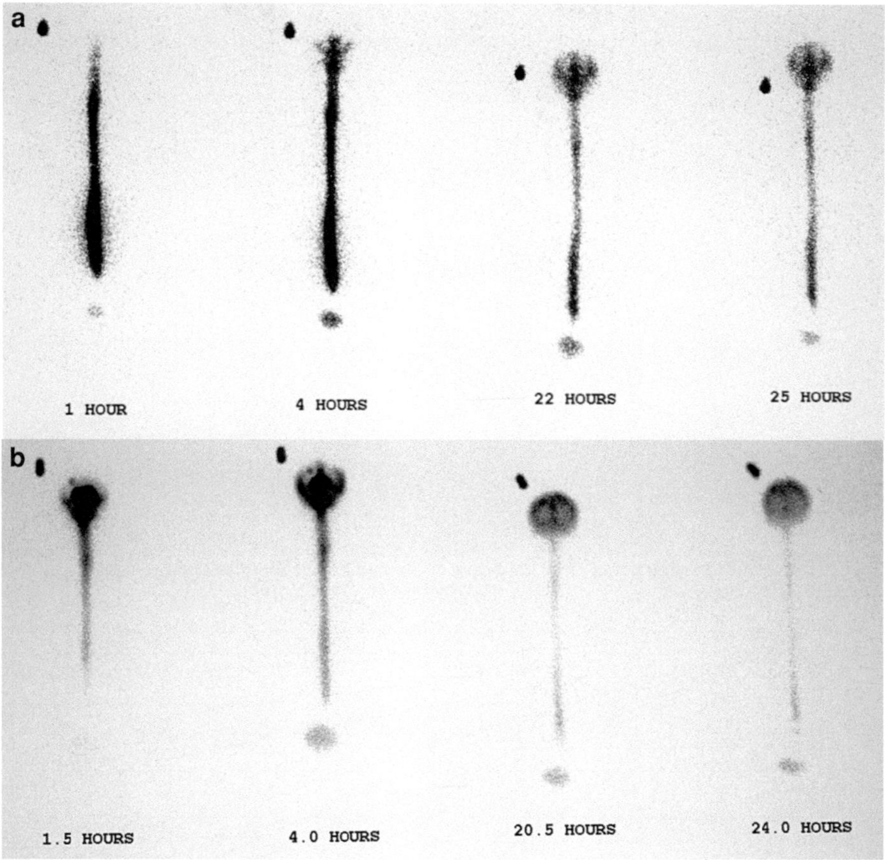

Fig. 4.1 (**a**) Whole-body imaging of In-111 in CSF after injection via lumbar puncture. (*F. Wong,* et al, *JNM 51 (Suppl 2), 378P, 2010*). (**b**) Whole-body imaging of In-111 in CSF after injection via Ommaya reservoir. (*F. Wong,* et al, *Eur. J. of Nucl. Med., 25(8):1075, 1998*)

in Figs. 4.2, 4.3, 4.4, 4.5, 4.6, 4.7, 4.8, 4.9, 4.10, 4.11 and 4.12. The CSF effective half-life (Te) with block or leaks from injection via Ommaya reservoir or lumbar puncture is listed in Table 4.2 [70]. Decreased tracer visualization on the side of the Ommaya reservoir (OM asymmetry) is noted in over 20% of patients although the Te is not significantly different from that seen in patients without OM asymmetry. Disposition of whether there are blocks or leaks was determined by the consensus of two nuclear physicians. When there is no block, no leak, nor OM asymmetry, Te is 15.3 h for Ommaya reservoir injection. With lumbar puncture, the Te is 15.4 h when there is no block nor leak. With blocks at the ventricular (V), cervical spine (C), or thoracic spine (T) level, Te is significantly larger than normal. Opening a closed VP shunt valve results in significantly lower Te with either Ommaya reservoir injection (7.1 ± 3.6 h) or lumbar puncture (8.5 ± 3.7 h). These lower but not significantly different Te's may be explained by the fact that when a VP shunt is in the open position,

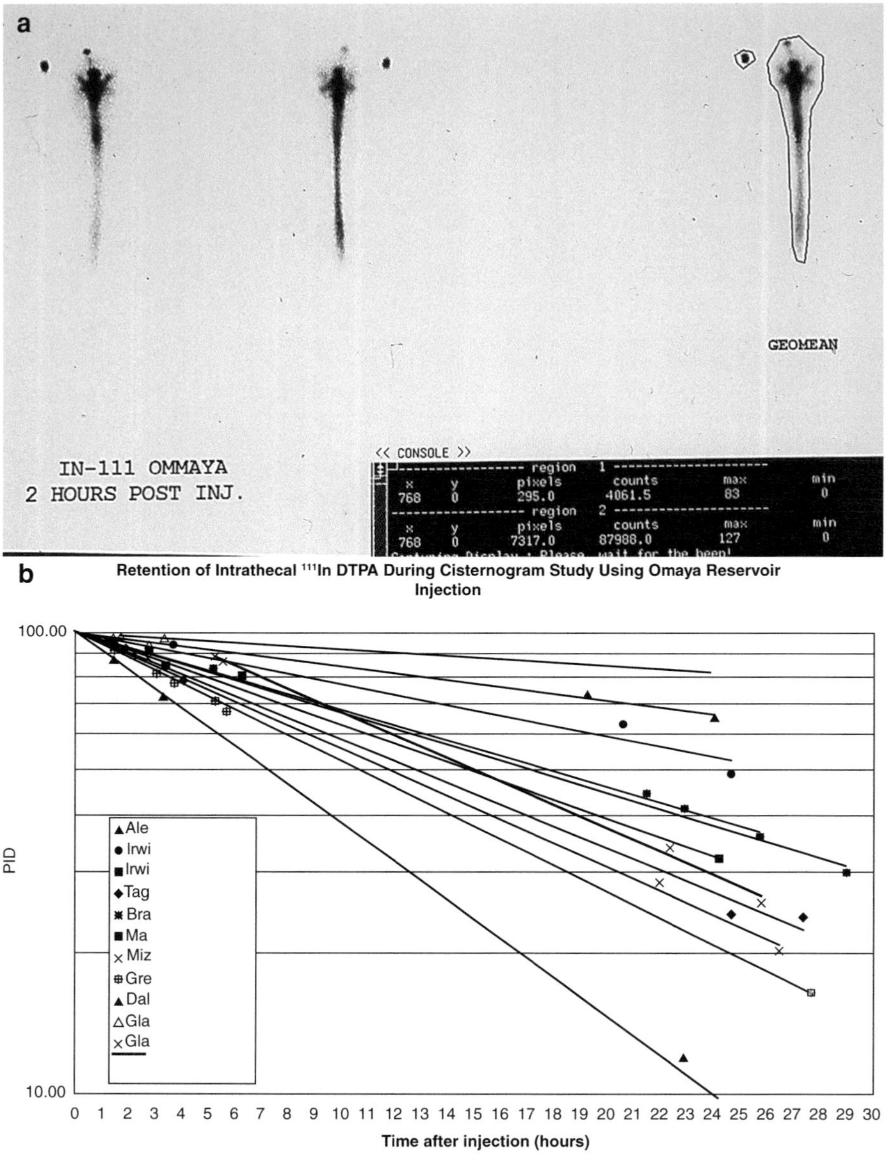

Fig. 4.2 (**a**) An example of deriving radioactivity counts from geometric-mean (GM) images. (**b**) Time–activity curve in semi-log scale of In-111 in the entire CSF pathways of 11 studies after Ommaya reservoir injection demonstrated monoexponential clearance

there is continuous drainage of CSF, in contrast to the intermittent leaks observed in studies of patients with rhinorrhea. When CSF block occurs and In-111 DTPA is injected via lumbar puncture, Te also decreases, which is a response different from that produced by injection via Ommaya reservoir.

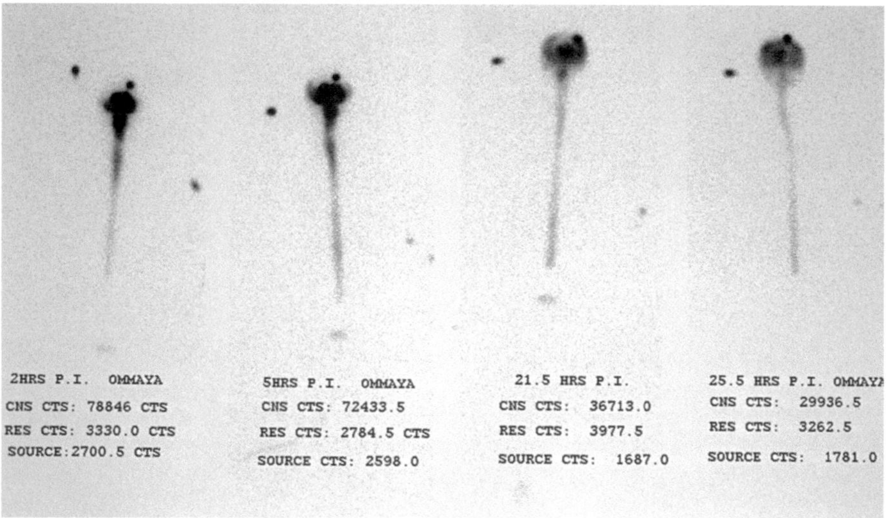

Fig. 4.3 In-111 DTPA Ommayogram of a patient with lung cancer LM with Te of 17.5H

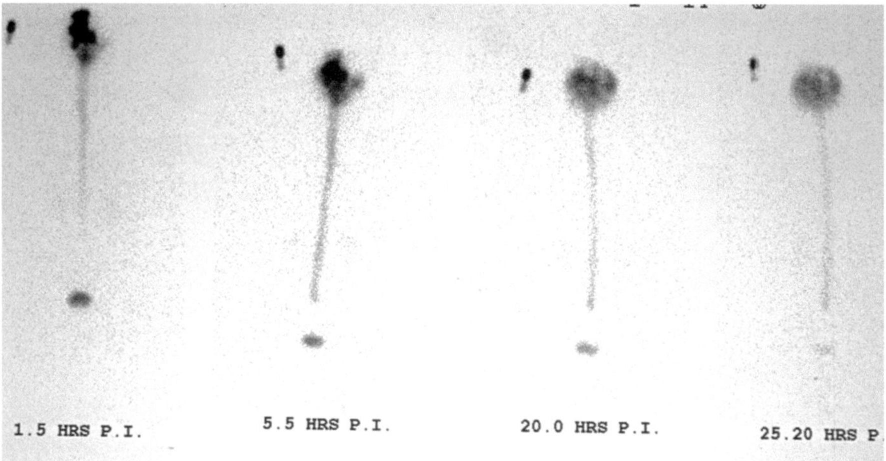

Fig. 4.4 Ommayogram in a patient with GBM after intracavitary injection of 0.5 mCi In-111 DTPA. In this patient, the Te of In-111 DTPA is 14.5 h for whole-body CSF and cavity (160 mL in the right temporal lobe)

Clearance of Tracer in Human CSF Space (Fig. 4.2a, b)

Since there is uneven depth of the spinal canal from the anterior and posterior body surface and from gamma camera detectors when a whole-body scan is performed, the geometric-mean images (generated from square root of products of the counts from

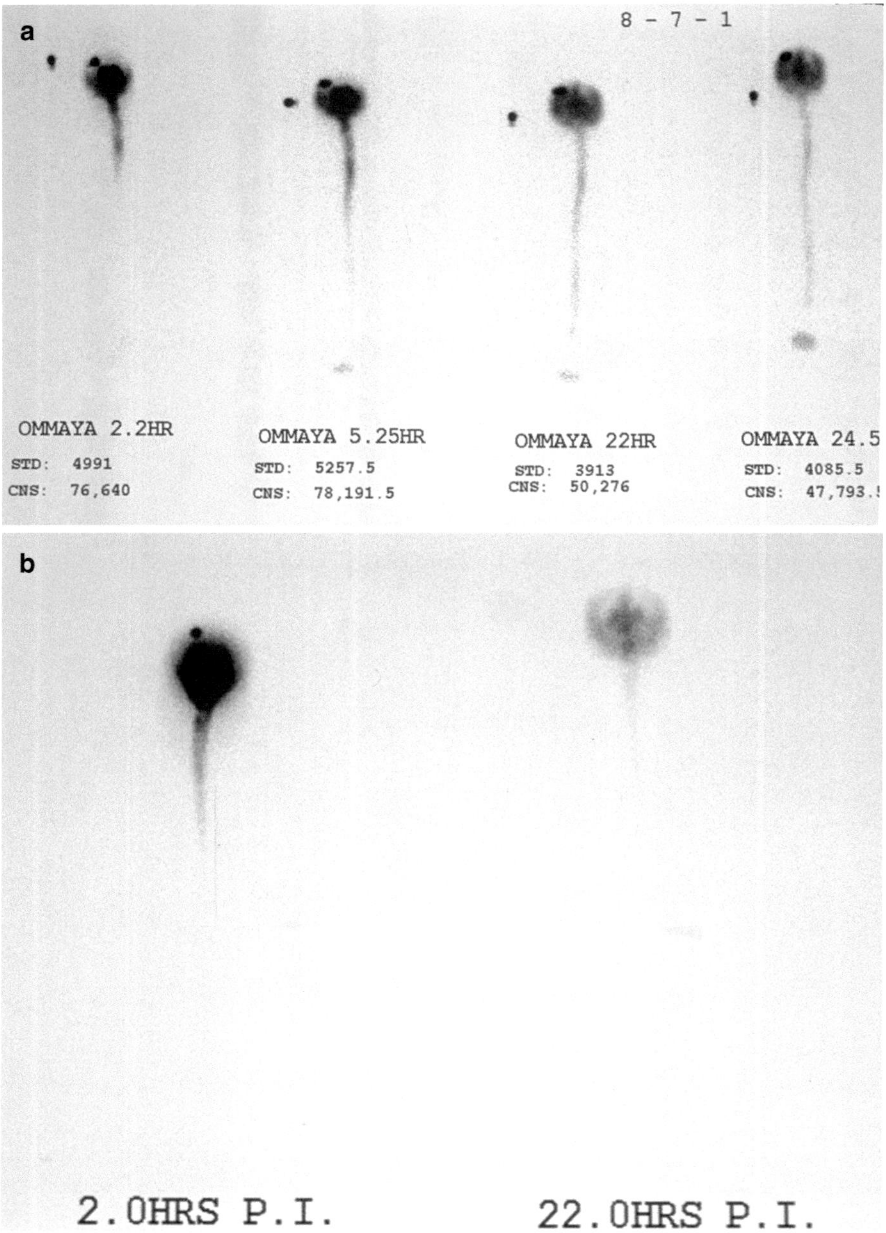

Fig. 4.5 (**a**) In-111 DTPA Ommayogram of a LM patient with T-spine block having a Te of 27 h. (**b**) Tc99m DTPA Ommayogram of a patient with T-spine block and Te of 5.5 h (off label use). (**c**) Asymmetric tracer distribution over the cerebral convexity in a patient with lung cancer, LM, and right parietal metastasis and Te of 17 h. External reference standard is placed in the left side

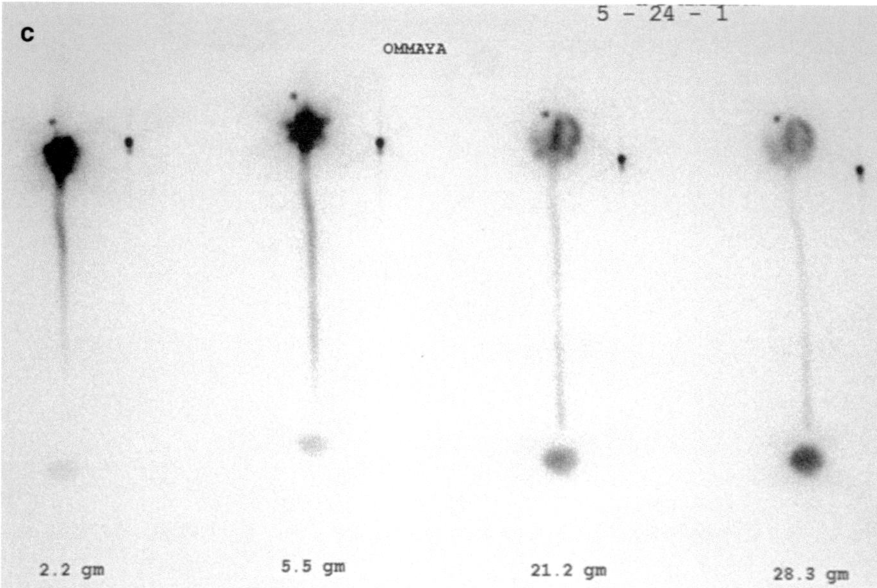

Fig. 4.5 (continued)

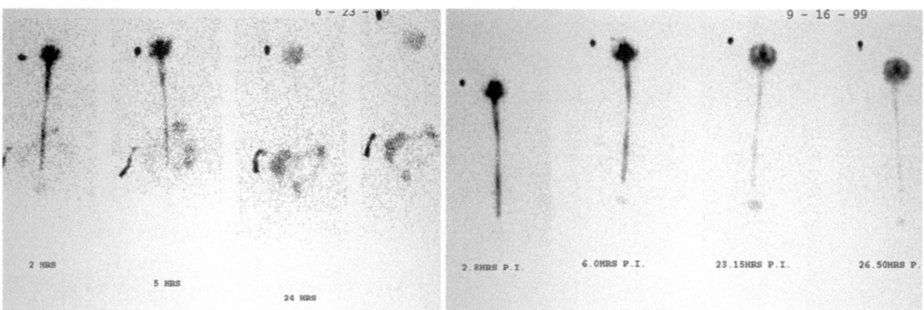

CSF Leak **After surgical repair, no CSF leak**

Fig. 4.6 A post-operative study of a meningioma patient with rhinorrhea using In-111 Cisternogram via lumbar injection showed leakage in the left nostril with left nasal pledget counts over 100,000 and pledget/serum count ratio of 2799, rapid and persistent GI activity, and Te of 6 h. After successful surgical repair, there is no more abdominal tracer activity; Te was normalized to 19 h and the left pledget/serum ratio was 0.88

the anterior camera and posterior camera) will give accurate assessment irrespective of the depth. An example is seen in Fig. 4.2a. An example of the time–activity curve of radioactivity in the CSF space is illustrated in 11 consecutive patient scans and shows a good linear relationship on the semi-log plot (Fig. 4.2b). Review of the images by two nuclear physicians was made to determine whether there is blockade, abnormal asymmetric uptake, leakage, or other anomalies. This retrospective study found

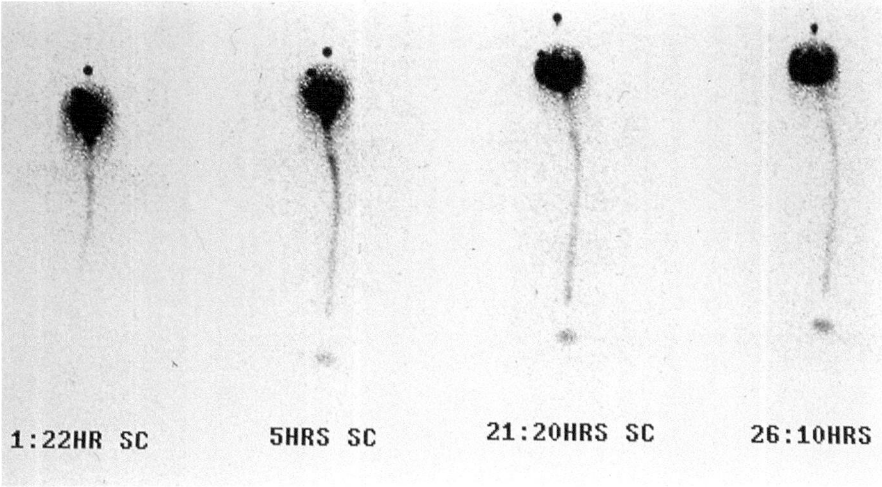

Fig. 4.7 Whole-body images to 26 h after intraventricular injection of Tc99m DTPA (off-label use)

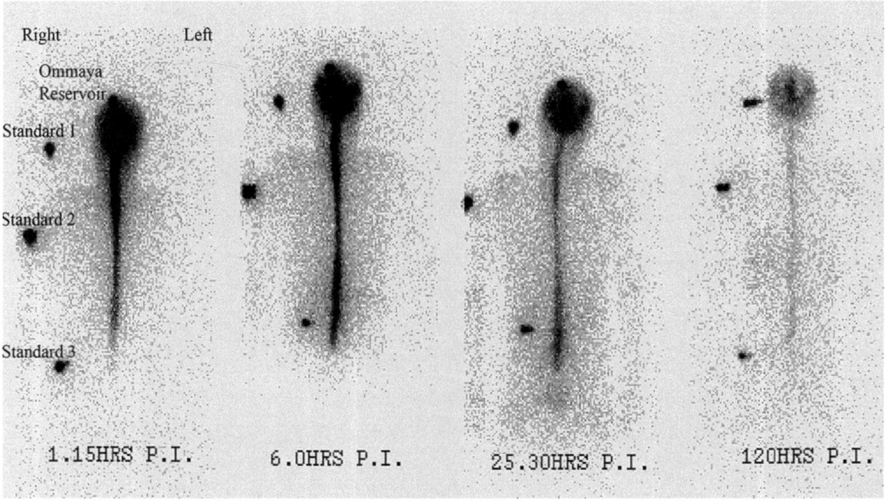

Fig. 4.8 Whole-body Ga-67 Ommayogram showing patent CSF pathways and persistent intrathecal retention to 120 h with low uptake outside of CSF (off-label use)

101 patient scans considered free of blockade, leakage, asymmetric distribution, or grossly delayed CSF transits by visual inspection from Ommaya reservoir injection. Similarly, 36 patient studies were included in which lumbar injection was used.

The effective half-life (Te) of In-111 DTPA is found to be 15.3 ± 4.3 h ($N = 101$) and 15.4 ± 8.5 h ($N = 36$) from injection to Ommaya reservoir and lumbar puncture, respectively, without statistical difference ($P = 0.95$) [70]. This finding is reasonable because either injection is into the same entire CSF space and thus, Te should

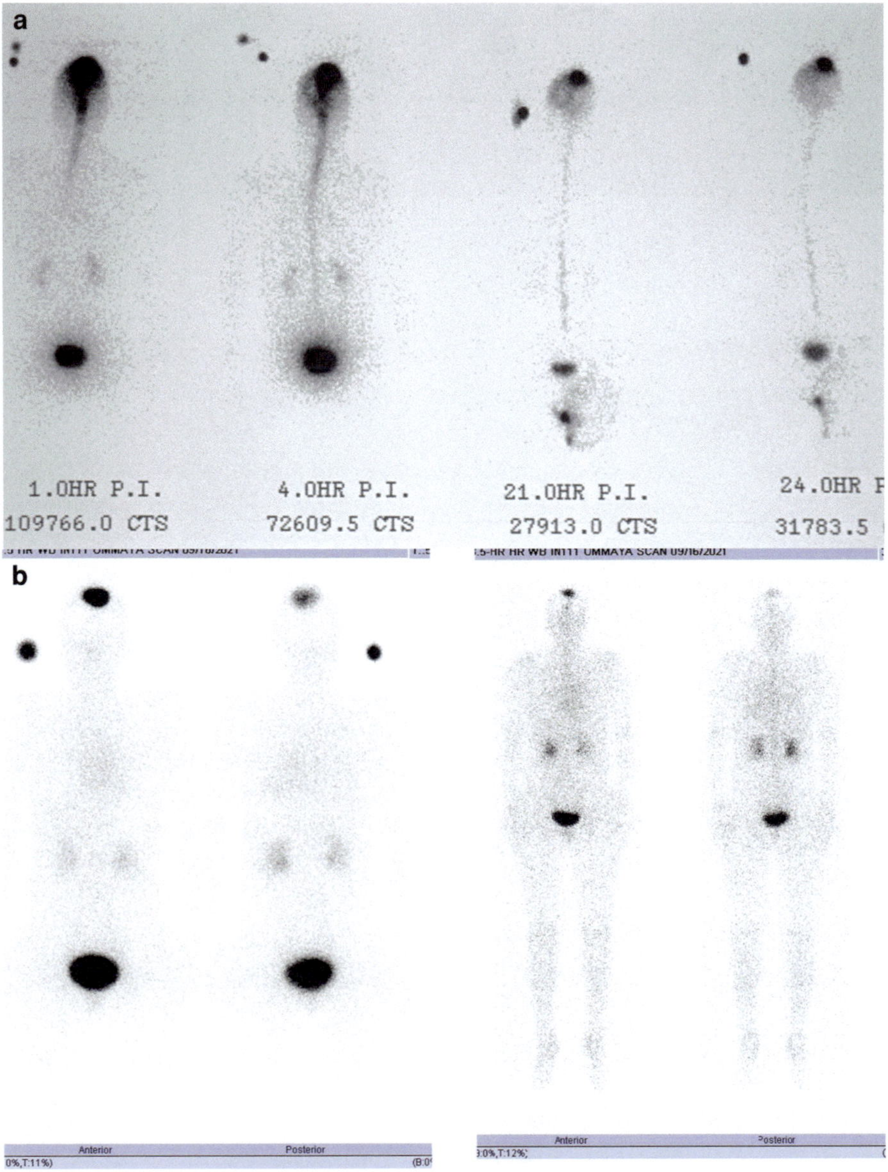

Fig. 4.9 (**a**) In-111 DTPA Ommayogram from inadvertent intraparenchymal injection resulting in rapid clearance of In-111 from CNS and Te of 7.5 h. (**b**) A 36-year-old female with triple-negative breast cancer and LM (+ HSV1 meningitis) underwent an Ommayogram using In-111 DTPA with anterior and posterior images at 1.5 and 3.5 h after injection. No tracer was seen in the ventricles but there was prompt clearance of In-111 (Te of 2 h) from the injection site and excretion of tracer to kidneys and urinary bladder. (**c**) SPECT-CT of head at 4 h after injection of In-111 DTPA into the Ommaya reservoir found a malpositioned catheter tip in the left caudate. Prompt clearance of In-111 DTPA is noted. The Ommaya reservoir was then surgically revised, while persistent adeno-carcinoma in the CSF was also confirmed

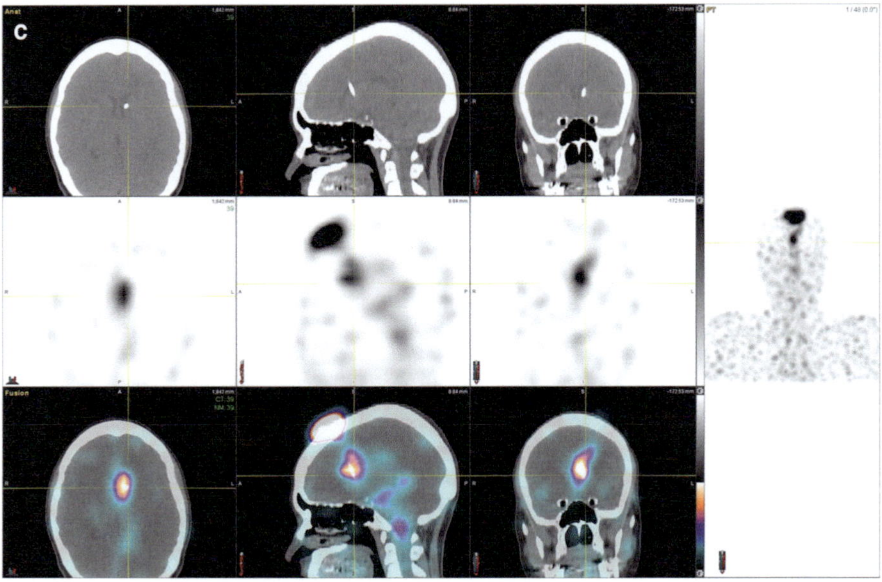

Fig. 4.9 (continued)

measure the same clearance from the CSF. These findings lend support for the adequacy of using a single CSF compartment model to derive clearance for In-111 as a surrogate for CSF bulk flow. For practical purposes, the Te from a LM patient scan is considered normal when Te is between 10 and 20 h, if no other abnormal scintigraphic findings are noted.

CSF Clearance of In-111 DTPA in LM (Figs. 4.3 and 4.4)

Examples of serial spinal fluid studies after intrathecal injection via an Ommaya reservoir (Ommayogram) are illustrated in Figs. 4.3 and 4.4. A typical study done for a patient with lung cancer and LM before the initiation of intrathecal chemotherapy was requested by a neuro-oncologist to assure patency of CSF flow. Serial images at 2, 5, 21.5, and 25.5 h show progressive drainage of tracer from the ventricles and down to the spinal cord then back over the cerebral convexity. There is also progressive decrease in radioactivity counts in the area over the CNS (brain and spine), reservoir (RES), and the external standard of 0.01 mCi in the right side of the head (source). No abrupt cessation of spinal fluid flow is noted from the anterior and posterior images and no abnormal inoculation of tracer is noted. The effective half-life of In111- DTPA (Te) in the CSF is 17.5 h. This is considered a normal study with patent CSF pathways allowing widespread distribution of intrathecal therapy.

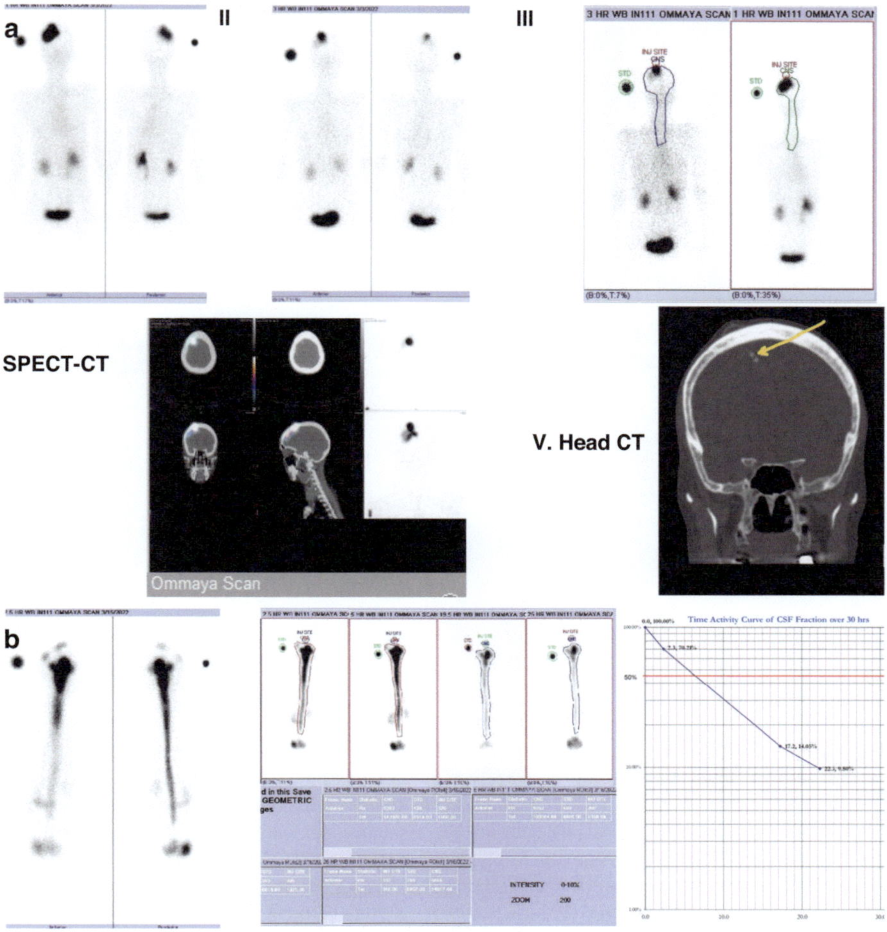

Fig. 4.10 (**a**) A 62-year-old female with LM had an Ommaya reservoir implanted and was found to have no tracer in the ventricle but prominent renal and bladder activities at 1 (I) and 3 (II) h post-injection. Attempt to access the reservoir for reinjection of tracer resulted in no CSF return. CSF Te was 1 h from geometric-mean images (III). SPECT-CT (IV) confirmed loculation at the injection site. A disconnection of the ventricular catheter was noted by 2-mm slice CT (V). (**b**) Following surgical revision with addition of a VP shunt, the Ommayogram shows prompt tracer transit from the reservoir to spine, peritoneal cavity, and urinary bladder at 2.5 h. Geometric-mean images (II) over 24 h are illustrated to demonstrate calculation of the effective half-life (Te) of 6.5 h from a semi-log time–activity curve (III)

In a study of spinal fluid flow from injection of In111- DTPA into a 160-mL postsurgical cavity via an Ommaya reservoir, clearance of tracer was also calculated with Te of 14.5 h from the cavity and 14.5 h from the entire CSF space (in the normal range) as illustrated in Fig. 4.4. There was immediate and continuous tracer in the ventricles and spinal cord further confirming that the postsurgical cavity was in direct communication with the CSF space. Therefore, intracavitary therapy by injection via ommaya reservoir would also result in exposure of leptomeninges to therapeutic agents and perhaps with a similar temporal profile.

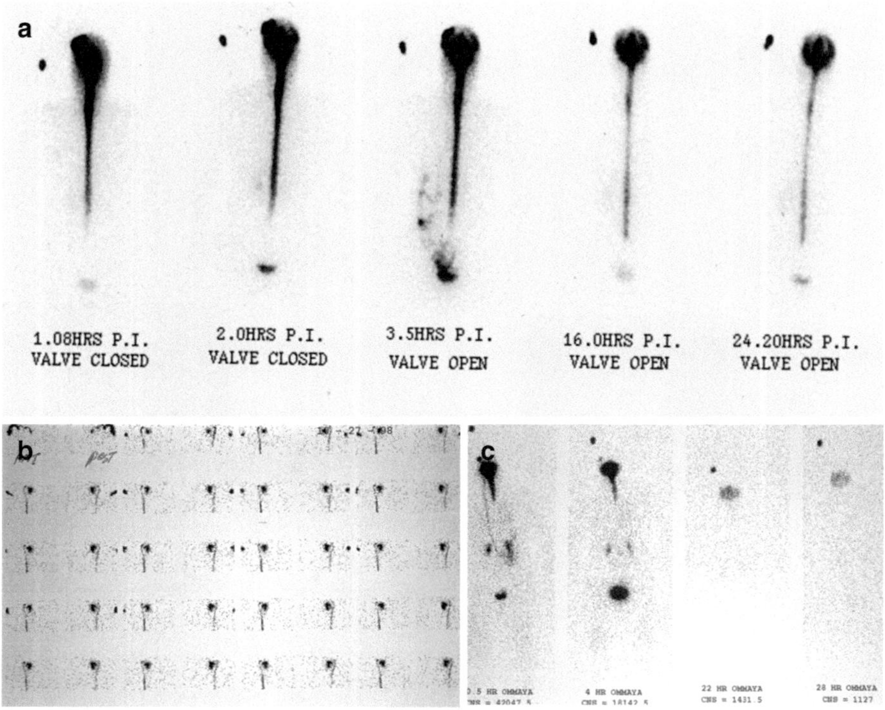

Fig. 4.11 (**a**) Whole-body imaging of In-111 DTPA in CSF after Ommaya reservoir injection in a patient with VP shunt valve closed showed Te of 50 h. Opening of the VP shunt valve at 3 h was followed by prompt transit and prompt clearance from the peritoneal cavity with Te of 10 h. (**b**) Serial (3 s frames) of anterior and posterior images of the head and neck to the VP shunt after injection of 0.5 mCi of In-111 DTPA into an Ommaya reservoir connected to the shunt in a patient with GBM. There is prompt transit of In-111 DTPA through the VP shunt. (**c**) Serial whole-body images of this patient with GBM showed thoracic spinal blockade and prompt transit of In-111 DTPA to the peritoneal cavity, and subsequent clearance to kidneys and urinary bladder. The Te was 4.5 h

Slow CSF Clearance with CSF Blockage (Fig. 4.5a, b)

When there is spinal blockade at the T level, slow spinal fluid flow of In-111 DTPA is demonstrated by the lack of tracer activity in the lumbar spine at 2.2 and 5.3 h in Fig. 4.5a. The effective half-life (Te) of tracer in the CSF is 27 h, greater than the range set forth in IIa. This Te together with an In-111 physical half-life of 67.2 h would result in a tracer biologic half-life of 45.1 h in the CSF space.

When Tc-99m DTPA was injected into the Ommaya reservoir, off-label (as is done in times of urgency and/or interruption of indium 111 DTPA supply), the lack of tracer in the lumbar spine is also noted at 20 and 22 h in Fig. 4.5b. The disadvantage of using Tc99m DTPA is also illustrated by the low count on the 22 h image. Calculation of the biologic half-life from the Te (5.5 h) and Tc-99m physical half-life yields a result of 64 h.

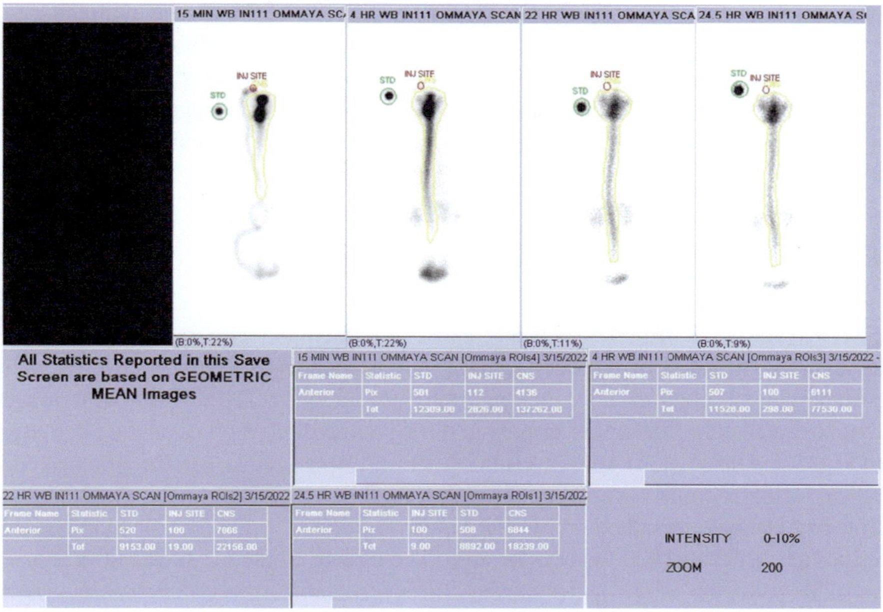

Fig. 4.12 A 42-year-old female with LM and an Ommaya reservoir connected to a VP programmable shunt with a progGav 2.0 setting at 10 (maximum at 20 indicating no drainage to peritoneum). Injection of In-111 DTPA for Ommayogram revealed the VP shunt and CSF in 15 min, and Te in CSF was 10 h

Table 4.2 Effective half-life of In-111 in CSF with blockage or leakage after Ommaya or lumbar injection

Te (hr)	CSF Te of In-111 DTPA in block or leak using T-test (bolded values are statistically significant)												
Route				Ommaya								Lumbar	
	Block or leak status	V C block no leak	T-block no leak	On diamox	Parenchymal inj	Leak no block	VP valve closed	VP open	OM Asymmetry	No block no leak no OM	No block no leak	Leak no block	Block ± leak
Studies (N)		8	16	3	7	3	15	14	28	101	36	36	7
Te mean		22.69	18.58	19.00	6.29	10.83	22.03	7.07	16.74	15.25	15.41	8.47	9.36
Te sd		5.74	5.79	1.73	3.09	3.82	11.16	3.64	6.63	4.33	4.55	3.70	5.83
Ommaya	V C block no leak	1.0000	0.1214										
	T-block no leak		1.0000										
	On diamox			1.0000									
	Parenchymal inj				1.0000								
	Leak no block					1.0000		**0.0001**				0.3978	
	VP valve closed						1.0000						
	VP open							1.0000					
	OM Asymmetry								1.0000				
*Normal	No block no leak no OM	**0.0077**	**0.0409**	**0.0454**	**0.0001**	0.1790	**0.0347**	**0.0000**	0.4263	1.0000	0.8472		
Lumbar	No block no leak										1.0000	**0.0000**	**0.0335**
	Leak no block											1.0000	
	Block ± leak												1.0000

The highest Te is noted with ventricular or cervical block. The lowest Te is associated with parenchymal injection. OM asymmetry denotes decreased visualization of tracer in the side with Ommaya reservoir implantation. When blocks, leaks, or OM asymmetry are excluded, the normal Te from Ommaya reservoir injection is found to be 15.25 ± 4.33 h. With lumbar puncture injection, normal Te is 15.41 ± 4.55 h and not different from that derived from Ommaya reservoir injection. Opening the VP shunt valve results in an instant exit of tracer and the Te is found to be 7.07 ± 3.64 h

Asymmetric trace distribution over the convexity may be observed in patients who have had recent Ommaya reservoir placement (OM Asym) or in patients with other underlying pathology, as demonstrated in Fig. 4.5c. A 41-year-old male with lung cancer and LM as well as cerebral metastasis to the right parietal lobe showed decreased tracer visualization and a Te of 17 h. A group of 28 patients with this pattern of asymmetric tracer uptake over the cerebral convexity (no leak nor spinal blocks) had a mean Te of 16.7 ± 6.6 h, a value that is not statistically significantly different from patients with no blocks nor leaks. These findings suggest that Te may not be sufficiently sensitive to detect blocks at the cerebral convexity.

Fast CSF Clearance with CSF Leakage (Fig. 4.6)

CSF leakage often occurs after head trauma or intracranial surgery including transsphenoidal resection of pituitary tumors. A postoperative cisternogram of a male patient with meningioma after lumbar drain injection of In111 DTPA and rhinorrhea demonstrated abnormal tracer activity in the right maxillary regions on the 5-h image of Fig. 4.6. There is also prompt visualization of tracer activities in the stomach and bowel resulting from swallowing of tracer leaked into the oropharynx. The standard tests of nasal pledget radioactivity count ratios (against 0.5 mL of whole blood) yield values greater than 1900 for both nostrils. The effective half-life of In111 DTPA in the CSF pathways is 6 h. After conservative management, repeated cisternograms show similar findings. The patient underwent open surgery to repair the meninges in the skull base. The follow-up study in 3 months revealed normal CSF flow pattern, no abnormal extrathecal tracer uptake and an effective half-life of 19 h.

Whole-Body CSF Imaging with Tc99m DTPA (Figs. 4.5b and 4.7)

In patients in whom Tc99m DTPA has been used as an alternative CSF imaging agent when In111 DTPA is not available, prolonged imaging becomes less sensitive because of low radioactivity counts from the short physical half-life of 6 h of Tc99m. With biological clearance from CSF flow, Te is expected to be than 6 h as seen in Fig. 4.5b. In order to visualize CSF, a larger amount of tracer activity is required as shown in Fig. 4.7; 10 mCi of Tc99m- DTPA was injected to allow imaging after decay of multiple half-lives at 26 h.

Whole-Body Ga-67 Scan Showed CSF Patency (Fig. 4.8)

During a winter storm in 1997, In111- DTPA supply was interrupted and a patient with melanoma and LM needed an Ommaya reservoir study before intrathecal therapy. With documented agreement between the attending nuclear physicians, attending neuro-oncologists and medical physicists, a dose of 0.5 mCi of Ga-67 citrate (a tumor-seeking agent typically used to detect lymphoma) was injected into the patient's Ommaya reservoir followed by serial whole-body imaging as prescribed in the In-111 DTPA protocol. This use of Ga-67 citrate to determine CSF patency from Ommaya reservoir injection was done on an off-label basis. As demonstrated in Fig. 4.8, there was prompt transit of tracer from the reservoir down to the spinal cord and back over the cerebral convexity. Patent CSF pathways were demonstrated, and only minimum tracer could be identified outside of the CSF throughout the study of 120 h. The multiple standards were placed in the right side of the patient for quantification. Images were acquired over the weekend for up to 120 h. This study demonstrated that an alternative radiopharmaceutical (Ga-67 citrate) with a physical half-life of 78.3 h (which is comparable to the physical half-life of 67.2 h for In-111) could allow prolonged evaluation of CSF.

Intraparenchymal Injection (Fig. 4.9a–c)

Inadvertent placement of the intraventricular catheter into the brain parenchyma can occur during or after initial surgical implantation despite immediate CT confirmation of appropriate catheter placement. There is prompt focal loculation of tracer in the brain and prompt absorption of tracer by the brain parenchyma resulting in less available injectate to the spinal fluid pathways as visualized in Fig. 4.9a. The resultant effective half-life (Te) is 7.5 h (less than the normal range of 10–20 h). There are also decreased tracer activities along the spinal cord and over the rest of the brain with increased excretion in the kidneys that collects in the urinary bladder during earlier scans, as seen in Fig. 4.7a. Because of earlier experience correlating intraparenchymal injection from visual inspection of the cisternogram and from Te calculation (Fig. 4.9b, with Te of 2 h), in this circumstance scans of subsequent time points are often cancelled to allow SPECT-CT confirmation of intraparenchymal position of catheter tip as seen in Fig. 4.9c. The catheter tip was indeed located within the left caudate nucleus on CT and the referring team was notified of the abnormality to allow them to withhold intrathecal therapy and proceed with revision of the intraventricular catheter placement.

Malfunction of Ommaya Reservoir (Fig. 4.10a, b)

Ommaya reservoirs provide an invaluable tool for accessing the ventricles [39]. They are surgically implanted over the skull and beneath the scalp, typically over the right frontal region to avoid potential damage to the cerebral cortex that controls language function. Connection of the reservoir to its ventricular catheter may be subject to mechanical failure. Other causes of Ommaya reservoir failure include scalp infection or excessive subgaleal fluid collection, usually from the concomitant presence of hydrocephalus. Such failure may not be readily detected by conventional methods of physical inspection or by difficulty of CSF aspiration. An In-111 DTPA Ommayogram (cisternogram via injection of the Ommaya reservoir) over at least 24 h will allow inspection of the initial CSF flow and delayed CSF distribution of tracer to determine patency of CSF flow.

Inadvertent intraparenchymal injection of chemotherapeutics may cause inflammation of the brain and is demonstrated in Fig. 4.9a–c. Failure of connection with the ventricular catheter can result in the accumulation of tracer in the subgaleal or subdural space resulting in prompt return of tracer to the general circulation and prompt renal excretion (Fig. 4.10a I–III). An attempt to access the reservoir for reinjection of tracer results in no CSF return further confirming reservoir malfunction. SPECT-CT revealed collection of tracer in the subdural region but no tracer reached the catheter. Catheter disconnection was also verified by high-resolution head CT (Fig. 4.10a V). Upon surgical revision and addition of a VP shunt, injection of In-111 DTPA into the Ommaya reservoir was followed by visualization of the abdomen at 2.5 h (Fig. 4.10b I). There is continuing circulation of tracer in the CSF and persistent tracer in the ventricle for 24 h (Fig. 4.10b II). The relatively fast effective half-life of 6.5 h (Fig. 4.10b III) is consistent with a patent VP shunt, while there is also circulation of tracer in the native CSF pathways.

Ventriculoperitoneal Shunt (Figs. 4.11a–c *and* 4.12)

Patients with leptomeningeal metastasis often have slow egress of CSF, likely related to arachnoiditis (from LM itself or from repeated intrathecal therapy) and loss of compliance of the arachnoid granulations on the parasagittal sinuses that allow resorption of CSF into the general circulation. The resultant increase in intracranial pressure (ICP) would manifest as hydrocephalus which is generally relieved by surgical implantation of ventriculoperitoneal shunts (VP). Many VP shunts have a valve to regulate exit of CSF in response to increased ICP. The VP shunt and the Ommaya reservoir may be implanted at different times but can also be integrated into one surgical session. Intrathecal chemotherapy can be instilled via an Ommaya reservoir that is connected to a VP shunt with an adjustable or on-off valve). Multiple issues can arise in such a setting including patency of the VP shunt itself (that is required for relief of increased ICP) and patency of the Ommaya reservoir (delivering injectate to the ventricle to enable flow to the rest of the CSF space).

After the valve of the VP shunt was closed for injection of tracer (In111- DTPA), serial images demonstrate tracer transit to the ventricle, down to the spinal cord, and back over the cerebral convexity during the first 2 h in Fig. 4.11a. Upon opening of the valve of the VP shunt at 3.5 h, there is prompt transit of tracer from the upper portion of the VP shunt down to the abdomen. Even with the shunt valve in the open position, every little tracer exit can be visualized via that VP shunt for 16 and 24 h. While the valve was closed, the Te was 50 h. Opening the VP shunt results in a normalized Te of 10 h. The relatively low Te is suggestive of CSF egress slowly over time, likely via the VP shunt.

An alternative way to test the VP shunt patency is to inject the tracer into the reservoir with the valve in the open position to observe tracer transit from the reservoir down to the peritoneal cavity, as demonstrated in the anterior/posterior dynamic image pairs every 3 s shown in Fig. 4.11b. Prompt visualization of tracer in the VP shunt flowing from its upper segment down to the abdomen within a few minutes will confirm patency of the VP shunt.

In this patient with glioblastoma and thoracic spine CSF blockade (Fig. 4.11c), although the VP shunt is patent and effectively reducing ICP by allowing CSF flow down to the abdomen, no tracer collected in the ventricle could transit beyond the upper thoracic spine. Further imaging to 28 h showed effectively complete exit of tracer from the CSF pathways with Te of 4 h, again demonstrating effectiveness of the VP shunt. These images also indicated inadequacy of intrathecal therapy to treat the spinal LM had it been instilled.

Programmable valve settings of VP shunts are used to drain CSF during periods of higher intracranial pressure (than the preset target ICP value). The proGav 2.0 has a pressure setting scale of 10–20 (at the setting of 20 it will not allow drainage unless the ICP exceeds 20 cm of water). For a patient with LM from lung adenocarcinoma and Ommaya reservoir connected with a VP shunt and proGav setting at 10, an Ommayogram was performed revealing prompt tracer transit to the peritoneal cavity and to the CSF detected at 15 min following injection. Based on the geometric-mean images (Fig. 4.12), the CSF Te was 10 h and was consistent with intermittent drainage of CSF through the VP shunt. There is also persistent tracer retention in the ventricles and slow ascent of tracer to the convexity indicating slow but patent CSF transit and slow draining of CSF from VP during intervalss of a higher ICP than was targeted by the shunt valve's occlusion setting.

SPECT-CT of Cisternograms

The use of single photon emission computed tomography (SPECT) allows 3-dimensional evaluation revealing distribution of tracer in different parts of the CSF compartment 24 h after tracer injection. Detailed anatomic distribution of tracer can be further evaluated by co-registered SPECT-CT images from contemporaneously acquired SPECT and CT in the same scanner [55]. While SPECT-CT is still subject to limitations of quantification methodology, serial SPECT-CT is also subject to limitations of repeated exposure to CT radiation. Nevertheless, qualitative findings from SPECT-CT on selected CSF regions and at selected time points still provide invaluable confirmation of tracer localization, such as in cases of intraparenchymal injection (Fig. 4.9c), Ommaya reservoir malfunction (Fig. 4.10a), or CSF leakage.

Discussion

Intrathecal Radiopharmaceuticals

The current state of the art of cisternography using In-111 DTPA can aptly evaluate the bulk flow of CSF from one compartment to another compartments within the CSF space, and can quantify the rate at which bulk flow is leaving the CSF space. No other reliable LM-specific functional information nor molecular information can be derived.

Until better biomarkers are derived from molecular imaging or in vitro analysis, the imaging diagnosis of LM and monitoring of LM progression or improvement may be better deferred to contrast-enhanced MRI which can provide more succinct functional as well as anatomic details, as described in Chap. 2.

Many diagnostic and therapeutic pharmaceuticals have been administered as intrathecal medications including anions, cations, nucleosides, steroids, cytokines, opioids, neurotransmitters, antibodies, peptides, and proteins. Compared with intravenous medications, there are heightened quality requirements for intrathecal medication including more stringent non-pyrogenicity (less than 2.5 EU in the LAL test, instead of less than 17 EU for intravenous medication). After being radiolabeled with diagnostic or therapeutic radionuclides, candidate study radiopharmaceuticals may be used to investigate intrathecal pharmacokinetics or pharmacodynamics as long as regulations of radiation safety are enforced. Intrathecal studies of LM using known diagnostic or therapeutic radiopharmaceuticals (Tables 3.2, 3.3, and 3.5 in Chap. 3) have the additional advantage that systemic biodistribution and low systemic toxicity have already been established. The use of Tc99m DTPA is a common alternative strategy when there is an unmet clinical need to assess CSF flow but In-111 DTPA is not available (Figs. 4.5b and 4.7). The technical limitation of Tc99m is that the radioactivity counts will be low overnight because of its short physical half-life of 6 h, and hence its even shorter effective half-life. Under the previously mentioned IRB-approved retrospective chart review, an Ommaya reservoir study of a patient with LM requiring intrathecal therapy using Ga-67 citrate as alternative radiopharmaceutical during In-111 shortage is reviewed and illustrated in Fig. 4.8. The patency of CSF flow was indeed illustrated using that radiotracer. Its longer physical half-life of 78.3 h indeed provided adequate visualization of CSF pathways up to 5 days after an 0.5 mCi injection. The prolonged retentiol of Ga-67 in the CSF and lack of Ga-67 distribution outside of the CSF compartments raises interesting dosimetry implications that will be further discussed in Chap. 12.

All radiopharmaceuticals in Table 4.1 have been applied in human intrathecal studies, in the USA and in other countries. In the USA, many of them were used in clinical trials before full enactment of FDA Modernization Act (FDAMA) in 2007. Radiopharmaceuticals without FDA approval for intrathecal use such as the known renal imaging agent Tc99m- DTPA (which has a physical half-life of 6 h for a same-day scan) and rarely, the tumor imaging agent Ga-67 citrate, have been used on an off-label basis for cisternography when In-111 DTPA is not available. Currently, the off-label use of radiopharmaceuticals is subject to strict institutional oversight, and falls under both state and federal jurisdiction. Before the FDAMA in 1997, medical use of RAM was only under regulation of National Radiation Council. Since the full enactment of FDAMA in 2007, the use of all radiopharmaceuticals has been under FDA jurisdiction in the same way as other pharmaceutical agents, in addition to being governed by NRC regulations. Therefore, off-label use of radiopharmaceuticals is expected to come under more stringent scrutiny than it did before 2007 and to be regulated more closely than are non-radioactive pharmaceuticals. The intricate oversight networks for the use of radiopharmaceuticals by departmental and institutional oversight, municipal rules, state regulation, and federal laws are further reviewed in Chap. 11.

Effective Half-Life (Te) of Radiopharmaceuticals in CSF

The effective half-life (Te) of a pharmaceutical in the entire CSF, when it is taken as one compartment, can be derived from the geometric-mean images derived from whole-body anterior and posterior images. It certainly can provide an additional objective parameter for cisternograms in addition to direct imaging findings that allow localization of tracer. As demonstrated throughout this chapter, the use of In-111 DTPA to image the hydraulic flow of CSF in LM patients has been aided by the estimation of Te of In-111 in the CSF. Te from LM patients may be higher than in patients without LM because of the potential impediment to CSF reabsorption caused by the tumor-induced inflammatory processes affecting physical compliance of the cristae villa of the arachnoid.

In clinical settings, four serial time points from four CSF imaging sessions of 30 min each in 24 h are perhaps justifiable and practical given the considerations of patient comfort or discomfort. With a limiting number of four images, the simplification of the kinetic model to one compartment may be also justified based on the linearity of semi-log time–activity curves over 24 h as shown in Fig. 4.2b. The correlation between CSF leakage and fast Te (below 10 h) has been reported [60]. While the clearance of In-111 DTPA varies by the different site of blockade [71], study of focal CSF blockade at the spinal level using Te also appears promising. However, when blockade is related to intraparenchymal injection or extravasation at the Ommaya reservoir, fast kinetics (smaller values of Te) are noted and may be explained by the interstitial clearance in soft tissues. Nevertheless, CSF Te may be also used to correlate with the patency of VP shunts and to predict small molecule pharmacokinetics. As demonstrated in Fig. 4.12, evaluation of Te can allow discretionary decisions on the feasibility of intrathecal therapy even when there is focal blockade of CSF flow or blockade of VP shunts. One important consideration is whether the relative surface area of the intracranial subarachnoid space will be sufficiently exposed to the therapeutics to receive therapeutic benefit. More clinical studies will be needed to establish the utility of CSF Te in a single-compartment model.

Since In-111 DTPA pharmacokinetics have been demonstrated to parallel those of methotrexate [68], the exposure of meninges including LM to methotrexate (a non-radioactive drug with no physical decay) correlate with the biological half-life (Tb) of In-111 DTPA. Therefore, intrathecal methotrexate dose adjustment can be made according to Te when there is CSF incomplete obstruction, presence of a ventriculoperitoneal shunt (with its valve in the open or closed position), or when a CSF leak is present. The translation of Te to Tb for In-111 is: Tb = Te/(1–0.01488*Te). A goal of normal Te = 15.5 is equivalent to a Tb of 20.2 h. A hypothetical partial obstruction without anatomic blockade with image-based Te of 22 h would have a Tb of 32.7 h. To provide the same drug exposure, the dose of methotrexate should be normalized by a factor of 20.2/32.7 = 0.62, or a 38% reduction. Conversely, in a patient with CSF leak or with a VP shunt with an open valve having Te of 9, Tb would be 10.39 h. In such a patient the dose should be adjusted by a factor or 20.2/10.39 or 1.94, or increased by 94%. These types of dose adjustment can only be made by assuming that other toxicity effects such as accumulation of peritoneal methotrexate are negligible/acceptable.

Whole-Body Scans and Radiation Dosimetry

Whole-body scans allow localization and visualization of radiopharmaceutical distribution in the body and CSF. When stringent quantification schemes are conducted, quantification of radiopharmaceuticals is possible and allows estimation of radiation absorbed doses in each CSF compartment and each visualized organ. Using serial imaging sessions over multiple effective half-lives and residence times as in Fig. 4.10, the areas under the curve of radioactivity in each CSF compartment and each organ can be used to derive radiation dosimetry according to established algorithms. When such image-based dosimetry principles and imaging schemes (Chap. 10) are applied to study serial cisternograms, the radiation dosimetry of CSF compartments and vital organs can be derived to contrast with those from simulations (Chap. 9). Depth dosimetry (radiation dose across the distance from the CSF–meninges interface) can also be derived from established anthropomorphic models (Chap. 9). Resulting radiation dosimetry for radiopharmaceuticals would allow estimation of safety (low toxicity to critical organs, commonly bone marrow) and efficacy (high radiation absorbed dose to CSF compartments and meninges) to guide and refine radionuclide therapy trials to treat LM. Less stringent quantification (more convenient in the settings of clinical service) with normalization of radioactivity counts to initial injected activity may also yield useful parameters including effective half-life, in addition to routine qualitative assessment.

Acknowledgments The authors are grateful to E. Edmund Kim MD, Professor of Radiology in the University of California at Irvine for his participating in reading scintigraphic scans of CSF flows of protocol DR10-0344.

References

1. Bering EA Jr. Circulation of the cerebrospinal fluid. Demonstration of the choroid plexuses as the generator of the force for flow of fluid and ventricular enlargement. J Neurosurg. 1962;19:405–13.
2. Sakka L, Coll G, Chazal J. Anatomy and physiology of cerebrospinal fluid. Eur Ann Otorhinolaryngol Head Neck Dis. 2011;128(6):309–16.
3. Dreha-Kulaczewski S, et al. Respiration and the watershed of spinal CSF flow in humans. Sci Rep. 2018;8(1):5594.
4. Enzmann DR, Pelc NJ. Normal flow patterns of intracranial and spinal cerebrospinal fluid defined with phase-contrast cine MR imaging. Radiology. 1991;178(2):467–74.
5. Levy LM, Di Chiro G. MR phase imaging and cerebrospinal fluid flow in the head and spine. Neuroradiology. 1990;32(5):399–406.
6. Price RA, Johnson WW. The central nervous system in childhood leukemia. I. The arachnoid. Cancer. 1973;31(3):520–33.
7. Gilbert MR. Neoplastic meningitis: a unique disease process or a 'test tube' for evaluating cancer treatments? Curr Oncol Rep. 2003;5(1):11–4.
8. Hartmann K, et al. First in vivo visualization of the human subarachnoid space and brain cortex via optical coherence tomography. Ther Adv Neurol Disord. 2019;12:1756286419843040.

9. Doge H, Hliscs R. Intrathecal therapy with 198Au-colloid for meningosis prophylaxis. Eur J Nucl Med. 1984;9(3):125–8.
10. Morin RL, Brookeman VA. 169Yb-DTPA distribution and dosimetry in cisternography. J Nucl Med. 1974;15(9):786–96.
11. Enzmann DR, et al. Metrizamide and radionuclide cisternography in communicating hydrocephalus. Radiology. 1979;130(3):681–6.
12. Li H, et al. Value of (18)F-FDG hybrid PET/MR in differentiated thyroid cancer patients with negative (131)I whole-body scan and elevated thyroglobulin levels. Cancer Manag Res. 2021;13:2869–76.
13. Wu Y, et al. Whole-body parametric imaging of FDG PET using uEXPLORER with reduced scan time. J Nucl Med. 2022;63(4):622–8.
14. Burns R, et al. Optimization of whole-body 2-[(18)F]FDG-PET/MRI imaging protocol for the initial staging of patients with myeloma. Eur Radiol. 2022;32(5):3085–96.
15. Green MA, et al. In vivo quantitative whole-body perfusion imaging using radiolabeled copper(II) bis(thiosemicarbazone) complexes and positron emission tomography (PET). Methods Mol Biol. 2022;2393:751–71.
16. Lehnert W, et al. Whole-body biodistribution and radiation dosimetry of [(18)F]PR04.MZ: a new PET radiotracer for clinical management of patients with movement disorders. EJNMMI Res. 2022;12(1):1.
17. Rashidi A, et al. Diagnostic accuracy of 2-[(18)F]FDG-PET and whole-body DW-MRI for the detection of bone marrow metastases in children and young adults. Eur Radiol. 2022;32(7):4967–79.
18. Toyonaga T, et al. Deep learning-based attenuation correction for whole-body PET—a multi-tracer study with (18)F-FDG, (68) Ga-DOTATATE, and (18)F-fluciclovine. Eur J Nucl Med Mol Imaging. 2022;49(9):3086–97.
19. Grossman SA, et al. Cerebrospinal fluid flow abnormalities in patients with neoplastic meningitis. An evaluation using 111indium-DTPA ventriculography. Am J Med. 1982;73(5):641–7.
20. Goodwin DA, et al. Preparation, physiology, and dosimetry of 111 In-labeled radiopharmaceuticals for cisternography. Radiology. 1973;108(1):91–8.
21. Wagner HN Jr, et al. A new radiopharmaceutical for cisternography: chelated ytterbium 169. Radiology. 1970;95(1):121–5.
22. Dichiro G, Reames PM, Matthews WB Jr. Risa-ventriculography and risa-cisternography. Neurology. 1964;14:185–91.
23. Di Chiro G, et al. Descent of cerevrospinal fluid to spinal subarachnoid space. Acta Radiol Diagn (Stockh). 1973;14(4):379–84.
24. Hosain F, Reba RC, Wagner HN Jr. Ytterbium-169 diethylenetriaminepentaacetic acid complex. A new radiopharmaceutical for brain scanning. Radiology. 1968;91(6):1294. passim.
25. Lette J, et al. A reproducible radionuclide procedure for measurement of cerebrospinal fluid shunt flow. Eur J Nucl Med. 1986;12(5–6):240–3.
26. de Rougemont J, et al. [Outflow in ventricular peritoneal derivations. Its determination with Na 131-I]. Neurochirurgie. 1970;16(4):307–18.
27. Wong FC, Groves M, Papadopulos N, Conrad C, Meyers C, Kim S, Puduvali V, Hsu S, Kim EE. Toxicity and efficacy profiles of intrathecal injection of I-131 NaI via intraventricular (IVent) or intralumbar (Ilumb) route for leptomeningeal metastases (LM) therapy. J Clin Oncol. 2006;24(18S):70s.
28. Rebischung C, et al. First human treatment of resistant neoplastic meningitis by intrathecal administration of MTX plus (125)IUdR. Int J Radiat Biol. 2008;84(12):1123–9.
29. Bergstrand G, et al. Positron emission tomography with 68Ga-EDTA in the diagnosis and localization of CSF fistulas. J Comput Assist Tomogr. 1982;6(2):320–4.
30. Maziere B, et al. [55Co]- and [64Cu]DTPA: new radiopharmaceuticals for quantitative tomocisternography. Int J Appl Radiat Isot. 1983;34(3):595–601.
31. Freesmeyer M, et al. High-resolution PET cisternography with 64Cu-DOTA for CSF leak detection. Clin Nucl Med. 2019;44(9):735–7.

32. Muriel FS, et al. Remission maintenance therapy for meningeal leukaemia: intrathecal methotrexate and dexamethasone versus intrathecal craniospinal irradiation with a radiocolloid. Br J Haematol. 1976;34(1):119–27.
33. Moseley RP, et al. Carcinomatous meningitis: antibody-guided therapy with I-131 HMFG1. J Neurol Neurosurg Psychiatry. 1991;54(3):260–5.
34. Lashford LS, et al. A pilot study of 131I monoclonal antibodies in the therapy of leptomeningeal tumors. Cancer. 1988;61(5):857–68.
35. Moseley RP, Benjamin JC, Ashpole RD. Carcinomatous meningitis: antibody-guided therapy with I-131 HMFG1. J Neurol Neurosurg Psychiatry. 1991;54(3):260–5.
36. Pandit-Taskar N, et al. Biodistribution and dosimetry of intraventricularly administered (124)I-omburtamab in patients with metastatic leptomeningeal tumors. J Nucl Med. 2019;60(12):1794–801.
37. Moseley RP, et al. Intrathecal administration of 131I radiolabelled monoclonal antibody as a treatment for neoplastic meningitis. Br J Cancer. 1990;62(4):637–42.
38. Iacoangeli M, et al. Intrathecal chemotherapy for treatment of overt meningeal leukemia: comparison between intraventricular and traditional intralumbar route. Ann Oncol. 1995;6(4):377–82.
39. Ommaya AK. Subcutaneous reservoir and pump for sterile access to ventricular cerebrospinal fluid. Lancet. 1963;2(7315):983–4.
40. Partain CL, et al. A multiregional kinetics model for cerebrospinal fluid. Radiology. 1978;127(3):705–11.
41. Chamberlain MC, Corey-Bloom J. Leptomeningeal metastases: 111indium-DTPA CSF flow studies. Neurology. 1991;41(11):1765–9.
42. Chamberlain MC, Kormanik P, Jaeckle KA. 111Indium-diethylenetriamine pentaacetic acid CSF flow studies predict distribution of intrathecally administered chemotherapy and outcome in patients with leptomeningeal metastases. Neurology. 1999;52(1):216–7.
43. James AE Jr, et al. Normal-pressure hydrocephalus. Role of cisternography in diagnosis. JAMA. 1970;213(10):1615–22.
44. Galli G, Troncone L, De Rossi G. 131-I-HSA cisternography and 131-I-HSA transfer from CSF to blood in normal pressure hydrocephalus. J Nucl Biol Med. 1973;17(2):64–70.
45. Larsson A, et al. Predictive value of quantitative cisternography in normal pressure hydrocephalus. Acta Neurol Scand. 1990;81(4):327–32.
46. Patten DH, Benson DF. Diagnosis of normal-pressure hydrocephalus by RISA cisternography. J Nucl Med. 1968;9(8):457–61.
47. Khan SH, Rather TA, Sinha S. Cerebral spinal fluid cisternography in normal pressure hydrocephalus of the elderly. Indian J Nucl Med. 2017;32(3):250–1.
48. Algin O, et al. MR cisternography: is it useful in the diagnosis of normal-pressure hydrocephalus and the selection of "good shunt responders"? Diagn Interv Radiol. 2011;17(2):105–11.
49. Andersson J, et al. Challenges in diagnosing normal pressure hydrocephalus: evaluation of the diagnostic guidelines. eNeurologicalSci. 2017;7:27–31.
50. Keong NC, et al. Imaging normal pressure hydrocephalus: theories, techniques, and challenges. Neurosurg Focus. 2016;41(3):E11.
51. Aunan-Diop JS, et al. Magnetic resonance elastography in normal pressure hydrocephalus-a scoping review. Neurosurg Rev. 2021;45(2):1157–69.
52. Oliveira LM, Nitrini R, Roman GC. Normal-pressure hydrocephalus: a critical review. Dement Neuropsychol. 2019;13(2):133–43.
53. Scully AE, et al. A systematic review of the diagnostic utility of simple tests of change after trial removal of cerebrospinal fluid in adults with normal pressure hydrocephalus. Clin Rehabil. 2018;32(7):942–53.
54. Hentschel SJ, et al. Subarachnoid-pleural fistula after resection of thoracic tumors. J Neurosurg. 2004;100(4 Suppl Spine):332–6.
55. Slart RH, et al. Persistent aseptic meningitis due to post-surgical spinal CSF leakage: value of fused (111m)In-DTPA SPECT-CT cisternography. Eur J Nucl Med Mol Imaging. 2006;33(7):856.

56. Jeffery PJ, et al. Bowel visualization during indium-111-labelled diethylene triamine pentaacetic acid cisternography due to massive cerebrospinal fluid leak. Case report and review of the literature. Eur J Nucl Med. 1990;17(6–8):365–8.
57. Kosuda S, et al. [Reassessment of a combination of cerebrospinal fluid scintigraphy and nasal pledget counts in patients with suspected rhinorrhea]. Kaku Igaku. 1998;35(6):435–41.
58. McKusick KA, et al. Radionuclide cisternography: normal values for nasal secretion of intrathecally injected 111In-DTPA. J Nucl Med. 1973;14(12):933–4.
59. Schicha H, Voth E, Emrich D. Detection of occult and intermittent rhinorrhea using 111In-DTPA. Eur J Nucl Med. 1985;11(2–3):76–9.
60. Wong F, McCutcheon I, Groves M, Kim E. Evaluation of CSF flow by whole-body scintigraphy. J Nucl Med. 2010;51:1789.
61. Glantz MJ, et al. Diagnosis, management, and survival of patients with leptomeningeal cancer based on cerebrospinal fluid-flow status. Cancer. 1995;75(12):2919–31.
62. Chamberlain MC, Kormanik PA. Prognostic significance of 111indium-DTPA CSF flow studies in leptomeningeal metastases. Neurology. 1996;46(6):1674–7.
63. Korkmaz M, et al. In-111 DTPA Ommayagrams in leptomeningeal carcinomatosis. Clin Nucl Med. 1995;20(7):610–2.
64. Eltobgy M, et al. Impact of cerebrospinal fluid flow study in patients undergoing intrathecal chemotherapy via ventricular catheter reservoir. J Neurooncol. 2021;153(1):161–7.
65. Hayden PW, Rudd TG, Shurtleff DB. Combined pressure-radionuclide evaluation of suspected cerebrospinal fluid shunt malfunction: a seven-year clinical experience. Pediatrics. 1980;66(5):679–84.
66. Gok B, et al. Radionuclide shunt patency study for suspected ventriculoatrial shunt malfunction. Clin Nucl Med. 2013;38(7):527–33.
67. Miller KT, Wilkinson DS. Pharmacokinetics of methotrexate in the cerebrospinal fluid after intracerebroventricular administration in patients with meningeal carcinomatosis and altered cerebrospinal fluid flow dynamics. Ther Drug Monit. 1989;11(3):231–7.
68. Mason WP, Yeh SD, DeAngelis LM. 111Indium-diethylenetriamine pentaacetic acid cerebrospinal fluid flow studies predict distribution of intrathecally administered chemotherapy and outcome in patients with leptomeningeal metastases. Neurology. 1998;50(2):438–44.
69. Chamberlain MC, et al. 111Indium-diethylenetriamine pentaacetic acid CSF flow studies predict distribution of intrathecally administered chemotherapy and outcome in patients with leptomeningeal metastases. Neurology. 1999;52(1):216–7.
70. Wong F. Effective half-life of in-111 DTPA in the CSF from whole-body Ommayogram/Cisternogram correlates with CSF leakage and blockade. J Nucl Med Mol Imaging. 2022;63 (Suppl 2):2917.
71. Wong F, Kim E, Groves M, McCutcheon E, Podoloff D. The clearance rates of In-111 DTPA from CSF vary with different types of CSF blockade. J Nucl Med. 2002;29(8):286.

Chapter 5
State of Art of LM Therapies: Intrathecal and Systemic Approaches

Hannah Culver and Morris D. Groves Jr

Introduction

Neoplastic meningitis and leptomeningeal metastasis (LM) refer to the dissemination of cancer to the pia mater, subarachnoid space, cerebrospinal fluid (CSF), and arachnoid membrane. LM is a metastatic manifestation of many different malignancies, especially adenocarcinomas, and it carries a poor prognosis. The current management of LM is multidisciplinary and requires the expertise of neuro-oncologists, medical oncologists, neurosurgeons, and radiation oncologists. Prognosis for patients with LM remains poor. The current goal of treatment is primarily palliation and prevention of neurologic deficits. Because of improvements in systemic treatment and survival for many cancers, LM may become more prevalent. This chapter will focus on treatment strategies for LM secondary to solid tumors, but many of the concepts are relevant to the diagnosis and treatment of leptomeningeal involvement in leukemia and lymphoma.

Intrathecal (IT) Chemotherapy

IT chemotherapy treats subclinical leptomeningeal deposits and tumor cells suspended in the CSF and may prevent further seeding of the leptomeninges. It is administered to circumvent the issues of drug delivery imposed by the blood–brain,

H. Culver (✉) · M. D. Groves Jr
Neuro-Oncology, Texas Oncology, Austin, TX, USA
e-mail: Hannah.culver@usoncology.com; morris.groves@usoncology.com

F. C. L. Wong (ed.), *Radiopharmaceuticals in the Management of Leptomeningeal Metastasis*, https://doi.org/10.1007/978-3-031-14291-8_5

blood–spine, and blood–CSF barriers [1]. There remains a debate regarding the benefit of IT chemotherapy over systemic chemotherapy. At least one report suggests IT chemotherapy increases toxicity without adding benefit versus radiation and systemic chemotherapy [2]. Another study arguing against IT chemotherapy showed better survival for patients treated with systemic rather than IT methotrexate [3].

Route of Administration of IT Chemotherapy

For patient comfort and better CSF distribution of chemotherapy, most patients have a ventricular reservoir placed for drug delivery. Intralumbar delivery of chemotherapy may result in drug placement outside of the thecal sac and increased variability of ventricular drug levels [4]. In CNS leukemia, chemotherapy delivery via ventricular reservoir appears to result in improved durability of remission as compared to intralumbar drug delivery [5, 6]. The reservoirs are usually well-tolerated but complications such as misplacement, catheter tip occlusion, or infection can occur in as many as 5% of patients [7–9].

Commonly Used IT Chemotherapies

Standard IT chemotherapies used in the treatment of LM include methotrexate (MTX), cytarabine (Ara-C), and thiotepa. Very few randomized trials have been performed to compare the efficacy of these drugs. In one study by Grossman et al., comparing IT MTX to IT thiotepa in 59 solid tumor patients, there was no difference in survival between the two groups [10]. In another study comparing IT MTX to IT MTX plus IT Ara-C there was no significant difference in outcomes in 44 patients [11].

MTX is the most commonly used IT drug for LM. It is a cell cycle phase-specific antimetabolite which acts primarily during S phase. Typical dosing schemes use MTX (10–12 mg) mixed with preservative-free normal saline and delivered IT twice per week for eight doses. If a response is noted with clearing of malignant cells from the CSF, then treatment is administered once per week for four doses, then twice monthly for four doses, then monthly treatments are given for a variable period of time. Intraventricular injections result in therapeutic concentrations (>1 μM) which persist for 48 h [4, 7]. Using MTX, along with radiation as needed, up to 50% of patients can stabilize or improve [7, 11–13]. MTX toxicities such as myelosuppression and mucositis can be prevented by the use of folinic acid which, conveniently, does not enter the CNS, leaving the MTX within the CNS unantagonized.

Thiotepa is an alkylating agent which has demonstrated responses in some patients [14]. It is usually administered in 10–15 mg doses, IT on a similar schedule as IT MTX. IT thiotepa was prospectively compared to IT MTX with no difference in efficacy noted between drugs, although thiotepa was more myelosuppressive [10].

Ara-C is a synthetic pyrimidine analog which is relatively S phase specific. It is used most commonly in patients with meningeal leukemia or lymphoma. The half-life of Ara-C in the CSF is much longer than that in the serum due to low levels of cytidine deaminase in the CSF. A long acting form of Ara-C, liposomal cytarabine, or DepoCyt®, was approved for use in lymphomatous meningitis based on improved CSF response rates and modest survival benefit. However, the drug was recently taken off the market in the USA. It continues to be available in selected European countries.

Even though combination chemotherapy improves outcomes in many systemic cancers, this same benefit has not been seen when combination IT chemotherapy has been tested for LM. Studies which combined MTX + thiotepa or Ara-C, MTX + thiotepa + Ara-C, and MTX + thiotepa + Ara-C + hydrocortisone have failed to improve response rates or survival percentages compared to single drug regimens [11, 15–17]. Two of these studies had increased degrees of myelosuppression or neurotoxicity over single drug regimens [16, 17]. A summarized list of standard IT chemotherapies can be found in Table 5.1.

Table 5.1 Standard IT chemotherapies

Drug	Reference first author	Disease (mixed, breast, etc.)	Dose	CSF response/notes
Methotrexate	Shapiro [4], Wasserstrom [13], Hitchins [11], Sause [12]	Mixed	10–12 mg IT twice per week × 8 doses, once per week × 4 doses, twice monthly × 4 doses, then monthly	MTX with radiation as needed up to 50% of patients stabilize or improve
Thiotepa	Gutin [14]	Mixed	10–15 mg similar schedule as MTX	Increased myelosuppression
Cytarabine (Ara-C)	Glantz [18]	Leukemia/ lymphoma; breast	25–100 mg similar schedule as MTX	Improved CSF response rates in liposomal cytarabine (DepoCyt®) and survival benefit; unavailable in the USA
IT MTX vs. IT thiotepa	Grossman [10]	Solid tumors	10 mg MTX vs. 10 mg thiotepa twice weekly	No difference in survival outcomes
IT MTX vs IT MTX + IT Ara-C	Hitchins [11]	Mixed	15 mg MTX vs. 15 mg MTX + 50 mg/m^2 Ara-C	No difference in survival outcomes

Experimental IT Treatments for LM

Temozolomide

An IT formulation of temozolomide, an orally bioavailable alkylator with activity against a variety of tumors, has been tested in an athymic rat model of leptomeningeal cancer with evidence of benefit and good tolerance of the therapy [19].

Topotecan

Topotecan is a water soluble semisynthetic camptothecin analog that inhibits topoisomerase I, causing single-strand DNA breaks. In primates, the concentration of the active lactone form is much higher with IT than systemic administration, making IT use of the drug logical [20, 21]. A phase I study of intrathecally delivered topotecan suggested IT topotecan may be active in leptomeningeal spread of leukemia and brain tumors. A phase II study showed the drug has roughly the same benefit (survival and CSF response) as the other agents.

Mafosfamide

Mafosfamide is a bifunctional alkylator, not requiring activation by hepatic microsomal enzymes, with a broad spectrum of activity in solid tumors. IT doses of 20 mg once or twice weekly have been used. A phase I study of mafosfamide in pediatric patients demonstrated some efficacy in meningeal leukemia [22], and a report of 16 children with LM from primary brain tumors treated with IT mafosfamide also shows promise [23]. In this report, 8 of 9 patients evaluable for response achieved complete responses, although all of the patients were simultaneously treated with systemic chemotherapy, so definitive evidence of efficacy could not be ascertained [23].

Diaziquone

Diaziquone (AZQ) is an alkylating agent which readily crosses the blood–brain barrier and has been tested as systemic therapy for primary brain tumors [24]. Cumulative myelosuppression precluded further evaluation of this compound for systemic use. Favorable pharmacokinetics resulted in the investigation of AZQ as a possible IT agent [25]. In a phase I/II study, the safety and efficacy of AZQ following IT administration were evaluated in 39 patients with refractory meningeal malignancies [26]. Dose-limiting toxicity consisting of headache, nausea, or vomiting occurred in only three patients at the highest dose. The overall response rate was 62%. Complete responses (CRs) occurred in 14 of 37 courses (38%) and partial responses (PRs) occurred in 9 of 37 courses (24%). Among patients with meningeal leukemia, CRs were observed in 11 of 26 courses (42%) and PRs in nine of 26 courses (35%). AZQ may merit further study for treatment of LM.

ACNU

ACNU is an alkylator which has shown activity when administered IT in a rat model of LM, although it did not penetrate as deeply into tumor masses as other drugs tested [27]. A phase I/II study of 27 patients with LM treated with IT ACNU demonstrated good drug tolerance; 8/21 (38%) patients who presented with positive cytology converted to negative cytology, with a range of response durations from 1 to 20+ months [28]. Two other patients had other indirect evidence of response to treatment. The authors concluded that IT ACNU was safe, had minimal toxicity, demonstrated efficacy in some patients with LM, and warranted further evaluation of alternative dosing and delivery approaches. ACNU has also been given via ventriculolumbar perfusion for CSF seeding from primary brain tumors with response rates and median survivals of: 17% and 12 months, 29% and 12 months, and 88% and 25 months for anaplastic glioma, glioblastoma multiforme, and PNET/medulloblastoma, respectively [29]. Further research on this molecule has been suspended at this time.

Immunotherapy

Immunotoxins

The use of monoclonal antibodies coupled to protein toxins to target tumor cell surface antigens is an attractive scheme to improve the selectivity of IT toxin delivery. Several animal models have been used to test this method of treatment. In a study by Gunther et al. [30], IT administered B43 (anti-CD19)-pokeweed antiviral protein (PAP) showed promise in a mouse model, however, has not been further studied. A human trial has been conducted using the immunotoxin, 454A12-rRA, delivered IT, in eight patients with LM. 454A12-rRA is a conjugate of a monoclonal antibody against the human transferrin receptor and recombinant ricin A chain, the enzymatically active subunit of the protein toxin ricin. The highest doses caused a CSF inflammatory response associated with headache, vomiting, and altered mental status responsive to steroids and CSF drainage. Four patients had a greater than 50% reduction of tumor cell counts in the lumbar CSF; however, no patient had their CSF cleared of tumor, and clinical or magnetic resonance imaging evidence of tumor progression was demonstrated in seven of the eight patients after treatment [31]. A phase I clinical trial that was completed in 2013 looked at the toxicity of intrathecal LMB-7 immunotoxin, a single-chain immunotoxin constructed from monoclonal antibody B3-Pseudomonas Exotoxin PE 38, in patients with leptomeningeal metastases (clinicaltrials.gov identifier: NCT00003020). In this trial that began in 1997, no significant antitumor activity was observed [32]. No further data were published.

Checkpoint Inhibitors

Given the remarkable response to immune checkpoint inhibitors (ICI) in many systemic malignancies, research is being done to evaluate their efficacy in the setting of LM [33]. The use of antibodies to block inhibitory signals through receptors such as cytotoxic T-lymphocyte antigen (CTLA)-4, programmed cell death (PD)-1, and programmed cell death like (PD-L)-1 is being utilized in metastatic melanoma, NSCLC, and renal cell carcinoma [34]. Two prospective, phase 2 trials have shown the efficacy of ipilimumab, an anti-CTLA-4 antibody, among patients with melanoma-associated brain metastasis [35, 36]. A phase 2 study of ipilimumab monotherapy resulted in a CNS response rate of 16% and a median overall survival of 7 months in patients with symptomatic brain metastases [35]. In a case report by Bot et al. [37], a patient with LM from melanoma received whole-brain radiotherapy (5 times 4 Gy) followed by four courses of ipilimumab 3 mg/kg every 3 weeks. A complete clinical and radiological response was observed, and patient survived for more than 1.5 years [37]. A study with nivolumab, a monoclonal antibody that blocks PD-1, demonstrated improvement in neurological symptoms (auditory hallucinations) and 7-month progression-free survival in an advanced NSCLC patient with LM after treatment administration [38]. In a prospective study by Hendriks et al. [39] patients with LM from NSCLC treated with an immune checkpoint inhibitor (nivolumab or pembrolizumab) had a median overall survival of 3.7 from the start of therapy. There was not a statistically significant difference in patients with poor or good prognosis based on NCCN criteria and 6-month and 12-month overall survival from start of ICI was 36.8% and 21.1%, respectively. Currently multiple clinical trials are underway to assess ICI efficacy in the setting of LM including pembrolizumab and combination ipilimumab and nivolumab for melanoma (clinicaltrials.gov identifier NCT02886585, ClinicalTrials.gov Identifier: NCT03091478, clinicaltrials.gov identifier NCT02939300).

Radiolabeled Monoclonal Antibodies

Tumor-specific monoclonal antibodies (Mabs) may improve delivery of radiotherapy to tumor cells, and numerous studies have demonstrated proof of principle of this concept. In several studies, small numbers of patients with LM have been treated with the IT ^{131}I-labeled monoclonal antibody, HMFG1. Clinical responses were seen, and a long term survivor (32 months) was seen, but aseptic meningitis, seizures, and myelosuppression were serious toxicities [40, 41]. ^{131}I-labeled antibodies directed toward tenascin and the proteoglycan chondroitin sulfate have been delivered IT to patients with some responses, maintenance of stable disease, and survival prolongation, and with little in the way of toxicity seen [42]. One study using tumor-specific Mabs in patients with diffuse LM achieved a clinical response rate of approximately 33%; better results were observed in more radiosensitive tumors [43].

To try and overcome the dose-limiting toxicity of myelosuppression caused by passage of the radioimmunoconjugate from the CSF to the blood compartment, repeated dosing of the radioimmunoconjugate was attempted. It was found that the therapeutic index of the radioimmunoconjugate was significantly increased by the development of an anti-mouse Ig response in the blood. The residence time of the radioimmunoconjugate in the blood was decreased due to the development of an anti-mouse IgG response in the blood. This resulted in less of an impact of the agent on the blood component with repeated dosing. This same effect was not seen in the CSF compartment, despite the presence of the anti-mouse immunoglobulins in the CSF. This differential effect created the therapeutic index [44]. In a large review of 40 LM patients who had failed conventional therapy and who were treated with IT ^{131}I-labeled Mabs, there was evidence of localization to tumor and minimal toxicity. The best results were seen in primitive neuroectodermal tumor ($n = 22$), where 53% of evaluable cases had responses and 11% had stable disease. Three exceptional survivals were recorded: one patient leads a normal life at 10 years 11 months, second patient is alive and normal at 3 years 2 months, and a third patient survived in good condition for 8 years. The mean survival of responders was 39 months and non-responders 4 months. In the total series, 50% of patients survived for at least 1 year with two long term survivors [45]. An active multicenter phase II/III clinical trial is examining the efficacy and safety of intracerebroventricular radioimmunotherapy using 131I-omburtamab (131I-8H9) for patients with neuroblastoma and central nervous system/leptomeningeal metastases. An approach using IT ^{131}I-labeled antibody specific for disialoganglioside (GD2) was used in five patients with GD2-positive LM with minimal side effects and a favorable CSF/blood ratio of ^{131}I. Tumors that are known to have GD2 expression and which might be possible candidates for this treatment include medulloblastoma/PNET, high-grade astrocytoma, malignant glioma, neuroblastoma, retinoblastoma, ependymoma, sarcoma, melanoma, and SCLC [46]. There is an ongoing phase 2 trial studying the side effects and how well IT iodine I 131 monoclonal antibody 3F8 works in treating patients with central nervous system cancer or leptomeningeal cancer (clinicaltrials.gov identifier NCT00445965). Phase 1 study demonstrated that the antibody reached therapeutic doses in the CSF, and 3 of 13 assessed patients achieved objective and/or cytologic responses [47]. Like other IT therapies this approach is limited by availability of tumor-specific antibodies as well as toxicities such as myelosuppression, aseptic meningitis, and increased ICP [33].

IT Immunotherapy

Because the subarachnoid space may serve as an immunologic sanctuary of tumor cells from antitumor immune reactions, treatments with immunomodulating cytokines might benefit patients with LM. Cytokines may enhance the immune response directed against some tumors. A small number of studies of patients with LM from melanoma, squamous cell carcinoma, and primary brain tumors have shown responses to interleukin-2 (IL-2) alone or combined with lymphokine-activated killer (LAK) cells, but overall the results of immunotherapy in LM have not been encouraging. The CSF in 12 of 12 patients treated with high-dose IT IL-2 could be made tumor cell free and would again respond to IT IL-2 at relapse [48]. Melanoma was the most responsive tumor, whereas NSCLC, medulloblastoma, and glioblastoma patients had no major responses. When IV IL-2 is used in combination with IT LAK cells, no significant improvement of responses is seen, although long term remissions are seen in small number of patients with LM from medulloblastoma and squamous cell carcinoma [49–51]. In a recent study of 42 patients with melanoma-associated LM who were treated with intrathecal IL-2, median survival was found to be 9.1 months (range 0.7–86.2) with 16% of patients surviving more than 24 months [52]. The side effects of IT IL-2 include fever, confusion, seizures, raised ICP, and there are marked interindividual variations in the immunological response [53]. Adoptive T-cell therapy using autologous tumor-infiltrating lymphocytes (TILs) has emerged as a promising therapy for advanced solid tumors. This is an immunological approach in which T cells are expanded ex vivo before being infused back into the patient [54]. Intrathecal autologous TILs in combination with intrathecal IL-2 were safe and feasible in an individual with refractory LM from melanoma who disease had progressed after monotherapy with IT IL-2 [55]. This patient received 3 doses of IT TILs which consisted of 96% $CD8^+$ T cells 1 week apart. On days 1 and 4 after IT TILs, IT IL-2 was administered [55]. Radiographic stabilization of leptomeningeal metastasis was observed after IT TIL therapy; however, parenchymal brain metastases were not controlled and progressed about 3 months after therapy [55].

Rituximab is a humanized monoclonal antibody against the CD-20 antigen expressed on most B-cell lymphomas. CSF levels of this large molecule are only 0.1% of the serum level after intravenous administration [56]. Several case reports demonstrating safety and possible benefits of intrathecal administration of rituximab led to a recently reported phase I study. In this study, the maximum tolerated dose of intrathecal rituximab was 25 mg twice weekly (9 doses total). Cytologic responses were seen in 6 of 10 patients; 4 patients experienced a complete response; 2 patients experienced improvement in intraocular lymphoma; and 1 patient's intraparenchymal lymphoma improved [57].

Gene Therapy

Because malignant cells in the thecal sac are bathed in CSF, this anatomic region presents an interesting system in which to evaluate gene therapy. The poor penetration of gene therapy vectors into nodular accumulations of tumor cells is an obvious

Table 5.2 Standard systemic therapies

Drug	Reference first author	Disease (mixed, breast, etc.)	Dose	CSF response/notes
IV MTX vs. IT MTX	Glantz [3]	Mixed	IV MTX—8 g/m^2 IT MTX—15 mg	Survival: 13.8 months IV MTX vs. 2.3 months IT MTX
Temozolomide	Segura [63]	Mixed	100 mg/m^2	Phase 2 trial stopped due to poor accrual—Median survival: 43 days
Capecitabine	Tham [64]	Breast	Metronomic dosing (500 mg three times a day continuously)	Case report of one patient; PFS of 23 months; patient still living at the time of report
Pemetrexed	Clinicaltrials. gov: NCT 00424242	Mixed	500 mg/m^2	Ongoing phase I trial
Bevacizumab	Wu [65], Chen [66], Sandler [67], Riess [68], Ariyasu [69]	Mixed	Varied	Can improve intra-tumor penetration of other chemotherapeutic agents when used in combination

obstacle. A phase I/II study was developed based on promising results, in terms of prolongation of survival and elimination of infiltrative tumor, which had emerged from studies on animal models of LM treated with the HSV-Tk/ganciclovir combination [58, 59]. A case report by Heiss et al. describes an LM patient that received intraventricular delivery of NIH3T3 producer cells expressing the thymidine kinase (HSV-Tk1) gene via a retroviral vector followed by intravenous ganciclovir. Although there was an apparent cytotoxic effect of ganciclovir on the vector producer cells, ultimately this treatment was insufficient to significantly reduce the extensive leptomeningeal tumor load or number of tumor cells in the CSF (seen in both MRI report and CSF cytology) [60]. Several other animal model systems have tested the applicability of gene therapy to LM and have suggested encouraging results [59, 61, 62]; however, there are no current human studies. Table 5.2 provides a condensed list of experimental systemic and IT treatments for reference.

Systemic Chemotherapy

Numerous studies have shown that systemic chemotherapy improves survival. It bypasses the administration issues of IT chemotherapy, treats the primary tumor, and is effective in treating bulky NM [70]. In a mouse model of LM from melanoma, it has been shown that the tight junctions of the new vessels within the tumor masses are penetrable by horseradish peroxidase and adriamycin. The leakiness of the blood vessels increases with increased time of tumor presence and growth. This suggests that systemic chemotherapy may have a role to play in the treatment of LM [71]. Choice of systemic treatment should be guided by the primary malignancy.

Currently utilized systemic therapies include high-dose MTX, high-dose cytarabine, capecitabine, thiotepa, bevacizumab, pemetrexed, and temozolomide. High-dose etoposide has also been utilized in patients with LM from small cell lung cancer [72]. There is retrospective evidence that systemic chemotherapy with or without IT chemotherapy may increase the likelihood of longer patient survival [73–75]. Therapeutic CSF levels of most systemically administered drugs are not generally considered to be achievable [76], although there is strong evidence that cytotoxic MTX levels (≥ 1 μM) can be achieved after high-dose administration [77]. One study supporting this concept compared high-dose IV to IT MTX, high-dose IV MTX was found to be more effective [3]. The differences in survival between the 2 groups were remarkable (13.8 months versus 2.3 months, IV versus IT MTX, respectively). Other groups have suggested that the toxicity of IV systemic therapies directed toward LM is less than that associated with IT chemotherapy, and that there is no loss of efficacy [2]. The use of high-dose IV MTX in LM may deserve further study.

Oral temozolomide may be a candidate for the treatment of LM due to its relatively mild toxicity, broad range of activity against human tumors and evidence that after systemic administration, CSF levels reach nearly 30% of plasma levels [78–80]. While case reports suggest possible efficacy against LM secondary to gliomas, paragangliomas, adenocarcinomas, SCLC, breast cancer, and melanoma, a trial of 31 children with gliomas by Broniscer et al. showed no impact on outcome [81, 82]. A phase II randomized controlled trial of 19 patients with LM from solid tumors was prematurely stopped due to poor accrual, with median time to progression of 28 days, median survival of 43 days, and only two patients completing the trial [63].

Capecitabine is a fluoropyrimidine carbamate designed as an oral alternative to 5-fluorouracil. It is enzymatically converted to 5-fluorouracil at the tumor site. The increased drug concentration at the tumor site may enhance its antitumor activity and reduce systemic toxicity [83]. There have been empirical observations of responses to the drug in patients with brain metastases as well as LM [84, 85]. Capecitabine has also resulted in responses in a few patients with recurrent brain metastases or LM even after previous capecitabine exposure [64, 85]. Based on the existing reports, capecitabine is now often used in patients with LM or brain metastases secondary to breast cancer.

Pemetrexed, a chemotherapeutic molecule similar to methotrexate, is a new generation multi-targeted ant-folate agent, which is approved for the treatment of NSCLC but has been shown to have broader antitumor activity [81]. As with methotrexate, CNS penetration of the drug is poor, with peak distribution reaching <5% of plasma concentrations. IT therapy has not been well explored but an active, ongoing phase I trial exploring IT pemetrexed is monitoring drug levels in serum and CSF as well as VEGF, and YKL 40 as markers of prognosis and response (clinicaltrials.gov Identifier NCT 00424242).

Bevacizumab is a systemically administered monoclonal antibody directed against VEGF. It is approved for use in colorectal, breast, and non-small cell lung cancers and glioblastoma multiforme. Recent reports have identified elevated VEGF levels in the CSF of the majority of patient with LM due to melanoma or breast or lung cancer [86–88]. Preliminary data suggest that in LM responders CSF VEGF levels fall and correlate with response [88]. Recent reports have shown that bevacizumab can improve intra-tumor penetration of other chemotherapeutic agents, such as etoposide and cisplatin in breast cancer [65, 66], carboplatin and paclitaxel in NSCLC [67, 68], and erlotinib in EGFR positive cancer [69], perhaps by normalizing tumor-related vessels. See Table 5.3 for summary of findings.

Table 5.3 Experimental IT and systemic treatments for LM

Drug	Reference first author	Disease (mixed, breast, etc.)	Phase of study	CSF response/notes
IT Topotecan	Groves [1]	Mixed	II	Similar response to other IT agents, limited toxicity
IT Mafosfamide	Slavc [23]	Pediatric primary brain tumors	N/A	Dose of 20 mg can be safely administered into the CSF and may produce responses and prolong remission of the leptomeningeal disease
IT Diaziquone	Berg [26]	Refractory meningeal malignancies (mixed)	I/II	39 patients; overall response rate = 62%; CR = 38%; PR = 24%
IT ACNU	Levin [28]	Mixed	I/II	27 patients; 8/21 patients (38%) seroconverted positive to negative CSF
IT 454A12-rRA	Laske [31]	Mixed	N/A	8 patients; 4 patients had greater than 50% reduction in tumor cell counts in CSF, 7/8 patients had tumor progression on imaging after treatment
IT LMB-7	Pastan [32]	Mixed	I	No significant antitumor activity seen
IT HMFG1	Moseley [40]	Mixed	N/A	1 long term survivor—32 months; serious toxicities include aseptic meningitis, seizures, and myelosuppression
IT ^{131}I labeled GD2	Kramer [46]	GD2 positive LM	N/A	5 patients; minimal side effects, favorable CSF/blood ratio
IT IL-2	Moser [48], Glitza [52]	Mixed	N/A	Melanoma the most responsive tumor; 42 patients with melanoma, 16% surviving 24 months or more, median survival 9.1 months
IT IL-2 + IT TILs	Glitza [55]	Refractory LM from melanoma	N/A	Radiographic stabilization of LM, however progression of brain metastases after 3 months
IT Rituxan	Rubenstein [57]	Lymphoma	I	Cytologic response in 6/10 patients; complete response in 4 patients

(continued)

Table 5.3 (continued)

Drug	Reference first author	Disease (mixed, breast, etc.)	Phase of study	CSF response/notes
IT HSV-Tk/ IV ganciclovir	Heiss	Mixed	N/A	Treatment insufficient to reduce the LM tumor load or number of tumor cells in CSF
Ipilimumab	Margolin [35], Bot [37]	Melanoma	II	Response rate of 16%, OS of 7 months; case report of one patient surviving 1.5 years after WBRT and ipilimumab monotherapy
Nivolumab	Gion [38], Hendriks [39]	Mixed (melanoma/ NSCLC)	N/A	Improvement in neurologic symptoms, 7-month PFS
Pembrolizumab or nivolumab	Hendriks [39]	Mixed (melanoma/ NSCLC)	N/A	6-month OS 36.8%; 12-month OS 21.1%

Hormonal Therapy

There is some evidence that hormonal therapy in conjunction with IT therapy may result in better overall survival in LM [74]. There are also case reports of hormonally responsive LM from breast cancer [89].

Targeted Therapies

The most common solid malignancies associated with leptomeningeal metastases are adenocarcinomas of the breast (12–35%), adenocarcinomas of the lung (10–26%), and melanoma (5–25%) [34]. Advances in molecular targeted systemic agents have prolonged survival especially in patients with lung cancer expressing epidermal growth factor receptor (EGFR) mutations and breast cancer patients harboring human epidermal growth factor receptor 2 (HER2) amplification [90].

Breast Cancer

IT Trastuzumab

HER2/neu-positive breast cancers are predisposed to have CNS involvement.

Trastuzumab can be intrathecally administered, either alone or in combination with different chemotherapy agents. It is generally well tolerated with minimal side effects. Several studies have been done examining combination therapy with trastuzumab including methotrexate and thiotepa with varying degrees of success [91, 92]. Intrathecal trastuzumab has been administered using different dosing ranges

(20–100 mg weekly, 100–150 mg biweekly) with no reported safety issues [34]. A prospective multi-institutional phase I/II dose escalation trial was recently published in abstract form evaluating the efficacy and safety (phase I) and the response rate (phase 2) of intrathecal trastuzumab in 34 patients. Intrathecal trastuzumab was well tolerated at the maximum dose level of 80 mg with no reported dose-limiting toxicities at the following dose schedule: 2×/week for 4 weeks, weekly for 4 weeks, and every 2 weeks thereafter. At a median follow-up of 9.1 months, the primary endpoint of a 25% response rate was not met, but 69% of patients showed a clinical benefit (stable disease or better) with a median OS of 12.1 months, exceeding historical controls [93].

A systematic review and pooled analysis of 13 articles evaluating 17 patients treated with intrathecal trastuzumab demonstrated clinical, cytologic, and radiographic responses in 69%, 67%, and 56% of cases, respectively [94]. In this same review those patients treated with intrathecal trastuzumab alone or in combination with chemotherapy had a median overall survival rate of 13.5 months (compared to previous historical data at 5.9 months) and a median CNS progression-free survival rate of 7.5 months.

A recent retrospective single institutional series reported significantly improved craniospinal progression-free survival with intrathecal trastuzumab compared to intrathecal chemotherapy or whole-brain radiotherapy alone [95].

Drug combinations are also being utilized in several studies. A phase 2 nonrandomized study examines the safety and efficacy of the combination of oral tucatinib, an experimental small molecular inhibitor of HER2, with IV trastuzumab, and oral capecitabine (clinicaltrials.gov identifier NCT03501979). There is an ongoing phase 1 trial for HER2-positive patients with LM that utilizes oral lapatinib, a small-molecule dual tyrosine kinase inhibitor (TKI) that targets HER2 and EGFR, in combination with capecitabine, an antimetabolite chemotherapeutic (clinicaltrials.gov identifier NCT02650752). In a single-arm phase 2 study, lapatinib plus capecitabine was active in managing brain metastases in patients with HER2-positive breast cancer who had not received previous whole-brain radiation therapy [96]. Conversely, in a phase III open-label study of lapatinib plus capecitabine versus IV trastuzumab plus capecitabine, there was no difference in the incidence of CNS metastases between the two combinations [97]. Currently, there is no evidence supporting the use of lapatinib, IV trastuzumab emtansine, or IV pertuzumab for managing LM in patients who have HER2-positive breast cancer [90].

At this time, intrathecal trastuzumab is the only targeted treatment that shows possible efficacy over conventional therapies for managing LM in HER2-positive breast cancer patients [90].

Lung Cancer

Many cases of LM arise in patients with non-small cell lung cancer (NSCLC) due to the prevalence of this disease. NSCLC can be categorized into numerous subtypes based on tumor genetic profile. Mutations in the *EGFR* gene and rearrangement of the *ALK* gene are the two most studied NSCLC genetic profiles [90]. Patient's with these mutations can be more effectively treated with *EGFR* tyrosine kinase inhibitor (TKI) and *ALK* inhibitors, respectively. In a study by Liao et al. [98] *EGFR*-mutated patients who received *EGFR* TKI therapy for LM showed longer overall survival compared to patients not so treated (10.9 months vs.2.3 months, $p < 0.001$). However poor penetration of these drugs through the blood–brain barrier (BBB) remains a significant issue. Previous studies and case series have shown some response using first generation TKIs oral erlotinib and oral gefitinib in the treatment of LM [99]. In a phase I study, high-dose gefitinib (750 or 1000 mg daily) resulted in neurologic symptom improvement in 57% of NSCLC patients who had shown prior response to *EGFR* TKI [100]. High dose or pulse administration of erlotinib proved to be effective and safe for managing LM in patients who failed to respond to standard-dose *EGFR TKI* [101]. Erlotinib, however, showed higher CSF concentration (28.7 vs. 3.7 ng/mL, $p = 0.0008$) and penetration levels (2.77% vs 1.13%, $p < 0.0001$) [102]. Some studies have suggested that dual therapy with oral afatinib, a second-generation EGFR-TKI, and IV cetuximab could provide benefit to patients with LM [103, 104]. Treatment with afatinib 40 mg and cetuximab 250 mg every 2 weeks results in clinical and radiographic improvement [103]. Benefit from combination therapy has also been reported in other studies including one utilizing erlotinib with IV pemetrexed cisplatin in patients that have failed gefitinib [105]. Oral osimertinib is a third generation TKI developed to target both EGFR-TKI sensitizing mutations and T790M. In recent studies it has shown superiority over first generation TKIs in untreated patients regardless of T790M status as well as T790M-positive disease that failed first line TKI [106, 107]. There is a recently completed phase 2 trial of tesevatinib, a BBB-penetrant oral TKI, in patients with EGFR-activating mutations and brain or leptomeningeal metastases (clinicaltrials.gov identifier NCT02616393). Early data suggests that tesevatinib has clinical activity in the CNS in EGFR mutant disease manifesting as LM in patients previously treated with erlotinib, gefitinib, or afatinib. An additional cohort of treatment-naïve patients is being added [108].

Anaplastic lymphoma kinase (ALK) rearrangements and MET mutations are found in 3–5% and 4% of NSCLC, respectively [109]. The presence of these genetic alterations confers sensitivity to ALK inhibitors. Oral crizotinib, the first targeted option for ALK-rearranged NSCLC patients, poorly penetrates the BBB, so the CNS remains a frequent site of relapse for ALK-positive patients treated with this drug [90]. In one case report, the CSF-to-plasma ratio of crizotinib was only 0.026 [110]. Initial studies of second-generation ALK inhibitors, such as oral ceritinib and oral alectinib, have shown increased CNS penetration, decreased radiological burden of metastases and LM, and improvement in symptoms [81]. Ceritinib is currently being studied in multiple Phase II and III studies including ASCEND-2, which treats crizotinib-resistant LM, ASCEND-3, which treats ALK-inhibitor naïve LM, ASCEND4 trial, where treatment is randomized to IV platinum plus pemetrexed doublet chemotherapy versus ceritinib, and ASCEND5 trial, where patients failing crizotinib are randomized to IV pemetrexed, IV docetaxel, or ceretinib [111]. To date, the ASCEND-2 and ASCEND-3 trial showed improved overall response rate (38.6% and 58.9%, respectively) and progression-free survival (5.7 months and 11.1 months, respectively). In a phase 2 study of alectinib in crizotinib-refractory ALK-rearranged NSCLC, a complete CNS response rate of 27% was observed [112]. Alectinib also resulted in an overall CNS response rate of 57% in study patients with measurable CNS metastases [112]. In a case series by Gainor et al. [113] alectinib 600 mg twice daily resulted in significant clinical and radiographic improvements in 3 out of 4 patients with crizotinib or ceritinib refractory LM. Other ALK inhibitors including oral lorlatinib and oral brigatinib may be used as well after progression under crizotinib according to expert opinion [109]. PF-06463922 is a new agent being investigated with purported superior potency against all known clinically acquired ALK mutations, including the highly resistant G1202R mutant, and is designed to minimize P-glycoprotein-mediated drug efflux and optimize penetration of the CNS [114].

Melanoma

Melanoma frequently metastasizes to the brain, with approximately 5% of cases spreading to the leptomeninges, the subarachnoid space, and cerebrospinal fluid (CSF). Only a few series of patients with LM from melanoma have been published with reported median overall survival of 8–10 weeks [115]. Approximately 50% of melanomas harbor an activating mutation in the v-Raf murine sarcoma viral oncogene homolog B (BRAF), most commonly BRAF V600E, which constitutively activates the mitogen-activated protein kinase (MAPK) pathway [33]. There are reports of response to BRAF inhibitors such as oral vemurafenib and oral dabrafenib in LM from melanoma but is less clear how great of a response in comparison to response in active brain metastases. In two patients with tumors containing BRAF V600 mutations, treatment with either vemurafenib alone or in sequence with whole-brain radiotherapy resulted in marked responses and long-term stabilization of LM [116, 117]. In one case study conducted by Schafer et al., a patient who was unresponsive to whole-brain radiotherapy was given vemurafenib at 960 mg twice per day, and after 12 weeks the patient had a complete resolution of clinical symptoms, achieved a cytological response in CSF, and had significant radiographic regression of the meningeal lesions on MRI [116]. Analyses of vemurafenib CSF concentration in patients with brain metastases have revealed low ratios of CSF to plasma concentration ($0.98 \pm 0.84\%$) and high rates of variability within a single patient [118]. Dabrafenib also does not cross an intact BBB but has similar intracranial and extracranial responses. However, observation after 4 weeks in one patient with LM from BRAF V600E-mutant melanoma treated with dabrafenib 150 mg twice a day revealed complete imaging and cytological response [119]. In a phase 2 trial evaluating dabrafenib in patients with active brain metastases from BRAF V600E or V600K-mutant melanoma complete + partial intracranial responses were 39.2% and 6.7%, respectively, in previously untreated disease [120]. It also should be noted that at least one case report to date of a patient treated with systemic dabrafenib for BRAF-mutant LM demonstrated ineffectiveness preventing disease progression [121].

Despite notoriously rapid and dramatic responses with single agents, most patients develop resistance with reactivation of the MAPK pathway (resulting from acquired NRAS and MEK mutations and BRAF-splice mutants) [54]. Combination of BRAF and MEK inhibitors such as dabrafenib-trametinib and now vemurafenib-cobimetinib limits resistance and increases overall survival (median overall survival 25.1 months) [122, 123]. There are emerging approaches that have shown promising results in the control of extracerebral disease in BRAF mutated tumors; however, only limited data are available on the efficacy of oral MEK inhibitors (trametinib, selumetinib, pimasertib, cobimetinib) or the combination of oral BRAF and oral MEK inhibitors (dabrafenib + trametinib, vemurafenib + cobimetinib) in patients with LM from melanoma.

Dabrafenib has also been utilized in the treatment of BRAF V600 E mutated gliomas with associated LM. In a retrospective analysis of three patients treated with 150 mg dabrafenib twice daily, all patients showed an impressive response after just 1 month of treatment radiographically and clinically despite their poor prognosis. One of the patients was still stable at 27 months after initiation of therapy [124]. There are ongoing trials evaluating the combined treatment with dabrafenib and trametinib in patients with brain tumors (ClinicalTrials.gov Identifier: NCT03919071, ClinicalTrials.gov Identifier: NCT02034110). See Table 5.4 for a summary of targeted treatments.

Table 5.4 Targeted treatments for LM

Drug	Reference first author	Disease (mixed, breast, etc.)	Dose	CSF response/notes
IT Trastuzumab	Zagouri [94]	Breast	20–100 mg weekly, 100–150 mg biweekly	17 patients—Systematic review, 69% clinical response; 67% cytologic response; 56% radiographic response
Lapatinib + capecitabine vs. IV trastuzumab + capecitabine	Pivot [97]	Breast	Lapatinib 1250 mg per day; capecitabine 2000 mg/m^2 per day Trastuzumab loading dose of 8 mg/kg followed by an infusion of 6 mg/kg every 3 weeks; capecitabine 2500 mg/m^2 per day	No difference in incidence of CNS metastases between the two combinations
Gefitinib	Jackman [100]	Lung	750 mg or 1000 mg daily	Neurologic symptom improvement in 57% of patients
Afatinib + cetuximab	Lin [103]	Lung	Afatinib 40 mg; cetuximab 250 mg every 2 weeks	Clinical and radiographic improvement
Tesevatinib	Berz [108]	Lung	300 mg daily	Six out of the seven patients had CNS symptom improvement, previously treated with erlotinib, gefitinib, or afatinib

Table 5.4 (continued)

Drug	Reference first author	Disease (mixed, breast, etc.)	Dose	CSF response/notes
Osimertinib vs. IV pemetrexed + carboplatin or cisplatin	Mok [106]	T790M positive lung	Osimertinib: 80 mg daily IV pemetrexed: 500 mg/m^2 + carboplatin AUC5 or cisplatin 75 mg/m^2	PFS in osimertinib was 10.1 months vs. 4.4 in combination therapy
Ceritinib	ASCEND-2	Crizotinib-resistant LM in ALK mutated lung	750 mg daily	Improved overall response rate 38.6%; PFS 5.7 months
Ceritinib	ASCEND-3	ALK-inhibitor naïve LM in lung	750 mg daily	Improved overall response rate 58.9%; PFS 11.1 months
Alectinib	Ou [112]	Crizotinib-resistant LM in ALK mutated lung	600 mg twice daily	Complete CNS response rate of 27%
Vemurafenib	Schafer [116]	BRAF V600E melanoma	960 mg twice daily	Case study of 1 patient complete resolution of clinical symptoms, cytologic response in CSF, and radiographic regression
Dabrafenib	Wilgenhof [119]	BRAF V600E melanoma	150 mg twice daily	Case report of 1 patient, complete imaging and cytologic response after 4 weeks
Dabrafenib + trametinib vs. dabrafenib + placebo	Long [122]	BRAF V600E melanoma	Dabrafenib: 150 mg twice daily + trametinib 2 mg once daily vs. Dabrafenib: 150 mg twice daily + placebo	Overall survival was 74% at 1 year and 51% at 2 years with dabrafenib + trametinib vs. 68% and 42%, respectively, with placebo
Vemurafenib + Cobimetinib vs. Vemurafenib + placebo	Larkin [123]	BRAF V600E melanoma	Vemurafenib: 960 mg twice daily + cobimetinib 60 mg once daily for 21 days on 7 days off vs. Vemurafenib: 960 mg twice daily + placebo	Median PFS in combination treatment was 9.9 months vs. 6.2 months with placebo
Dabrafenib	Burger [124]	BRAF V600E glioma + LM	150 mg twice daily	Retrospective analysis of 3 patients showed impressive response both radiographically and clinically; one patient still stable after 27 months

Conclusion

Research into new IT treatments for LM is few but with some encouraging findings in limited cases. More optimistically, the slow but steadily accruing evidence of the benefit of targeted oral agents (osimertinib, alectinib, etc.) in the appropriate LM patients [125], suggests that more research into drugs that engage an appropriate target and reach the leptomeninges and CSF in sufficient levels, will have an impact on survival for LM patients.

References

1. Groves MD, Glantz MJ, Chamberlain MC, et al. A multicenter phase II trial of intrathecal topotecan in patients with meningeal malignancies. Neuro-Oncology. 2008;10(2):208–15.
2. Bokstein F, Lossos A, Siegal T. Leptomeningeal metastases from solid tumors: a comparison of two prospective series treated with and without intra-cerebrospinal fluid chemotherapy. Cancer. 1998;82(9):1756–63.
3. Glantz MJ, Cole BF, Recht L, et al. High-dose intravenous methotrexate for patients with nonleukemic leptomeningeal cancer: is intrathecal chemotherapy necessary? J Clin Oncol. 1998;16(4):1561–7.
4. Shapiro WR, Young DF, Mehta BM. Methotrexate: distribution in cerebrospinal fluid after intravenous, ventricular and lumbar injections. N Engl J Med. 1975;293(4):161–6.
5. Bleyer WA, Poplack DG. Intraventricular versus intralumbar methotrexate for central-nervous-system leukemia: prolonged remission with the Ommaya reservoir. Med Pediatr Oncol. 1979;6(3):207–13.
6. Haghbin M, Galicich JH. Use of the Ommaya reservoir in the prevention and treatment of CNS leukemia. Am J Pediatr Hematol Oncol. 1979;1(2):111–7.
7. Shapiro WR, Posner JB, Ushio Y, et al. Treatment of meningeal neoplasms. Cancer Treat Rep. 1977;61(4):733–43.
8. Chamberlain MC, Kormanik P, Jaeckle KA, et al. 111Indium-diethylenetriamine pentaacetic acid CSF flow studies predict distribution of intrathecally administered chemotherapy and outcome in patients with leptomeningeal metastases. Neurology. 1999;52(1):216–7.
9. Chamberlain MC. Leptomeningeal metastases: a review of evaluation and treatment. J Neuro-Oncol. 1998;37(3):271–84.
10. Grossman SA, Finkelstein DM, Ruckdeschel JC, et al. Randomized prospective comparison of intraventricular methotrexate and thiotepa in patients with previously untreated neoplastic meningitis. Eastern Cooperative Oncology Group. J Clin Oncol. 1993;11(3):561–9.
11. Hitchins RN, Bell DR, Woods RL, et al. A prospective randomized trial of single-agent versus combination chemotherapy in meningeal carcinomatosis. J Clin Oncol. 1987;5(10):1655–22.
12. Sause WT, Crowley J, Eyre HJ, et al. Whole brain irradiation and intrathecal methotrexate in the treatment of solid tumor leptomeningeal metastases—a Southwest Oncology Group study. J Neurooncol. 1988;6(2):107–12.
13. Wasserstrom WR, Glass JP, Posner JB. Diagnosis and treatment of leptomeningeal metastases from solid tumors: experience with 90 patients. Cancer. 1982;49(4):759–22.
14. Gutin PH, Weiss HD, Wiernik PH, et al. Intrathecal N, N', N''-triethylenethiophosphoramide [thio-TEPA (NSC 6396)] in the treatment of malignant meningeal disease: phase I-II study. Cancer. 1976;38(4):1471–5.
15. Trump DL, Grossman SA, Thompson G, et al. Treatment of neoplastic meningitis with intraventricular thiotepa and methotrexate. Cancer Treat Rep. 1982;66(7):1549–51.

16. Giannone L, Greco FA, Hainsworth JD. Combination intraventricular chemotherapy for meningeal neoplasia. J Clin Oncol. 1986;4(1):68–73.
17. Stewart DJ, Maroun JA, Hugenholtz H, et al. Combined intraommaya methotrexate, cytosine arabinoside, hydrocortisone and thio-TEPA for meningeal involvement by malignancies. J Neuro-Oncol. 1987;5(4):315–22.
18. Glantz MJ, LaFollette S, Jaeckle KA, et al. Randomized trial of a slow-release versus a standard formulation of cytarabine for the intrathecal treatment of lymphomatous meningitis. J Clin Oncol. 1999;17(10):3110–6.
19. Sampson JH, Archer GE, Villavicencio AT, et al. Treatment of neoplastic meningitis with intrathecal temozolomide. Clin Cancer Res. 1999;5(5):1183–8.
20. Blaney SM, Cole DE, Balis FM, et al. Plasma and cerebrospinal fluid pharmacokinetic study of topotecan in nonhuman primates. Cancer Res. 1993;53(4):725–7.
21. Blaney SM, Cole DE, Godwin K, et al. Intrathecal administration of topotecan in nonhuman primates. Cancer Chemother Pharmacol. 1995;36(2):121–4.
22. Blaney S, Balis F, Murphy R, et al. A phase I study of intrathecal mafosfamide in patients with refractory meningeal malignancies. Proc Am Soc Clin Oncol 1993;34: Abstract.
23. Slavc I, Schuller E, Czech T, et al. Intrathecal mafosfamide therapy for pediatric brain tumors with meningeal dissemination. J Neurooncol. 1998;38(2–3):213–8.
24. Schold SCJ, Mahaley MSJ, Vick NA, et al. Phase II diaziquone-based chemotherapy trials in patients with anaplastic supratentorial astrocytic neoplasms. J Clin Oncol. 1987;5(3):464–71.
25. Zimm S, Collins JM, Curt GA, et al. Cerebrospinal fluid pharmacokinetics of intraventricular and intravenous aziridinylbenzoquinone. Cancer Res. 1984;44(4):1698–701.
26. Berg SL, Balis FM, Zimm S, et al. Phase I/II trial and pharmacokinetics of intrathecal diaziquone in refractory meningeal malignancies. J Clin Oncol. 1992;10(1):143–8.
27. Huang TY, Arita N, Hayakawa T, et al. ACNU, MTX and 5-FU penetration of rat brain tissue and tumors. J Neurooncol. 1999;45(1):9–17.
28. Levin VA, Chamberlain M, Silver P, et al. Phase I/II study of intraventricular and intrathecal ACNU for leptomeningeal neoplasia. Cancer Chemother Pharmacol. 1989;23(5):301–7.
29. Ushio Y, Kochi M, Kitamura I, et al. Ventriculolumber perfusion of 3-[(4-amino-2-methyl-5-pyrimidinyl)-methyl]-1-(2-chloroethyl-1-nitrosourea hydrochloride for subarachnoid dissemination of gliomas. J Neurooncol. 1998;38(2–3):207–12.
30. Gunther R, Chelstrom LM, Tuel-Ahlgren L, et al. Biotherapy for xenografted human central nervous system leukemia in mice with severe combined immunodeficiency using B43 (anti-CD19)-pokeweed antiviral protein immunotoxin. Blood. 1995;85(9):2537–45.
31. Laske DW, Muraszko KM, Oldfield EH, et al. Intraventricular immunotoxin therapy for leptomeningeal neoplasia. Neurosurgery. 1997;41(5):1039–49.
32. Pastan I, Hassan R, FitzGerald DJ, Kreitman RJ. Immunotoxin treatment of cancer. Annu Rev Med. 2007;58:221–37.
33. Wang N, Bertalan MS, Brastianos PK. Leptomeningeal metastasis from systemic cancer: review and update on management. Cancer. 2018;124(1):21–35.
34. Sahebjam S, Forsyth PA, Smalley KS, Tran ND. Experimental treatments for leptomeningeal metastases from solid malignancies. Cancer Control. 2017;24(1):42–6. https://doi.org/10.1177/107327481702400106.
35. Margolin K, Ernstoff MS, Hamid O, et al. Ipilimumab in patients with melanoma and brain metastases: an open-label, phase 2 trial. Lancet Oncol. 2012;13:459–65.
36. Di Giacomo AM, Ascierto PA, Pilla L, et al. Ipilimumab and fotemustine in patients with advanced melanoma (NIBIT-M1): an open-label, single-arm phase II trial. Lancet Oncol. 2012;13(9):879–86.
37. Bot I, Blank CU, Brandsma D. Clinical and radiological response of leptomeningeal melanoma after whole brain radiotherapy and ipilimumab. J Neurol. 2012;259:1976–8. https://doi.org/10.1007/s00415-012-6488-4.
38. Gion M, Remon J, Caramella C, Soria JC, Besse B. Symptomatic leptomeningeal metastasis improvement with nivolumab in advanced non-small cell lung cancer patient. Lung Cancer. 2017;108:72–4.

39. Hendriks LEL, Henon C, Auclin E, et al. Outcome of patients with non–small cell lung cancer and brain metastases treated with checkpoint inhibitors. J Thorac Oncol. 2019;14:1244–54.
40. Moseley RP, Benjamin JC, Ashpole RD, et al. Carcinomatous meningitis: antibody-guided therapy with I-131 HMFG1. J Neurol Neurosurg Psychiatry. 1991;54(3):260–5.
41. Moseley RP, Papanastassiou V, Zalutsky MR, et al. Immunoreactivity, pharmacokinetics and bone marrow dosimetry of intrathecal radioimmunoconjugates. Int J Cancer. 1992;52(1):38–43.
42. Bigner DD, Brown M, Coleman RE, et al. Phase I studies of treatment of malignant gliomas and neoplastic meningitis with 131I-radiolabeled monoclonal antibodies anti-tenascin 81C6 and anti-chondroitin proteoglycan sulfate Me1–14 F (ab')2—a preliminary report. J Neurooncol. 1995;24(1):109–22.
43. Papanastassiou V, Pizer BL, Chandler CL, et al. Pharmacokinetics and dose estimates following intrathecal administration of 131I-monoclonal antibodies for the treatment of central nervous system malignancies. Int J Radiat Oncol Biol Phys. 1995;31(3):541–52.
44. Kemshead JT, Hopkins K, Pizer B, et al. Dose escalation with repeated intrathecal injections of 131I-labelled MAbs for the treatment of central nervous system malignancies. Br J Cancer. 1998;77(12):2324–30.
45. Coakham HB, Kemshead JT. Treatment of neoplastic meningitis by targeted radiation using (131)I-radiolabelled monoclonal antibodies. Results of responses and long term follow-up in 40 patients. J Neurooncol. 1998;38(2–3):225–32.
46. Kramer K, Cheung NK, Humm JL, et al. Targeted radioimmunotherapy for leptomeningeal cancer using (131)I-3F8. Med Pediatr Oncol. 2000;35(6):716–8.
47. Kramer K, Humm JL, Souweidane MM, et al. Phase I study of targeted radioimmunotherapy for leptomeningeal cancers using intra-Ommaya 131-I-3F8. J Clin Oncol. 2007;25(34):5465–70.
48. Moser R, Bruner JM, Grimm EA. Biologic therapy for brain tumors. Cancer Bull. 1991;43:117–26.
49. Okamoto Y, Shimizu K, Tamura K, et al. An adoptive immunotherapy of patients with medulloblastoma by lymphokine-activated killer cells (LAK). Acta Neurochir. 1988;94(1–2):47–52.
50. Shimizu K, Okamoto Y, Miyao Y, et al. Adoptive immunotherapy of human meningeal gliomatosis and carcinomatosis with LAK cells and recombinant interleukin-2. J Neurosurg. 1987;66(4):519–21.
51. Silvani A, Salmaggi A, Parmiani G, et al. Successful adoptive immunotherapy with lymphokine-activated killer cells in the treatment of medulloblastoma disseminated via cerebrospinal fluid: case report. Neurosurgery. 1994;34(6):1078–80.
52. Glitza IC, Rohlfs M, Bassett R, et al. IMCT-07: therapeutic outcomes of intrathecal interleukin-2 in metastatic melanoma patients with leptomeningeal disease (LMD). Neuro Oncol. 2015;17(Suppl 5):v108. https://doi.org/10.1093/neuonc/nov218.07.
53. Salmaggi A, Dufour A, Silvani A, et al. Intrathecal immunotherapy in CNS tumors disseminating via CSF: preliminary evaluation using different treatment schedules. Ital J Neurol Sci. 1996;17(4):267–76.
54. Smalley KS, Fedorenko IV, Kenchappa RS, Sahebjam S, Forsyth PA. Managing leptomeningeal melanoma metastases in the era of immune and targeted therapy. Int J Cancer. 2016;139(6):1195–201. https://doi.org/10.1002/ijc.30147.
55. Glitza IC, Haymaker C, Bernatchez C, et al. Intrathecal administration of tumor-infiltrating lymphocytes is well tolerated in a patient with leptomeningeal disease from metastatic melanoma: a case report. Cancer Immunol Res. 2015;3(11):1201–6. https://doi.org/10.1158/2326-6066.CIR-15-0071.
56. Rubenstein JL, Combs D, Rosenberg J, Levy A, McDermott M, Damon L, Ignoffo R, Aldape K, Shen A, Lee D, Grillo-Lopez A, Shuman MA. Rituximab therapy for CNS lymphomas: targeting the leptomeningeal compartment. Blood. 2003;101(2):466–8. Accessed 18 Jul 2019. https://doi.org/10.1182/blood-2002-06-1636.
57. Rubenstein JL, Fridlyand J, Abrey L, et al. Phase I study of intraventricular administration of rituximab in patients with recurrent CNS and intraocular lymphoma. J Clin Oncol. 2007;25(11):1350–6.

58. Ram Z, Walbridge S, Oshiro EM, et al. Intrathecal gene therapy for malignant leptomeningeal neoplasia. Cancer Res. 1994;54(8):2141–5.
59. Vrionis FD, Wu JK, Qi P, et al. Tumor cells expressing the herpes simplex virus-thymidine kinase gene in the treatment of Walker 256 meningeal neoplasia in rats. J Neurosurg. 1996;84(2):250–7.
60. Heiss JD, Taha S, Oldfield EH, Ram Z. Intrathecal gene therapy for treatment of leptomeningeal carcinomatosis. J Neurooncol. 2011;104(1):365–9. https://doi.org/10.1007/s11060-010-0458-4.
61. Viola JJ, Ram Z, Walbridge S, et al. Adenovirally mediated gene transfer into experimental solid brain tumors and leptomeningeal cancer cells. J Neurosurg. 1995;82(1):70–6.
62. Rosenfeld MR, Bergman I, Schramm L, et al. Adeno-associated viral vector gene transfer into leptomeningeal xenografts. J Neurooncol. 1997;34(2):139–44.
63. Segura PP, Gil M, Balana C, Chacon I, Langa JM, Martin M, Bruna J. Phase II trial of temozolomide for leptomeningeal metastases in patients with solid tumors. J Neuro-Oncol. 2012;109:137–42. https://doi.org/10.1007/s11060-012-0879-3.
64. Tham YL, Hinckley L, Teh BS, et al. Long-term clinical response in leptomeningeal metastases from breast cancer treated with capecitabine monotherapy: a case report. Clin Breast Cancer. 2006;7(2):164–6.
65. Wu PF, Lin CH, Kuo CH, Chen WW, Yeh DC, Liao HW, Huang SM, Cheng AL, Lu YS. A pilot study of bevacizumab combined with etoposide and cisplatin in breast cancer patients with leptomeningeal carcinomatosis. BMC Cancer. 2015;15:299. https://doi.org/10.1186/s12885-015-1290-1.
66. Chen IC, Lin CH, Jan IS, Cheng AL, Lu YS. Bevacizumab might potentiate the chemotherapeutic effect in breast cancer patients with leptomeningeal carcinomatosis. J Formos Med Assoc. 2016;115:243–8. https://doi.org/10.1016/j.jfma.2015.03.005.
67. Sandler A, Gray R, Perry MC, Brahmer J, Schiller JH, Dowlati A, Lilenbaum R, Johnson DH. Paclitaxel-carboplatin alone or with bevacizumab for non-small-cell lung cancer. N Engl J Med. 2006;355:2542–50. https://doi.org/10.1056/NEJMoa061884.
68. Riess JW, Nagpal S, Iv M, Zeineh M, Gubens MA, Ramchandran K, Neal JW, Wakelee HA. Prolonged survival of patients with non-small-cell lung cancer with leptomeningeal carcinomatosis in the modern treatment era. Clin Lung Cancer. 2014;15:202–6. https://doi.org/10.1016/j.cllc.2013.12.009.
69. Ariyasu R, Horiike A, Koyama J, Saiki M, Sonoda T, Kawashima Y, Takano N, Oguri T, Nishikawa S, Kitazono S, Yanagitani N, Ohyanagi F, Nishio M. Efficacy of bevacizumab and erlotinib combination for leptomeningeal carcinomatosis after failure of erlotinib. Anti-Cancer Drugs. 2017;28:565–7. https://doi.org/10.1097/CAD.0000000000000489.
70. Batool A, Kasi A. Leptomeningeal carcinomatosis. In: StatPearls. Treasure Island (FL): StatPearls Publishing; 2018. [Updated 2018 Oct 27]. https://www.ncbi.nlm.nih.gov/books/NBK499862/.
71. Siegal T, Sandbank U, Gabizon A, et al. Alteration of blood-brain-CSF barrier in experimental meningeal carcinomatosis. A morphologic and adriamycin-penetration study. J Neurooncol. 1987;4(3):233–42.
72. Postmus PE, Haaxma-Reiche H, Berendsen HH, et al. High dose etoposide for meningeal carcinomatosis in patients with small cell lung cancer. Eur J Cancer Clin Oncol. 1989;25:377–8.
73. Grant R, Naylor B, Greenberg HS, et al. Clinical outcome in aggressively treated meningeal carcinomatosis. Arch Neurol. 1994;51(5):457–61.
74. Boogerd W, Hart AA, van der Sande JJ, et al. Meningeal carcinomatosis in breast cancer. Prognostic factors and influence of treatment. Cancer. 1991;67(6):1685–95.
75. Jayson GC, Howell A, Harris M, et al. Carcinomatous meningitis in patients with breast cancer. An aggressive disease variant. Cancer. 1994;74(12):3135–41.
76. Zachariah B, Zachariah SB, Varghese R, et al. Carcinomatous meningitis: clinical manifestations and management. Int J Clin Pharmacol Ther. 1995;33(1):7–12.

77. Tetef ML, Margolin KA, Doroshow JH, et al. Pharmacokinetics and toxicity of high-dose intravenous methotrexate in the treatment of leptomeningeal carcinomatosis. Cancer Chemother Pharmacol. 2000;46(1):19–26.
78. Friedman HS. Temozolomide in early stages of newly diagnosed malignant glioma and neoplastic meningitis. Semin Oncol. 2000;27(3 Suppl 6):35–40.
79. Raymond E, Izbicka E, Soda H, et al. Activity of temozolomide against human tumor colony-forming units. Clin Cancer Res. 1997;3(10):1769–74.
80. Marzolini C, Decosterd LA, Shen F, et al. Pharmacokinetics of temozolomide in association with fotemustine in malignant melanoma and malignant glioma patients: comparison of oral, intravenous, and hepatic intra-arterial administration. Cancer Chemother Pharmacol. 1998;42(6):433–40.
81. Nayar G, Ejikeme T, Chongsathidkiet P, et al. Leptomeningeal disease: current diagnostic and therapeutic strategies. Oncotarget. 2017;8(42):73312–28. Published 2017 Aug 16. https://doi.org/10.18632/oncotarget.20272.
82. Broniscer A, Chintagumpala M, Fouladi M, Krasin MJ, Kocak M, Bowers DC, Iacono LC, Merchant TE, Stewart CF, Houghton PJ, Kun LE, Ledet D, Gajjar A. Temozolomide after radiotherapy for newly diagnosed high-grade glioma and unfavorable low-grade glioma in children. J Neuro-Oncol. 2006;76:313–9. https://doi.org/10.1007/s11060-005-7409-5.
83. Groves MD. New strategies in the management of leptomeningeal metastases. Arch Neurol. 2010;67:305–12.
84. Giglio P, Tremont-Lukats IW, Groves MD. Response of neoplastic meningitis from solid tumors to oral capecitabine. J Neurooncol. 2003;65(2):167–72.
85. Ekenel M, Hormigo AM, Peak S, DeAngelis LM, Abrey LE. Capecitabine therapy of central nervous system metastases from breast cancer. J Neurooncol. 2007;85(2):223–7.
86. Groves MD, Hess KR, Puduvalli VK, et al. Biomarkers of disease: cerebrospinal fluid vascular endothelial growth factor (VEGF) and stromal cell derived factor (SDF)-1 levels in patients with neoplastic meningitis (NM) due to breast cancer, lung cancer and melanoma. J Neurooncol. 2009;94(2):229–34.
87. Stockhammer G, Poewe WF, Burgstaller SF, et al. Vascular endothelial growth factor in CSF: a biological marker for carcinomatous meningitis. Neurology. 2000;54(8):1670–6.
88. Herrlinger U, Wiendl H, Renninger M, Forschler H, Dichgans J, Weller M. Vascular endothelial growth factor (VEGF) in leptomeningeal metastasis: diagnostic and prognostic value. Br J Cancer. 2004;91(2):219–24.
89. Boogerd W, Dorresteijn LD, van Der S, et al. Response of leptomeningeal metastases from breast cancer to hormonal therapy. Neurology. 2000;55(1):117–9.
90. Lee DW, Lee KH, Kim JW, Keam B. Molecular targeted therapies for the treatment of leptomeningeal carcinomatosis: current evidence and future directions. Int J Mol Sci. 2016;17(Suppl. 7):E1074. https://doi.org/10.3390/ijms17071074.
91. Stemmler HJ, Mengele K, Schmitt M, et al. Intrathecal trastuzumab (Herceptin) and methotrexate for meningeal carcinomatosis in HER2-overexpressing metastatic breast cancer: a case report. Anti-Cancer Drugs. 2008;19(8):832–6. https://doi.org/10.1097/CAD.0b013e32830b58b0.
92. Ferrario C, Davidson A, Bouganim N, Aloyz R, Panasci LC. Intrathecal trastuzumab and thiotepa for leptomeningeal spread of breast cancer. Ann Oncol. 2009;20(4):792–5. https://doi.org/10.1093/annonc/mdp019.
93. Kumthekar P, Gradishar W, Lin N, Pentsova E, Groves M, Jeyapalan S, Melisko M, Grimm S, Lassman A, Raizer J. CMET-22. Intrathecal (IT) Trastuzumab (T) for the treatment of leptomeningeal metastases (LM) in patients (pts) with human epidermal growth factor receptor 2-positive (HER2 +) cancer: a multicenter phase 1/2 study. Neuro Oncol. 2018;20(Suppl 6):vi58. https://doi.org/10.1093/neuonc/noy148.234.
94. Zagouri F, Sergentanis TN, Bartsch R, Berghoff AS, Chrysikos D, de Azambuja E, Dimopoulos MA, Preusser M. Intrathecal administration of trastuzumab for the treatment of meningeal carcinomatosis in HER2-positive metastatic breast cancer: a systematic review and pooled analysis. Breast Cancer Res Treat. 2013;139(1):13–22. https://doi.org/10.1007/s10549-013-2525-y.

95. Figura NB, Rizk VT, Mohammadi H, Evernden B, Mokhtari S, Yu HM, Robinson TJ, Etame AB, Tran ND, Liu J, Washington I, Diaz R, Czerniecki BJ, Soliman H, Han HS, Sahebjam S, Forsyth PA, Ahmed KA. Clinical outcomes of breast leptomeningeal disease treated with intrathecal trastuzumab, intrathecal chemotherapy, or whole brain radiation therapy. Breast Cancer Res Treat. 2019;127:841–4. https://doi.org/10.1007/s10549-019-05170-7.
96. Bachelot T, Romieu G, Campone M, Diéras V, Cropet C, Dalenc F, et al. Lapatinib plus capecitabine in patients with previously untreated brain metastases from HER2-positive metastatic breast cancer (LANDSCAPE): a single-group phase 2 study. Lancet Oncol. 2013;14:64–71. https://doi.org/10.1016/s1470-2045(12)70432-1.
97. Pivot X, Manikhas A, Zurawski B, et al. CEREBEL (EGF111438): a phase III, randomized, open-label study of lapatinib plus capecitabine versus trastuzumab plus capecitabine in patients with human epidermal growth factor receptor 2-positive metastatic breast cancer. J Clin Oncol. 2015;33:1564–73.
98. Liao B-C, Lee J-H, Lin C-C, et al. Epidermal growth factor receptor tyrosine kinase inhibitors for non–small-cell lung cancer patients with leptomeningeal carcinomatosis. J Thorac Oncol. 2015;10(12):1754–61. https://doi.org/10.1097/jto.0000000000000669.
99. Chen J, Soudy H. Osimertinib in the treatment of leptomeningeal disease in T790M-negative, epidermal growth factor receptor-mutated non-small cell lung cancer: a case report. Chin Clin Oncol. 2019;8(3):29. https://doi.org/10.21037/cco.2019.02.02.
100. Jackman DM, Cioffredi LA, Jacobs L, et al. A phase I trial of high dose gefitinib for patients with leptomeningeal metastases from non-small cell lung cancer. Oncotarget. 2015;6(6):4527–36. https://doi.org/10.18632/oncotarget.2886.
101. Kawamura T, Hata A, Takeshita J. High-dose erlotinib for refractory leptomeningeal metastases after failure of standard-dose EGFR-TKIs. Cancer Chemother Pharmacol. 2015;75:1261–6.
102. Togashi Y, Masago K, Masuda S. Cerebrospinal fluid concentration of gefitinib and erlotinib in patients with non-small cell lung cancer. Cancer Chemother Pharmacol. 2012;70:399–405.
103. Lin CH, Lin MT, Kuo YW, Ho CC. Afatinib combined with cetuximab for lung adenocarcinoma with leptomeningeal carcinomatosis. Lung Cancer. 2014;85(3):479–80. https://doi.org/10.1016/j.lungcan.2014.06.002.
104. Janjigian YY, Smit EF, Groen HJ, et al. Dual inhibition of EGFR with afatinib and cetuximab in kinase inhibitor-resistant EGFR-mutant lung cancer with and without T790M mutations. Cancer Discov. 2014;4(9):1036–45. https://doi.org/10.1158/2159-8290.CD-14-0326.
105. Yang H, Yang X, Zhang Y, Liu X, Deng Q, Zhao M, et al. Erlotinib in combination with pemetrexed/cisplatin for leptomeningeal metastases and cerebrospinal fluid drug concentrations in lung adenocarcinoma patients after gefitinib failure. Target Oncol. 2015;10(1):135–40.
106. Mok TS, Wu YL, Ahn MJ, Garassino MC, Kim HR, Ramalingam SS, Shepherd FA, He Y, Akamatsu H, Theelen WS, et al. Osimertinib or platinum-pemetrexed in EGFR T790M-positive lung cancer. N Engl J Med. 2017;376:629–40.
107. Soria JC, Ohe Y, Vansteenkiste J, Reungwetwattana T, Chewaskulyong B, Lee KH, Dechaphunkul A, Imamura F, Nogami N, Kurata T, et al. Osimertinib in untreated EGFR-mutated advanced non-small-cell lung cancer. N Engl J Med. 2018;378:113–25.
108. Berz D, et al. P2.03b-016 tesevatinib in NSCLC patients with EGFR activating mutations and brain metastases (BM) or leptomeningeal metastases (LM). J Thorac Oncol. 12(1):S942–3.
109. Le Rhun E, Weller M, Brandsma D, Van den Bent M, de Azambuja E, Henriksson R, Boulanger T, Peters S, Watts C, Wick W, Wesseling P, Rudà R, Preusser M, On behalf of the EANO Executive Board and ESMO Guidelines Committee. EANO–ESMO clinical practice guidelines for diagnosis, treatment and follow-up of patients with leptomeningeal metastasis from solid tumours. Ann Oncol. 2017;28(Suppl_4):iv84–99. https://doi.org/10.1093/annonc/mdx221.
110. Costa DB, Kobayashi S, Pandya SS, Yeo WL, Shen Z, Tan W, et al. CSF concentration of the anaplastic lymphoma kinase inhibitor crizotinib. J Clin Oncol. 2011;29(15):e443–5.

111. Facchinetti F, Tiseo M, Di Maio M, et al. Tackling ALK in non-small cell lung cancer: the role of novel inhibitors. Transl Lung Cancer Res. 2016;5(3):301–21. https://doi.org/10.21037/tlcr.2016.06.10.
112. Ou SH, Ahn JS, De Petris L, et al. Alectinib in crizotinib-refractory ALK-rearranged non-small-cell lung cancer: a phase II global study. J Clin Oncol. 2016;34:661–8. https://doi.org/10.1200/JCO.2015.63.9443.
113. Gainor JF, Sherman CA, Willoughby K, et al. Alectinib salvages CNS relapses in ALK-positive lung cancer patients previously treated with crizotinib and ceritinib. J Thorac Oncol. 2015;10(2):232–6. https://doi.org/10.1097/JTO.0000000000000455.
114. Zou HY, Friboulet L, Kodack DP, et al. PF-06463922, an ALK/ROS1 inhibitor, overcomes resistance to first and second generation ALK inhibitors in preclinical models. Cancer Cell. 2015;28(1):70–81. https://doi.org/10.1016/j.ccell.2015.05.010.
115. Foppen M, Geukes H, Brandsma D, Blank CU, van Thienen JV, Haanen JB, Boogerd W. Targeted treatment and immunotherapy in leptomeningeal metastases from melanoma. Ann Oncol. 2016;27(6):1138–42. https://doi.org/10.1093/annonc/mdw134.
116. Schafer N, Scheffler B, Stuplich M, Schaub C, Kebir S, Rehkamper C, et al. Vemurafenib for leptomeningeal melanomatosis. J Clin Oncol. 2013;31:e173–4. https://doi.org/10.1200/JCO.2012.46.5773.
117. Lee JM, Mehta UN, Dsouza LH, Guadagnolo BA, Sanders DL, Kim KB. Long-term stabilization of leptomeningeal disease with whole-brain radiation therapy in a patient with metastatic melanoma treated with vemurafenib: a case report. Melan Res. 2013;23:175–8. https://doi.org/10.1097/CMR.0b013e32835e589c.
118. Sakji-Dupre L, et al. Cerebrospinal fluid concentrations of vemurafenib in patients treated for brain metastatic BRAF-V600 mutated melanoma. Melanoma Res. 2015;25:302–5. https://doi.org/10.1097/CMR.0000000000000162.
119. Wilgenhof S, Neyns B. Complete cytologic remission of V600E BRAF-mutant melanoma-associated leptomeningeal carcinomatosis upon treatment with dabrafenib. J Clin Oncol. 2015;33(28):e109–11. https://doi.org/10.1200/JCO.2013.48.7298.
120. Long GV, Trefzer U, Davies MA, et al. Dabrafenib in patients with Val600Glu or Val600Lys BRAF-mutant melanoma metastatic to the brain (BREAK-MB): a multicentre, open-label, phase 2 trial. Lancet Oncol. 2012;13:1087–95.
121. Simeone E, De Maio E, Sandomenico F, et al. Neoplastic leptomeningitis presenting in a melanoma patient treated with dabrafenib (a V600EBRAF inhibitor): a case report. J Med Case Rep. 2012;6:131. Published 2012 May 17. https://doi.org/10.1186/1752-1947-6-131.
122. Long GV, Stroyakovskiy D, Gogas H, Levchenko E, de Braud F, Larkin J, Garbe C, Jouary T, Hauschild A, Grob JJ, Chiarion-Sileni V, Lebbe C, et al. Overall survival for dabrafenib and trametinib versus dabrafenib and placebo in V600 BRAF-mutant melanoma: a multi-center, double-blind, phase 3 randomised controlled trial. Lancet. 2015;386(9992):444–51.
123. Larkin J, Ascierto PA, Dreno B, Atkinson V, Liszkay G, Maio M, Mandala M, Demidov L, Stroyakovskiy D, Thomas L, de la Cruz-Merino L, Dutriaux C, et al. Combined vemurafenib and cobimetinib in BRAF-mutated melanoma. N Engl J Med. 2014;371:1867–76.
124. Burger MC, Ronellenfitsch MW, Lorenz NI, et al. Dabrafenib in patients with recurrent, BRAF V600E mutated malignant glioma and leptomeningeal disease. Oncol Rep. 2017;38(6):3291–6. https://doi.org/10.3892/or.2017.6013.
125. Thomas KH, Ramirez RA. Leptomeningeal disease and the evolving role of molecular targeted therapy and immunotherapy. Ochsner J. 2017;17(4):362–78.

Chapter 6
Radiation Therapy for Leptomeningeal Disease

Samantha M. Buszek and Caroline Chung

Introduction

Leptomeningeal disease (LMD), also known as neoplastic meningitis, leptomeningeal carcinomatosis, or carcinomatous meningitis, is a rare cancer complication that was first diagnosed in 1870 by Eberth et al. [1]. This condition occurs in approximately 5% of all cancer patients, presenting most commonly in primary diagnoses of breast cancer (41%), lung cancer (24%), gastrointestinal tract malignancies (13%), and melanoma (12%) [2–4]. However, incidence continues to rise with continuous improvements in systemic therapies that allow patients diagnosed with cancer to live longer, as well as improvements in both technology and availability of imaging of the neuroaxis leading to continued increases in diagnosis [3].

LMD can be found incidentally on routine follow-up imaging or present with signs and symptoms of CSF flow obstruction or local invasion of tumor. Ultimately, a high index of suspicion is often required to make an early diagnosis of LMD. Diagnostic studies include imaging of the entire neuroaxis (brain and cervical, thoracic, and lumbar spine) as well as lumbar puncture, performed after imaging to avoid false positives on MRI. Following diagnosis, standard treatments for LMD include neuroaxis directed therapies in addition to optimal systemic therapy for the primary and extra-CNS disease. Radiation therapy (RT) is commonly incorporated as a part of the multimodal approach in the treatment of LMD and has traditionally been recommended for patients with bulky or symptomatic metastatic sites of LMD to provide symptom relief, CSF flow correction, or for debulking of

S. M. Buszek · C. Chung (✉)
Department of Radiation Oncology, University of Texas MD Anderson Cancer Center, Houston, TX, USA
e-mail: cchung3@mdanderson.org

F. C. L. Wong (ed.), *Radiopharmaceuticals in the Management of Leptomeningeal Metastasis*, https://doi.org/10.1007/978-3-031-14291-8_6

disease to facilitate further systemic therapy [4–9]. Several RT techniques have been utilized for the treatment of LMD, including involved-field RT, whole brain RT, and craniospinal irradiation.

Regardless of systemic and local control of the primary disease, prognosis in the setting of LMD is very poor, with reported average survivals of approximately 2–4 months, even with treatment [10–13]. There are currently no standardized guidelines for the treatment of LMD, and many clinicians are hesitant to treat patients with clinically advanced neoplastic meningitis given the high risk of toxicity and unknown value of treatment. Furthermore, in the modern era of immunotherapy, it is unclear if the incidence or prevalence of LMD is increasing.

Indications for Radiotherapy

Radiation therapy (RT) is commonly incorporated as a part of the multimodal approach in the treatment of LMD and has traditionally been recommended for patients with bulky or symptomatic metastatic sites of LMD to provide symptom relief, CSF flow correction, or for debulking of disease to facilitate further systemic therapy [4–9]. The timing, dose, and technique of RT used, however, currently depend on the clinical characteristics of the patient, the location and extent of the LMD, and the clinical judgment of the treating physician. Patients can often be stratified by their risk status to aid in the treatment decision-making process [14].

Good Risk LMD

Patients with LMD can be defined as Good Risk if they have all of the following characteristics: Karnofsky Performance Status (KPS) ≥60, no major neurologic deficits, minimal systemic disease, and if they have a reasonable systemic treatment option should they need them. Patients in this category are typically diagnosed with LMD based on routine imaging and are being evaluated on an outpatient basis. Ultimately, the level of aggressiveness of the treatment provided should include a discussion with the patient and their wishes. Patients with Good Risk LMD may also be treated with palliative and/or best supportive care if they decline more intensive treatment options [14].

RT is typically included in the multimodal treatment of patients with Good Risk LMD. Typical treatment options for this classification include involved-field RT to bulky disease and/or symptomatic sites (e.g. whole brain RT or involved-site RT to the spine), consideration for clinical trials, and/or consideration of systemic therapy with targeted therapies or immune checkpoint inhibitors for special patient populations.

Poor Risk LMD

In contrast to Good Risk LMD, patients with LMD can be defined as Poor Risk if they have any of the following characteristics: KPS <60, multiple, serious, or major neurologic deficits, extensive systemic disease with few treatment options, bulky central nervous system (CNS) disease, or encephalopathy. Some exceptions to these symptoms, where a patient may still be considered for a more aggressive treatment course, include patients with exceptionally chemosensitive tumors (e.g. small cell lung cancer, lymphoma) [14].

Involved-site RT or whole brain RT to symptomatic sites may be used in the treatment of Poor Risk LMD, along with the best supportive care.

Radiotherapy Details and Techniques

The optimal treatment of LMD is multimodal in nature and should be discussed in multidisciplinary setting. Once a treatment regimen is determined, symptomatic patients should be considered for dexamethasone treatment to improve their symptoms in the acute setting, along with any further therapies. A single patient may be considered for any of the following RT techniques, either simultaneously, or in sequence, depending on the patient's clinical presentation, cancer histology, and natural history of cancer-related events. Once the timing of RT has been established in concordance with systemic or intrathecal treatment options, the patient may be prepared for their course of RT. It is important to note that symptomatic sites may not have radiographic correlation; however, localized RT to the suspected site of disease in these patients is reasonable (e.g. RT to lumbosacral spine in a patient with progressive cauda equine syndrome). General palliative dosing regimens of 30 Gy in 10 fractions, 20 Gy in 5 fractions, or 8 Gy in 1 fraction are appropriate.

Involved-Field Radiotherapy

The term involved-field RT (IFRT) comes from the lymphoma radiation oncology literature and describes the fields' progression of shrinking their RT field from all lymph node regions (total lymphoid RT) to the involved lymph node regions (IFRT). IFRT specifically involves treating the involved area of disease, along with the surrounding field (e.g. involved lymph node and that lymph node region); however, in the treatment of LMD, the term IFRT refers to treating the area of known or suspected disease, with margin to ensure full treatment of the area thought to be causing symptoms. Therefore, IFRT in the treatment of LMD involves treating one spinal vertebral body up and down from the visualized disease. Other terms used to describe this technique include focal spine RT and localized spine RT (Fig. 6.1).

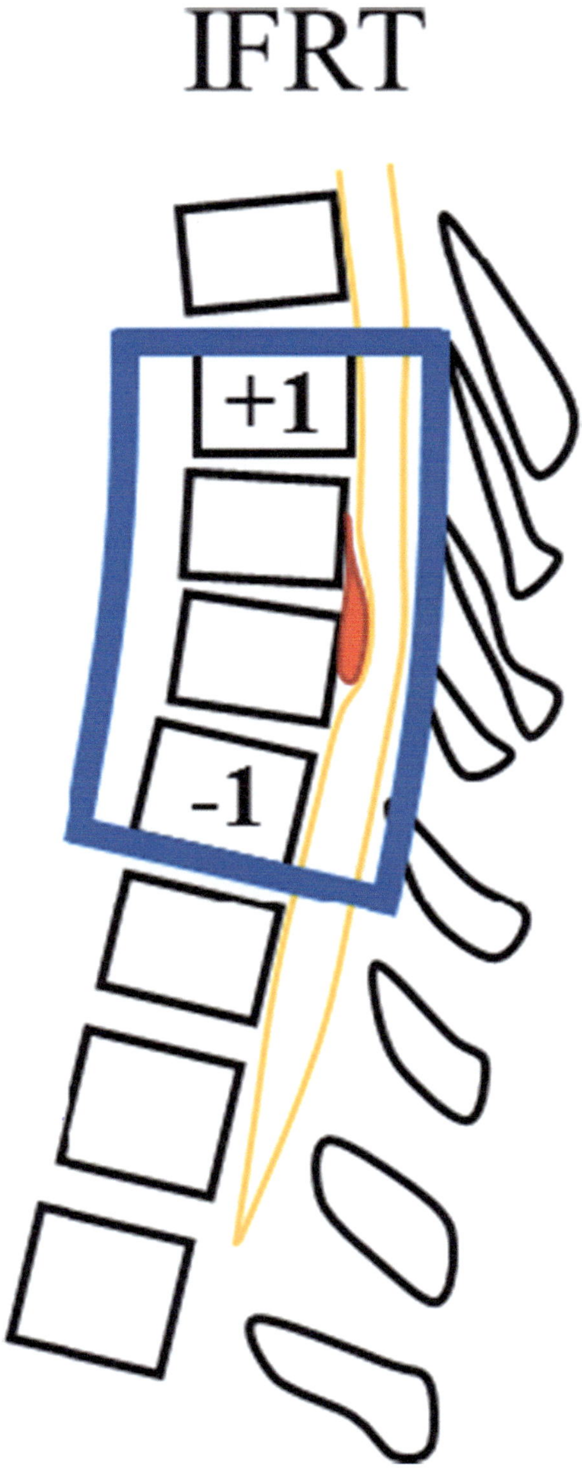

Fig. 6.1 Involved-field radiotherapy. Example radiation treatment field encompassing one vertebral body up and down from bulky LMD seen on imaging

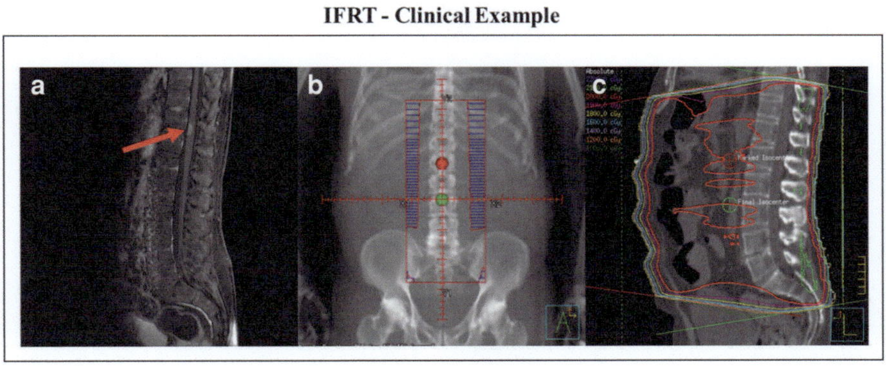

Fig. 6.2 Involved-field radiotherapy clinical example. (**a**) Sagittal view of T1-post gadolinium enhanced MRI of the thoracic and lumbar spine with arrow indicating area of intramedullary metastatic disease at T11. (**b**) Anterior–posterior IFRT field and block drawn to encompass T10 through the sacrum. (**c**) Sagittal view of radiation isodose lines

For the majority of LMD histologies, IFRT is preferred over craniospinal irradiation (CSI) to avoid excess myelosuppression and other toxicities such as fatigue, diarrhea, nausea, vomiting, and esophagitis.

In cases of cauda equina syndrome, which involves the compression of spinal nerve roots causing progressive leg pain and saddle anesthesia prior to the development of bowel and/or bladder incontinence, the entire lumbosacral region may be targeted with RT.

Clinical Vignette A middle-aged male with a history of nasopharynx cancer presented to the emergency center with a lower extremity fracture from a fall and decreased sensation in his bilateral groin, thighs, and buttocks, as well as progressive urinary incontinence for the past 3 weeks. MRI of his spine revealed multiple enhancing lesions along the surface of his thoracic and lumbar spinal cord, as well as along his cauda equina, representing leptomeningeal metastases, with an intramedullary lesion at T11 (Fig. 6.2). The patient was classified as poor risk LMD given his extensive systemic disease and progressive neurologic symptoms and was treated with palliative IFRT to his spine (T10 through the sacrum) with 20 Gy in 5 fractions. The patient reported improvement in sensation of his thighs and buttocks and was discharged to hospice care with a Foley catheter.

Whole Brain Radiotherapy

Whole brain radiotherapy (WBRT) is used to treat patients with focal or disseminated collections of LMD (Fig. 6.3) causing hydrocephalus or isolated cranial neuropathies. The use of WBRT in patients with LMD has been shown to have a potential survival benefit, especially if the patient has other parenchymal brain metastases [15, 16]. Patients are typically treated with 30 Gy in 10 fractions to the

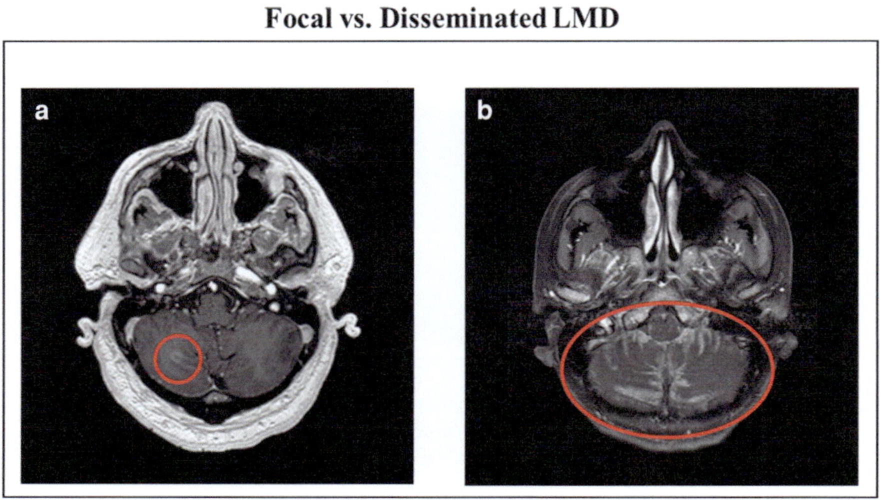

Fig. 6.3 Focal vs. disseminated LMD. (**a**) Focal LMD of the cerebellum. (**b**) Disseminated LMD of the cerebellum. Both cases were treated with WBRT

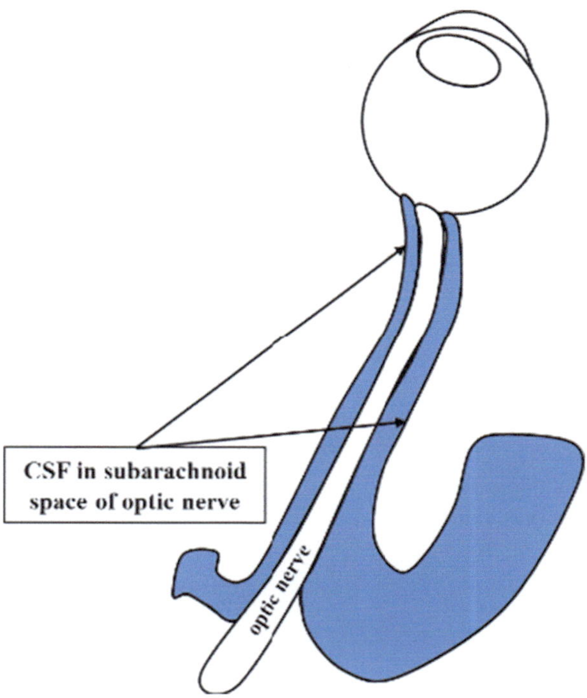

Fig. 6.4 Cerebral fluid in subarachnoid space of optic nerve. (Image modified from Killer, Jaggi [17])

entire brain, with margin to ensure coverage of all locations of cerebral spinal fluid (CSF). This includes extension of the field to incorporate the first two cervical vertebral bodies, as well as the back portion of the orbits to ensure full coverage of the subarachnoid space of the optic nerve, which contains CSF (Fig. 6.4) [17].

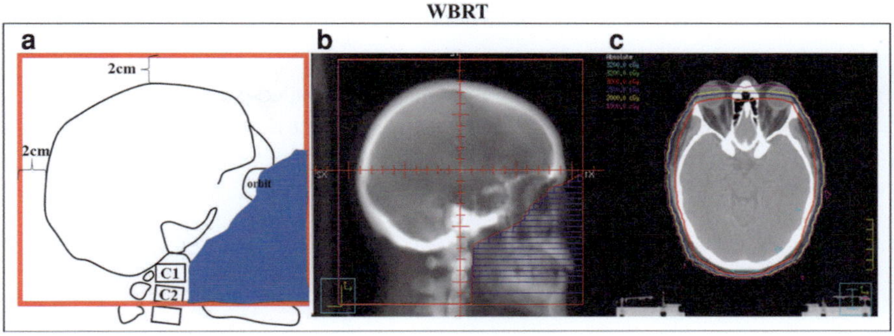

Fig. 6.5 Whole brain radiation field. (**a**) Schematic of WBRT field. (**b**) Sagittal view of WBRT field and blocks. (**c**) Axial view of WBRT isodose lines to include the back of the orbits. In the treatment of LMD, the RT field traditionally includes the first two cervical vertebral bodies and flashes the back of the orbits

WBRT is performed using two opposed lateral beams. A block is created to expose the back of the orbit, cribriform plate, and the first two cervical vertebral bodies. The edges of the beam are placed 2 cm from the skull edge to ensure adequate coverage of the brain (Fig. 6.5).

Craniospinal Irradiation

Craniospinal Irradiation (CSI) is a technique used to treat the entire craniospinal axis with radiation. It has a high rate of success in the treatments of a few specific primary CNS diseases (e.g. medulloblastoma and germinoma) but is much less commonly used in the treatment of LMD given the risk of toxicity (e.g. myelosuppression preventing further systemic therapy, severe fatigue, diarrhea, nausea, esophagitis, etc.) associated with this treatment, except in a few specific histologies [11, 18–20]. CSI involves a technically complex set-up of one to two spine RT fields, depending on the height of the patient, matched with a whole brain field with the goal of treating the entire craniospinal axis in a homogenous fashion. This technique can be performed with the patient in the prone or supine position and can be delivered with photon or proton RT. Detailed explanations of each technique have been previously published [11, 21–24]. To reduce toxicity from this technique, clinicians should consider the use of intensity-modulated radiotherapy (IMRT) or protons.

CSI may be considered in patients with breast cancer, leukemia, or lymphoma primary histologies, as an alternative to high-dose methotrexate.

Special Histologic Considerations

A systematic review for the use of RT in LMD that included patients of any age with a diagnosis of LMD who had RT as a part of their treatment regimen was recently published with treatment recommendations separated by primary histologic subtypes of cancer. The following findings were adapted from Buszek et al. [25].

Mixed Histologies

A total of 19 studies reported on patients with LMD from a mix of histologies [6, 11, 15, 26–41]. Eighteen of these studies were observational in nature and included patients with breast ($n = 375$), melanoma ($n = 68$), lung ($n = 469$), bladder ($n = 2$), prostate ($n = 1$), ovarian ($n = 3$), solid tumors not otherwise specified (NOS; $n = 59$), gastrointestinal NOS ($n = 12$), colon ($n = 2$), gastric ($n = 12$), kidney ($n = 2$), adult brain tumors ($n = 51$), unknown primary ($n = 69$), leukemia/lymphoma ($n = 111$), and pediatric brain tumors ($n = 6$). The median age of these patients ranged from 13 to 65 years. Patients were treated with any combination of whole brain radiotherapy (WBRT), craniospinal irradiation (CSI), focal brain RT (FBRT; fractionated or stereotactic radiosurgery [SRS]), focal spine radiotherapy (FSRT), intrathecal chemotherapy (ITC), intraventricular radioisotope, systemic chemotherapy (C), and best supportive care (BSC). Reported OS for the cohorts ranged from 1.4 to 10 months. Additionally, Coakham et al. reported their use of I-131 radiolabeled monoclonal antibodies to treat neoplastic meningitis in pediatric and adult patients between 1984 and 1993 and reported a mean survival of 39 months in therapy responders and 4 months in non-responders [39]. They concluded that these results are sufficiently encouraging to stimulate further attempts at cerebrospinal fluid therapy with I-131 monoclonal antibodies; however, this is very little reported use of this technique in the treatment of LMD in the literature since that time. Overall, the included studies involving mixed histologies leading to LMD reported a variety of conclusions, with an overall consensus that any treatment had a lower risk of death than supportive care alone. Patients who were able to complete a course of WBRT lived longer, and those who received combined modality treatment had the longest survival.

A National Cancer Database (NCDB) analysis reported the results of patients treated for LMD from any histology from 2005 to 2014. Patients were diagnosed with lung cancer ($n = 334$), breast cancer ($n = 96$), GI cancer NOS ($n = 39$), leukemia/lymphoma ($n = 19$), and unknown primary ($n = 3$). Of the cohort, 52 patients were treated with RT alone, 88 patients were treated with RT + C, 232 patients were treated with C alone, and 147 patients were treated with the BSC. Of the patient's that received RT, 85% were treated with WBRT, 14% with focal brain RT (FBRT), and 1% with WBRT and focal spine RT (FSRT). Median OS for the entire cohort was 3 months (2.7–3.3 months). Treated patients exhibited a higher median OS compared to BSC and patients treated with C + RT revealed the highest median OS of 5 months (3.5–6.5 months) followed by patients treated with RT alone who had a median OS of 3 months (1.7–4.3 months). The authors concluded that patients with LMD have poor outcomes overall, but those who had a good performance status and normal CSF levels had a more favorable prognosis upon active treatment [42].

Breast Cancer

Nine studies included patients with a primary histology of breast cancer [43–52]. Of these, seven studies were observational studies, and a single study reported the results of guideline recommendations, and a randomized controlled trial. The observational studies included a total of 764 patients treated with RT for LMD in sample sizes ranging from 8 to 187 per study. These patients were treated from 1986 to 2015 and ranged in age from 23 to 80 years. Patients were treated with WBRT ($n = 243$), FSRT ($n = 47$), C ($n = 220$), ITC ($n = 434$), or BSC ($n = 20$), with multiple patients receiving combinations of these treatments; however, exact numbers were not reported. The OS for patients treated in these studies ranged from 3.8 to 7.5 months. Longer survival was associated with hormone receptor positive tumors, limited prior therapy for systemic disease, and LMD as the site of first metastasis, with mixed conclusions on the impact of improvement when RT is added to C/ITC. A positive correlation was noted between improved quality of life and treatment with RT in the single study that evaluated this endpoint [48]. Any treatment was associated with longer survival when compared to BSC alone. Interestingly, a high burden of disease at the time of LMD diagnosis was not found to be associated with worse survival [51]. Overall, studies supported inclusion of RT as a part of the multimodality treatment approach in LMD of breast cancer.

Boogerd et al. published a randomized controlled trial to determine the relevance of ITC for LMD in breast cancer [52]. Patients were randomized to ITC ($n = 17$) or non-ITC treatment ($n = 18$). Appropriate systemic therapy and RT were given in each group (35% of patients in the ITC arm received focal RT and 2 patients received WBRT; 50% of patients in the non-ITC arm received focal RT, and 4 received WBRT). The authors found that standard systemic chemotherapy with focal RT for LMD is feasible. The addition of ITC did not lead to a survival benefit or improved neurological response and was associated with an increased risk of neurotoxicity.

Pediatric Central Nervous System Disease

Three observational studies included pediatric patients with central nervous system (CNS) disease [53–55]. These series evaluated 34 patients (ages 1–34) treated from 1977 to 2012 with diagnoses of astrocytoma ($n = 6$), medulloblastoma ($n = 9$), ependymoma ($n = 3$), ATRT ($n = 4$), PNET ($n = 3$), and other ($n = 9$). Patients received treatment for their LMD with FSRT (*n* = 28), CSI (*n* = 6), and FBRT (*n* = 6). The median OS was not reached in two studies. In patients with astrocytoma receiving FSRT, the median OS was 7 months. In patients with either medulloblastoma, ependymoma, PNET, or other treated with FSRT, the 12 month OS was 68%; patients with PNET had a median OS of 9.2 months. For patients with primary CNS disease, NOS, the mean OS was 25.7 months with salvage CSI. The authors concluded that RT in the treatment of LMD is beneficial with minimal toxicity.

Gastrointestinal Cancer

Seven observational studies incorporated patients with gastrointestinal (GI) malignancies and LMD [56–62]. These studies included 127 patients treated from 1944 to 2010 with the diagnoses of gastric cancer (*n* = 99), esophageal cancer (*n* = 7), and GI NOS (*n* = 21). Patients were treated with RT alone NOS (*n* = 30), WBRT (*n* = 19), FSRT (*n* = 1), ITC (*n* = 15), RT + ITC (*n* = 48), C (*n* = 8), RT + C (*n* = 3), or BSC (*n* = 7). The median OS ranged from 1 to 3 months. The authors concluded that ITC improved survival on multivariate analysis and cytological negative conversion was predictive of a relatively longer survival.

Adult CNS Gliomas

Seven observational studies incorporated patients with LMD from adult gliomas [63–69]. These studies incorporated 101 patients treated between 1978 and 2015, with diagnoses of glioblastoma (GBM, *n* = 77), World Health Organization (WHO) grade II glioma (*n* = 1), WHO grade III astrocytoma (*n* = 14), and oligodendrogliomas (*n* = 7). Patients were treated with FBRT (*n* = 5), BSC (*n* = 5), C (*n* = 16), C + CSI (*n* = 4), C + FBRT+FSRT (*n* = 3), C + FBRT (*n* = 2), C+ whole spine RT (*n* = 1), and surgical resection (*n* = 2). The median OS from the diagnosis of LMD ranged from 2.8 to 10.2 months, with 32 months for oligodendrogliomas NOS. The series that included non-GBMs reported longer survival outcomes. The authors concluded that patients treated with a combination of C + RT had significantly prolonged survival compared to either therapy alone or the BSC. Patients with no symptoms from LMD and better performance status at presentation had longer survival with no difference in outcomes between patients with large volume versus small volume LMD disease.

Non-small Cell Lung Cancer

A total of eight observational studies of 893 patients treated from 1986 to 2014 for LMD from non-small cell lung cancer were included [16, 70–76]. Patients were treated with WBRT (*n* = 389), FSRT (*n* = 10), C (*n* = 39), targeted therapy (TT;

$n = 278$), ITC ($n = 7$), or BSC ($n = 31$). Overall survival ranged from 3 to 8.7 months for all patients. There were conflicting findings on whether WBRT or tyrosine-kinase inhibitors (TKIs) improved survival for patients; survival was improved for selected patients who received ITC. Similar to other histologies, patients with good performance status at the time of LMD diagnosis had better outcomes.

Melanoma

Three observational studies reviewed patients with a diagnosis of LMD from melanoma [77–79]. These authors reviewed 140 patients treated from 1944 to 2015 with FSRT ($n = 26$), FBRT ($n = 2$), WBRT ($n = 42$), FSRT + FBRT ($n = 9$), C ($n = 54$), immunotherapy ($n = 8$), ITC, ($n = 53$), and surgical resection ($n = 3$). The median OS ranged from 2.3 to 5.2 months with the longest survival seen in the most modern series that included immunotherapy [78]. The authors concluded that survival is improved with the introduction of anti-PD-1 antibodies and BRAF inhibitors and that multimodality therapy combined with these new techniques may be required to obtain the best control of neurologic symptoms and improve survival.

Leukemia/Lymphoma

Two observational series included patients with leukemia or lymphoma [80, 81]. A total of 47 patients were treated between 1988 and 2016 with diagnoses of chronic lymphocytic leukemia (CLL; $n = 3$) and diffuse large B-cell lymphoma (DLBCL; $n = 44$). Patients were treated with FBRT ($n = 4$), WBRT ($n = 42$), and CSI ($n = 1$). The three patients with CLL had an OS of 8 months, 3 months, and still alive at censorship at 6 months. The median OS of the patients with DLBCL was 7 months. The authors concluded that patients with CLL and LMD involvement of their optic nerve had improved survival with focal RT and that RT provides high response rates in DLBCL and can contribute to long-term disease free survival.

Gynecologic Cancer

Two observational studies included patients with gynecologic cancer leading to a diagnosis of LMD [82, 83]. These studies included 15 patients treated between 1996 and 2010 with diagnoses of ovarian cancer ($n = 12$) and cervical/endometrial cancer ($n = 3$). Patients were treated with WBRT ($n = 8$), FBRT ($n = 1$), FSRT ($n = 5$), C ($n = 1$), and BSC ($n = 1$). The median overall survival was 3.6 months for patients with ovarian cancer, and 2, 4, and 7 months for the three patients with cervical/endometrial cancer. The authors concluded that RT can provide a partial or complete response to LMD, although with recurrence likely.

Esthesioneuroblastoma

One observational study included patients with esthesioneuroblastoma [84]. In this study, Chamberlain et al. included four patients ranging in age from 47 to 58 years treated in 2002 with FSRT (n = 2), WBRT (n = 3), and C (n = 4). The patients had OS of 4, 11, 12, and 13 months, respectively. The authors concluded that LMD from esthesioneuroblastoma is treatable with acceptable toxicity.

Pediatric Rhabdomyosarcoma

One observational series included patients with rhabdomyosarcoma and LMD [85]. The authors included 13 pediatric patients with LMD (age from 1 to 34 years) treated from 1999 to 2016 with FBRT (n = 1), WBRT (n = 5), CSI (n = 10), C (n = 4), surgery (n = 2). The median OS was 5 months and the authors concluded that treatment with CNS directed RT should be considered; however, outcomes were poor.

Treatment Related Toxicities

The use of RT in the treatment of LMD may be associated with both acute and long term toxicities; although these are sometimes difficult to differentiate from the effects of other aspects of therapy, or from the disease itself. In the treatment of LMD, where RT doses are palliative, the treatments are generally very well tolerated with mild transient acute toxicities.

Involved-Field Radiation Therapy

When IFRT is used in the treatment of LMD, the patient may only experience side effects in the treatment field, meaning the location of the spine where the radiation was delivered. The potential acute and long term toxicities are dependent on the length of the cord irradiated, the fraction size of RT, and the addition of systemic or intrathecal chemotherapy. Additionally, possible acute toxicities are dependent on which portion of the spine receives RT.

In the acute setting, if the cervical spine is irradiated, the patient may experience transient esophagitis, sore throat, or neck stiffness; if the thoracic spine is irradiated, the patient may experience transient esophagitis or possibly radiation pneumonitis (occurs 1–3 months following RT); if the lumbar spine is irradiated, the patient may experience transient diarrhea; and if the sacrum is irradiated, the patient may experience transient diarrhea or increased bladder frequency with possible pain with urination.

Rare, but potential long term toxicities of radiation to the spinal canal include radiation-induced myelopathy. Transient radiation-induced myelopathy, although rare with an incidence of 4–14% in patients treated for head and neck cancer (these patients receive a much higher RT dose than that given for LMD), may develop 2–6 months following spinal irradiation. This side effect, known as Lhermitte's Sign, typically presents as an electric shock-like sensation in the spine and extremities, exacerbated by neck flexion. It is caused by reversible demyelination of ascending sensory neurons following RT of the cervical or thoracic spine and is unlikely to occur with the dose regimens recommended for the treatment of LMD [86–89].

Whole Brain Radiation Therapy

The possible acute side effects from radiation to the brain may include: fatigue, hair loss, transient and self-limited neurologic deterioration, and headaches. In the long term, patients treated with WBRT may experience neuroendocrine sequelae such as hypothyroidism and disturbances in the secretion of growth hormone, memory difficulty, personality changes, or secondary malignancies. These symptoms, however, are much more common in patients who receive higher doses of RT than typically given for WBRT.

Craniospinal Irradiation

As previously mentioned, CSI may cause significant myelosuppression from the volume of active bone marrow that is irradiated with this technique [20]. Additionally, depending on the patient set-up (supine versus prone) and the RT technique utilized (2D, 3D, IMRT, or protons), the patient may experience additional gastrointestinal side effects, such as nausea, vomiting, diarrhea, and esophagitis.

Furthermore, the possible acute and long-term side effects of WBRT also apply to patients who are treated with CSI, as this technique includes a WBRT field. Therefore, patients may also exhibit fatigue, neuroendocrine sequelae, neuropsychological sequelae, and secondary malignancies; however, given the natural history of disease of LMD and the median overall survival of months, the majority of patients will not experience any long-term side effects from these treatments.

Conclusions

LMD is an important and devastating complication of cancer that leads to significant morbidity and mortality. Since its initial discovery in the 1800s, the incidence of this condition has continued to increase as our methods of diagnosis continue to improve and numerous cancer histologies are seeing longer disease free intervals and survival in the modern era of targeted therapy. The optimal management of this condition remains unknown, with limited data to guide standard of care treatment.

Traditionally, radiotherapy has been recommended for patients with bulky metastatic disease, regardless of clinical symptoms, or for sites of disease causing symptoms [4–9]. In our own clinical experience, radiotherapy for the treatment of LMD is consistently considered and discussed in the multidisciplinary setting. The treatment of RT is often recommended for patients with bulky disease seen on imaging or causing symptoms to prevent further neurologic compromise, or for asymptomatic patients with LMD seen on brain MRI who have well-controlled extracranial disease.

Three main techniques of RT can be considered for patients with LMD, including IFRT, WBRT, and CSI. The choice of a single technique or combination of techniques should be decided based upon the patient's risk status and the location of their symptoms/imaging findings.

References

1. Eberth. Zur Entwicklung des Epitheliomas (Cholesteatomas) dur Pia under der Lungs. Virchows Arch. 1870;49:51–63.
2. Fauci AS, Braunwald E, Kasper DL, et al. Harrison's principles of internal medicine. 17th ed. McGraw Hill; 2008.
3. Nugent JL, et al. CNS metastases in small cell bronchogenic carcinoma: increasing frequency and changing pattern with lengthening survival. Cancer. 1979;44(5):1885–93.
4. Shapiro WR, et al. Treatment of meningeal neoplasms. Cancer Treat Rep. 1977;61(4):733–43.
5. Theodore WH, Gendelman S. Meningeal carcinomatosis. Arch Neurol. 1981;38(11):696–9.
6. Wasserstrom WR, Glass JP, Posner JB. Diagnosis and treatment of leptomeningeal metastases from solid tumors: experience with 90 patients. Cancer. 1982;49(4):759–72.
7. Chamberlain MC. Leptomeningeal metastases: a review of evaluation and treatment. J Neurooncol. 1998;37(3):271–84.
8. Kaplan JG, et al. Leptomeningeal metastases: comparison of clinical features and laboratory data of solid tumors, lymphomas and leukemias. J Neurooncol. 1990;9(3):225–9.
9. Olson ME, Chernik NL, Posner JB. Infiltration of the leptomeninges by systemic cancer. A clinical and pathologic study. Arch Neurol. 1974;30(2):122–37.
10. Chamberlain MC, et al. Diagnostic tools for neoplastic meningitis: detecting disease, identifying patient risk, and determining benefit of treatment. Semin Oncol. 2009;36(4 Suppl 2):S35–45.
11. Hermann B, Hultenschmidt B, Sautter-Bihl ML. Radiotherapy of the neuroaxis for palliative treatment of leptomeningeal carcinomatosis. Strahlenther Onkol. 2001;177(4):195–9.
12. Hitchins RN, et al. A prospective randomized trial of single-agent versus combination chemotherapy in meningeal carcinomatosis. J Clin Oncol. 1987;5(10):1655–62.
13. Waki F, et al. Prognostic factors and clinical outcomes in patients with leptomeningeal metastasis from solid tumors. J Neurooncol. 2009;93(2):205–12.
14. Network, N.C.C. Central nervous system cancers. 2019. [cited 2019 7/9/2019]. https://www.nccn.org/professionals/physician_gls/pdf/cns.pdf.
15. Brower JV, et al. Management of leptomeningeal metastases: prognostic factors and associated outcomes. J Clin Neurosci. 2016;27:130–7.
16. Ozdemir Y, Yildirim BA, Topkan E. Whole brain radiotherapy in management of non-small-cell lung carcinoma associated leptomeningeal carcinomatosis: evaluation of prognostic factors. J Neurooncol. 2016;129(2):329–35.

17. Killer HE, et al. Cerebrospinal fluid dynamics between the intracranial and the subarachnoid space of the optic nerve. Is it always bidirectional? Brain. 2007;130(Pt 2):514–20.
18. Schiopu SR, et al. Craniospinal irradiation using helical tomotherapy for central nervous system tumors. J Radiat Res. 2017;58(2):238–46.
19. Tsang DS, et al. Craniospinal irradiation for treatment of metastatic pediatric low-grade glioma. J Neurooncol. 2017;134(2):317–24.
20. Kumar N, et al. Impact of acute hematological toxicity on treatment interruptions during cranio-spinal irradiation in medulloblastoma: a tertiary care institute experience. J Neurooncol. 2017;134(2):309–15.
21. Zong-Wen S, et al. Radiotherapy for adult medulloblastoma: evaluation of helical tomotherapy, volumetric intensity modulated arc therapy, and three-dimensional conformal radiotherapy and the results of helical tomotherapy therapy. Biomed Res Int. 2018;2018:9153496.
22. Wang K, et al. Plan quality and robustness in field junction region for craniospinal irradiation with VMAT. Phys Med. 2018;48:21–6.
23. Seravalli E, et al. Dosimetric comparison of five different techniques for craniospinal irradiation across 15 European centers: analysis on behalf of the SIOP-E-BTG (radiotherapy working group)(). Acta Oncol. 2018;57(9):1240–9.
24. Farace P, et al. Supine craniospinal irradiation in pediatric patients by proton pencil beam scanning. Radiother Oncol. 2017;123(1):112–8.
25. Buszek S, Chung C. Radiotherapy in leptomeningeal disease: a systematic review of randomized and non-randomized trials. Front Oncol. 2019;9:1224. https://doi.org/10.3389/fonc.2019.01224.
26. Passarin MG, et al. Leptomeningeal metastasis from solid tumors: a diagnostic and therapeutic challenge. Neurol Sci. 2015;36(1):117–23.
27. Gani C, et al. Outcome after whole brain radiotherapy alone in intracranial leptomeningeal carcinomatosis from solid tumors. Strahlenther Onkol. 2012;188(2):148–53.
28. Clarke JL, et al. Leptomeningeal metastases in the MRI era. Neurology. 2010;74(18):1449–54.
29. Oechsle K, et al. Prognostic factors and treatment options in patients with leptomeningeal metastases of different primary tumors: a retrospective analysis. J Cancer Res Clin Oncol. 2010;136(11):1729–35.
30. Kwon J, et al. Impact of multimodality approach for patients with leptomeningeal metastases from solid tumors. J Korean Med Sci. 2014;29(8):1094–101.
31. Sause WT, et al. Whole brain irradiation and intrathecal methotrexate in the treatment of solid tumor leptomeningeal metastases—a Southwest Oncology Group study. J Neurooncol. 1988;6(2):107–12.
32. Chamberlain MC, Kormanik PA. Prognostic significance of coexistent bulky metastatic central nervous system disease in patients with leptomeningeal metastases. Arch Neurol. 1997;54(11):1364–8.
33. Herrlinger U, et al. Leptomeningeal metastasis: survival and prognostic factors in 155 patients. J Neurol Sci. 2004;223(2):167–78.
34. Chamberlain MC, Kormanik PA. Prognostic significance of 111indium-DTPA CSF flow studies in leptomeningeal metastases. Neurology. 1996;46(6):1674–7.
35. Sakaguchi M, et al. Patient outcomes of whole brain radiotherapy for brain metastases versus leptomeningeal metastases: a retrospective study. Asia Pac J Clin Oncol. 2017;13(5):e449–57.
36. Pan Z, et al. Concurrent radiotherapy and intrathecal methotrexate for treating leptomeningeal metastasis from solid tumors with adverse prognostic factors: a prospective and single-arm study. Int J Cancer. 2016;139(8):1864–72.
37. Bokstein F, Lossos A, Siegal T. Leptomeningeal metastases from solid tumors: a comparison of two prospective series treated with and without intra-cerebrospinal fluid chemotherapy. Cancer. 1998;82(9):1756–63.
38. Wolf A, et al. Stereotactic radiosurgery for focal leptomeningeal disease in patients with brain metastases. J Neurooncol. 2017;134(1):139–43.
39. Coakham HB, Kemshead JT. Treatment of neoplastic meningitis by targeted radiation using (131)I-radiolabelled monoclonal antibodies. Results of responses and long term follow-up in 40 patients. J Neurooncol. 1998;38(2–3):225–32.

40. Du C, et al. Leptomeningeal metastasis from solid tumors: a single center experience in Chinese patients. J Neurooncol. 2013;115(2):285–91.
41. Chamberlain MC. Pediatric leptomeningeal metastases: outcome following combined therapy. J Child Neurol. 1997;12(1):53–9.
42. Hyun JW, et al. Leptomeningeal metastasis: clinical experience of 519 cases. Eur J Cancer. 2016;56:107–14.
43. Feyer P, et al. DEGRO practical guidelines for palliative radiotherapy of breast cancer patients: brain metastases and leptomeningeal carcinomatosis. Strahlenther Onkol. 2010;186(2):63–9.
44. Chamberlain MC, Kormanik PR. Carcinomatous meningitis secondary to breast cancer: predictors of response to combined modality therapy. J Neurooncol. 1997;35(1):55–64.
45. Kingston B, et al. Treatment and prognosis of leptomeningeal disease secondary to metastatic breast cancer: a single-centre experience. Breast. 2017;36:54–9.
46. Le Rhun E, et al. Prolonged survival of patients with breast cancer-related leptomeningeal metastases. Anticancer Res. 2013;33(5):2057–63.
47. Le Rhun E, et al. A retrospective case series of 103 consecutive patients with leptomeningeal metastasis and breast cancer. J Neurooncol. 2013;113(1):83–92.
48. Niwinska A, Rudnicka H, Murawska M. Breast cancer leptomeningeal metastasis: the results of combined treatment and the comparison of methotrexate and liposomal cytarabine as intra-cerebrospinal fluid chemotherapy. Clin Breast Cancer. 2015;15(1):66–72.
49. Niwinska A, et al. Determinants of prolonged survival for breast cancer patient groups with leptomeningeal metastasis (LM). J Neurooncol. 2018;138(1):191–8.
50. Yu H, et al. Meningeal carcinomatosis in patients with breast cancer: report of 8 patients. Breast Cancer. 2001;8(1):74–8.
51. Yust-Katz S, et al. Breast cancer and leptomeningeal disease (LMD): hormone receptor status influences time to development of LMD and survival from LMD diagnosis. J Neurooncol. 2013;114(2):229–35.
52. Boogerd W, et al. The relevance of intraventricular chemotherapy for leptomeningeal metastasis in breast cancer: a randomised study. Eur J Cancer. 2004;40(18):2726–33.
53. Kandt RS, et al. Cerebrospinal metastases in malignant childhood astrocytomas. J Neurooncol. 1984;2(2):123–8.
54. Ray GL, et al. Definitive treatment of leptomeningeal spinal metastases in children. Pediatr Blood Cancer. 2013;60(11):1839–41.
55. Wei RL, et al. Salvage craniospinal irradiation with an intensity modulated radiotherapy technique for patients with disseminated neuraxis disease. Pract Radiat Oncol. 2012;2(4):e69–75.
56. Giglio P, et al. Neoplastic meningitis in patients with adenocarcinoma of the gastrointestinal tract. Cancer. 2005;103(11):2355–62.
57. Kim M. Intracranial involvement by metastatic advanced gastric carcinoma. J Neurooncol. 1999;43(1):59–62.
58. Lee JL, et al. Leptomeningeal carcinomatosis in gastric cancer. J Neurooncol. 2004;66(1–2):167–74.
59. Tomita H, et al. Leptomeningeal carcinomatosis associated with gastric cancer. Int J Clin Oncol. 2012;17(4):361–6.
60. Kim NH, et al. Leptomeningeal carcinomatosis from gastric cancer: single institute retrospective analysis of 9 cases. Ann Surg Treat Res. 2014;86(1):16–21.
61. Oh SY, et al. Gastric leptomeningeal carcinomatosis: multi-center retrospective analysis of 54 cases. World J Gastroenterol. 2009;15(40):5086–90.
62. Lukas RV, et al. Leptomeningeal carcinomatosis in esophageal cancer: a case series and systematic review of the literature. Dis Esophagus. 2015;28(8):772–81.
63. Cohen ZR, et al. Intractable vomiting from glioblastoma metastatic to the fourth ventricle: three case studies. Neuro Oncol. 2002;4(2):129–33.
64. Mandel JJ, et al. Leptomeningeal dissemination in glioblastoma; an inspection of risk factors, treatment, and outcomes at a single institution. J Neurooncol. 2014;120(3):597–605.

65. Vertosick FT Jr, Selker RG. Brain stem and spinal metastases of supratentorial glioblastoma multiforme: a clinical series. Neurosurgery. 1990;27(4):516–21; discussion 521–2.
66. Burger MC, et al. Addition of anti-angiogenetic therapy with bevacizumab to chemo- and radiotherapy for leptomeningeal metastases in primary brain tumors. PLoS One. 2016;11(6):e0155315.
67. Dardis C, et al. Leptomeningeal metastases in high-grade adult glioma: development, diagnosis, management, and outcomes in a series of 34 patients. Front Neurol. 2014;5:220.
68. Endo H, et al. Leptomeningeal dissemination of cerebellar malignant astrocytomas. J Neurooncol. 2003;63(2):191–9.
69. Roldan G, et al. Leptomeningeal disease in oligodendroglial tumors: a population-based study. J Neurooncol. 2011;104(3):811–5.
70. Morris PG, et al. Leptomeningeal metastasis from non-small cell lung cancer: survival and the impact of whole brain radiotherapy. J Thorac Oncol. 2012;7(2):382–5.
71. Kuiper JL, et al. Treatment and survival of patients with EGFR-mutated non-small cell lung cancer and leptomeningeal metastasis: a retrospective cohort analysis. Lung Cancer. 2015;89(3):255–61.
72. Lee SJ, et al. Leptomeningeal carcinomatosis in non-small-cell lung cancer patients: impact on survival and correlated prognostic factors. J Thorac Oncol. 2013;8(2):185–91.
73. Liao BC, et al. Epidermal growth factor receptor tyrosine kinase inhibitors for non-small-cell lung cancer patients with leptomeningeal carcinomatosis. J Thorac Oncol. 2015;10(12):1754–61.
74. Chamberlain MC, Kormanik P. Carcinoma meningitis secondary to non-small cell lung cancer: combined modality therapy. Arch Neurol. 1998;55(4):506–12.
75. Xu Q, et al. Treatment and prognostic analysis of patients with leptomeningeal metastases from non-small cell lung cancer. Thorac Cancer. 2015;6(4):407–12.
76. Li YS, et al. Leptomeningeal metastases in patients with NSCLC with EGFR mutations. J Thorac Oncol. 2016;11(11):1962–9.
77. Chamberlain M, Kormanik P. Leptomeningeal metastases due to melanoma. Int J Oncol. 1996;9(3):505–10.
78. Arasaratnam M, et al. Leptomeningeal melanoma-a case series in the era of modern systemic therapy. Pigment Cell Melanoma Res. 2018;31(1):120–4.
79. Harstad L, Hess KR, Groves MD. Prognostic factors and outcomes in patients with leptomeningeal melanomatosis. Neuro Oncol. 2008;10(6):1010–8.
80. Currie JN, et al. Optic neuropathy in chronic lymphocytic leukemia. Arch Ophthalmol. 1988;106(5):654–60.
81. Milgrom SA, et al. Radiation therapy as an effective salvage strategy for secondary CNS lymphoma. Int J Radiat Oncol Biol Phys. 2018;100(5):1146–54.
82. Teckie S, et al. Radiation therapy for epithelial ovarian cancer brain metastases: clinical outcomes and predictors of survival. Radiat Oncol. 2013;8:36.
83. Asensio N, et al. Meningeal carcinomatosis and uterine carcinoma: three different clinical settings and review of the literature. Int J Gynecol Cancer. 2009;19(1):168–72.
84. Chamberlain MC. Treatment of intracranial metastatic esthesioneuroblastoma. Cancer. 2002;95(2):243–8.
85. De B, et al. Central nervous system relapse of rhabdomyosarcoma. Pediatr Blood Cancer. 2018;65(1):e26710.
86. Jones A. Transient radiation myelopathy (with reference to Lhermitte's sign of electrical paraesthesia). Br J Radiol. 1964;37:727–44.
87. Lim DC, et al. Lhermitte's sign developing after IMRT for head and neck cancer. Int J Otolaryngol. 2010;2010:907960.
88. St Clair WH, et al. Spinal cord and peripheral nerve injury: current management and investigations. Semin Radiat Oncol. 2003;13(3):322–32.
89. Leung WM, et al. Lhermitte's sign among nasopharyngeal cancer patients after radiotherapy. Head Neck. 2005;27(3):187–94.

Chapter 7
Neurophysiology Evaluation in Leptomengeal Metastasis Disease

Sudhakar Tummula

Introduction

Various neurophysiological tests are available to assess the central nervous and peripheral nervous system. Most of these include application of stimulus along the known sensory or motor neural pathways and recording multiple potentials as stimulus travels in a predictable manner. The recorded potentials are summated responses and compared to normal values. Potentials are generally measured with regard to the latency (time from stimulus to the response at a given site), interpotential latency, and amplitude of the responses. For therapeutic applications tests could assess toxicity (prolongation of latency or decrease in amplitude). Having a baseline before intervention would be a reliable patient's own control to follow. It is to be recognized that reliable baseline responses (waveforms) might be absent in cancer patients. This could be due to the location of patient's cancer including LMD or iatrogenic toxicity. For example, spinal cord tumor or radiation sequale to the spinal cord could result in inadequate recording of ascending sensory signals along the posterior columns—SSEP or inadequate recording of descending motor signals along the corticospinal pathways—TMS. Neurotoxicty from prior chemotherapy (peripheral neuropathy) and radiation (plexopathy) could result in poor or absent baseline responses. Underlying medical conditions like diabetes, nutritional deficiencies, degenerative spine disease could also affect the signals. These clinical aspects need to be taken into consideration as leptomeningeal dissemination of cancer is generally a late manifestation in patients battle with cancer. There is a good possibility of inability to obtain baseline responses. Experienced neurophysiology team is recommended in achieving good baselines, maintaining the same standards

S. Tummula (✉)
University of Texas M. D. Anderson Cancer Center, Houston, TX, USA
e-mail: stummala@mdanderson.org

F. C. L. Wong (ed.), *Radiopharmaceuticals in the Management of Leptomeningeal Metastasis*, https://doi.org/10.1007/978-3-031-14291-8_7

and testing methodology for repetitive assessments following initial treatment, repeated dosing, or dose escalation. Few tests geared towards spinal cord function like SSEP and TMS could be useful for intrathecal treatments either given via lumbar puncture or via ommaya. No established publications exist in application of these methodologies in leptomeningeal disease management. However, these methodologies are widely used in cancer patients, during surgical resection of cranial and spinal cord tumors and metastais [1]. These tests are also used in suspected neurotoxicity from chemotherapy [2], other neurotoxic disorders [3], and other conditions that cause leptomeningeal pathology like infectious meiningitis [4]. We feel these tests are applicable when treatments are undertaken for leptomeningeal disease given there could be underlying spinal cord dysfunction, central or peripheral neural pathway dysfunction if reliable signals were present at baseline. Changes in baseline responses obtained in a given patient could be from progression of leptomeningeal disease or neurotoxicity resulting from intrathecal treatment. SSEP examples in our experience are shared in Figs. 7.1 and 7.2. SSEP and TMS investigate central pathways, BAER (brain stem auditory evoked pathways) and VEP (visual evoked pathways) measure the respective auditory and visual pathways. Neurotoxicity is broadly characterized into demyelinating and axonal. Demyelinating pathology is generally reversible resulting in responses with prolonged latency.

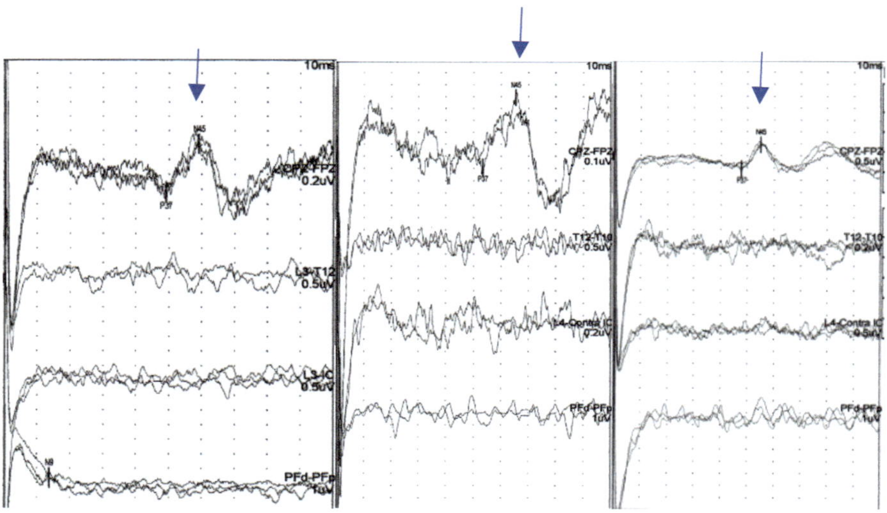

Fig. 7.1 Left Tibial SSEP responses obtained at baseline (left) and sequentialy every 3 weeks (middle and right) after intrathecal therapy via lumbar puncture for LMD. P37/N45 responses (arrow) at baseline seen at 48/59 ms improved to 47/55 ms 6 weeks after treatment corresponding to clinical improvement. Findings are reassuring for lack of immediate iatrogenicity

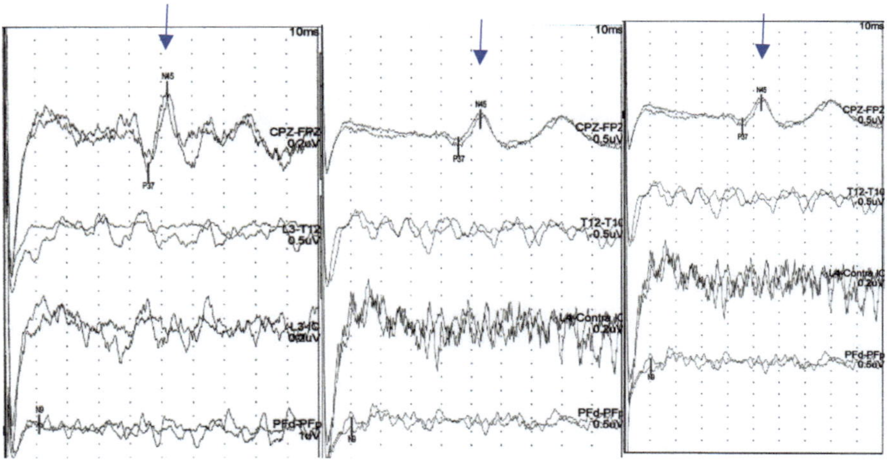

Fig. 7.2 Right Tibial responses show similar improvement of the P37/N45 responses. Baseline responses were seen at 46/52 ms (first arrow), improving to 45.6/53 ms (third arrow) at 6 weeks

Axonal pathology could result in irreversible injury with responses that are low in amplitude or none.

Various methods will be briefly described. Test or combination of tests [5] could be chosen based on the most affected tumor site or anticipated injury from treatment, and available resources. As leptomeningeal disease treatments are given intrathecally, spinal cord evaluation with SSEP & TMS could be most useful [6]. In patients with predominant involvement of cranial nerves from leptomeningeal diseases, VEP, BAER, routine audiological assessment, ophthalmological evaluation could be considered in tandem. Neurophysiological testing when available is noninvasive and generally tolerable making them applicable for baseline testing and sequential assessments after treatment.

EEG (electroencephalogram) has been widely used in cancer patients to help in the diagnosis and management of seizures. Leptomeningeal metastasis with or without intraparenchymal tumor metastasis could result in seizures and cerebral dysfunction [4]. EEG abnormalities include background slowing, focal slowing, epileptiform discharges, or frank electrographic seizures that do not have clinical correlates like tonic or clonic body movements. Altered mental status in leptomeningeal disease patients including after therapeutic intervention would require evaluation with EEG. Leptomeningeal disease can increase intracranial pressure due to alteration in CSF flow (poor absorption or blockage). The ensuing CSF plateau waves result in transient patient unresponsivess and could be confused with seizures [7, 8]. EEG could be helpful with nonspecific but characteristic delta slowing (Figs. 7.3, 7.4, and 7.5).

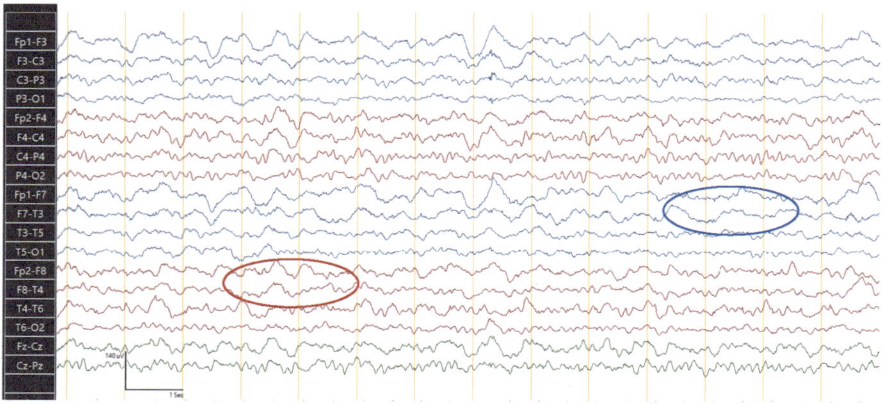

Fig. 7.3 EEG—Frontal and temporal region paroxysmal delta, left (blue temporal area) more prominent than right (red temporal area) opening pressure-26, WBC-247/μL; protein-65 mg/dL, glucose-46 mg/dL, cytology— + malignant cells, MRI—extensive LMD, no intracranial lesions

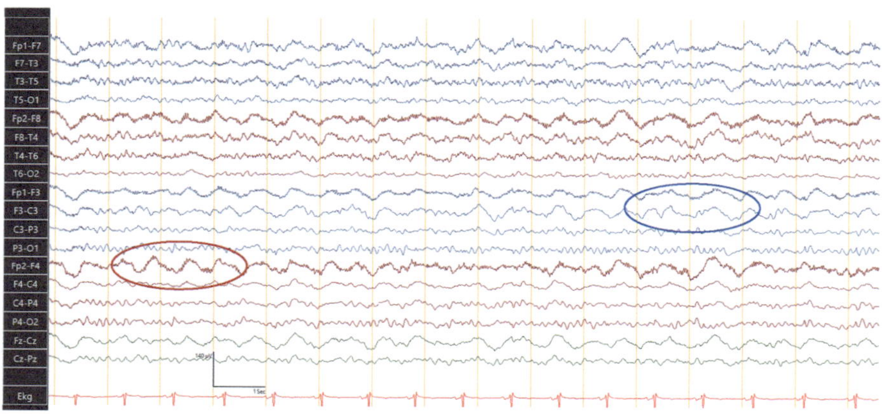

Fig. 7.4 EEG: Patient following commands and oriented. Background is normal with frontal paronxysmal delta activity. Opening pressure from ommaya reservoir—46, WBC-24/μL, protein 24 mg/dL, cytology— + malignant cells. MRI—extensive LMD

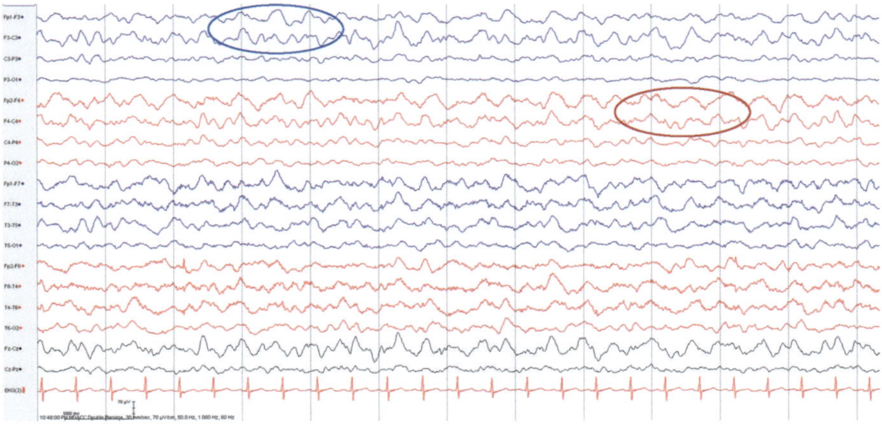

Fig. 7.5 EEG—Frontal region shows paroxysmal delta paroxysmal delta, left (blue frontal area), right (red frontal area) known brain metastasis, stable. ICP 25

Evoked Potentials (SSEP, BAER, VEP, TMS)

Potential	Stimulus site	Recording	Obligatory major responses	Measured useful responses	Comments
SSEP upper extremity	Median or ulnar nerve	Erb's point, cervical spine, cortical	N9, N11/N13, N20/P25	Latency ±, interwave latency, amplitude	Useful for cervical spine and brain stem monitoring
SSEP lower extremity	Tibial nerve	Popliteal fossa, lumbar spine, cervical spine, cortical	LP, P31/N34, P37/N45	Latency, interwave latency, ± amplitude	Useful for entire spine and brain stem monitoring
BAER	EAR	Mastoid and cortical	Wave I, II, III, V	Latency, interwave latency amplitude	Useful for auditory pathways
VEP	EYE	Occipital cortex	P 100	Latency and amplitude. Inter eye latency	Useful for visual pathways
TMS	Cortical—Motor homunculus	Hand, leg, and foot	Motor responses	Latency	Useful for descending motor pathways

EMG, NCS: These tests are useful for peripheral nerve and plexus evaluation. Routine chemoneurotoxicity includes peripheral neuropathy. If leptomeningeal treament is given along with systemic chemotherapy these tests could be useful to assess tandem neurotoxicity. Peripheral neuropathy can result in abnormal SSEP responses as well. Late nerve conduction responses like H waves that include reflex arc within the spinal cord could have some utility in spinal cord evaluation. Obtaining nerve conductions like SSEP at baseline will be patient's own control which could be followed over time to assess neurotoxicity.

References

1. Park J, Cho YE, Park M, Lee J, Kim D, Park YG. Correlation between preoperative somatosensory evoked potentials and intraoperative neurophysiological monitoring in spinal cord tumors. J Clin Monit Comput. 2020;35:979–99. https://doi.org/10.1007/s10877-020.
2. Palomar García V, Abdulghani Martínez F, Bodet Agustí E, Andreu Mencía L, Palomar Asenjo V. Drug-induced ototoxicity: current status. Acta Otolaryngol. 2001;121(5):569–72.
3. Aminoff M, Albers J. Electrophysiological techniques in the evaluation of patients with suspected neurotoxic disorders. In: Aminoff's electrodiagnosis in clinical neurology. 6th ed. Elsevier Inc.
4. Arulprakash S, Verma SP, Bhardwaj VK, Mishra SS, Chansoria M. Brain stem auditory evoked responses and visual evoked responses in children with tubercular meningitis. Indian Pediatr. 2006;43(7):631–4.
5. Rivera Lara L, Püttgen HA. Multimodality monitoring in the neurocritical care unit. Continuum (Minneap Minn). 2018;24(6):1776–88.
6. Kobayashi M, Pascual-Leone A. Transcranial magnetic stimulation in neurology. Lancet Neurol. 2003;2(3):145–56.
7. Zima LA, Tulpule S, Samson K, Shonka N. Seizure prevalence, contributing factors, and prognostic factors in patients with leptomeningeal disease. J Neurol Sci. 2019;403:19–23. https://doi.org/10.1016/j.jns.2019.05.032.
8. Gold CA, Odom N, Srinivasan S, Schaff L, Haggiagi A, Odia Y. Electrographic correlates of plateau waves in patients with leptomeningeal metastases. Neurohospitalist. 2016;6(4):161–6.

Chapter 8
Radionuclide Leptomeningeal Metastasis Therapy Trials

Franklin C. L. Wong

Introduction: Rationale for Intrathecal Radionuclide Therapy Trials (Table 8.1)

It has been demonstrated that intraventricular injection of chemotherapy would result in higher rate of complete response (88% versus 33%) and lower rate of relapse (0% versus 50%) and more long-term disease-free survivors (33% versus 8%) when compared with lumbar injection in patients treated for actual lymphoblastic leukemia [1]. Since Ommaya reservoir and similar devices allow repeated direct access to ventricles after initial percutaneous injection into the reservoir, the intraventricular approach has been used in most of radionuclide LM therapy trials.

Currently, In-111 DTPA is the only FDA-approved radiopharmaceutical for intrathecal application [2]. Multiple other radiopharmaceuticals have been studied via intrathecal injection in humans [3–19] as in Table 8.1. Most of them can be used at low dose for diagnostic purposes and perhaps at high doses for therapy. Important concerns would be efficacy and potential toxicity. These concerns can be guided by reliable and accurate radiation dosimetry, either derived from simulation or derived from nuclear imaging. The following radiopharmaceuticals have been formally studied and published in the literature.

F. C. L. Wong (✉)
Department of Nuclear Medicine, University of Texas M. D. Anderson Cancer Center, Houston, TX, USA
e-mail: fwong@mdanderson.org

F. C. L. Wong (ed.), *Radiopharmaceuticals in the Management of Leptomeningeal Metastasis*, https://doi.org/10.1007/978-3-031-14291-8_8

Table 8.1 Intrathecal radiopharmaceuticals for diagnosis and therapy

Intrathecal radiopharmaceutical	Radionuclide	Tp1/2 (hr)	Molecular class	Radiation emission(s)	Detection	Source
Nonspecific solution:						
In-111 DTPA **(FDA approval)**	In-111	67.2	Chelate	Electrons, photons	Gamma camera/SPECT	Grossman [2]
In-111 EDTA	In-111	67.2	Chelate	Electrons, photons	Gamma camera	Goodwin [3]
In-111 transferrin	In-111	67.2	Protein	Electrons, photons	Gamma camera	Goodwin [3]
Tc99m DTPA	Tc99m	6.0	Chelate	Photons	Gamma camera	Larson [6]
Tc99m pertechnetate	Tc99m	6.0	Anion	Photons	Gamma camera	Lette [4]
Yb-169 DTPA	Yb-169	768.6	Chelate	Photons	Gamma camera	Hosain [5]
I-125 iododeoxyuridine (IUDR)	I-125	1425.6	Nucleoside	Electrons	Radioactivity count	Rebischung [7]
I-131 Sodium iodide (NaI)	I-131	193.7	Anion	Electrons, photons	Radioactivity count	de Rougemont [8]
I-131 Sodium iodide (NaI)	I-131	193.7	Anion	Electrons, photons	Gamma camera	Wong [9]
I-131 Human serum albumin	I-131	193.7	Protein	Electrons, photons	Gamma camera	Di Chiro [10]
Ga-67 citrate	Ga-67	78.3	Cation	Electrons, photons	Gamma camera	Wong (2022) (Chap. 4, Fig. 4.8)
Ga-68 EDTA	Ga-68	1.1	Chelate	Positron, photons	PET	Bergstran [11]
Co-55 DTPA	Co-55	17.5	Chelate	Positron, photons	PET	Maziere [12]
Cu-64 DOTA	Cu-64	12.7	Chelate	Positron, photons	PET	Freesmeyer [13]
Nonspecific Colloids:						
P-32 chromic phosphate	P-32	343.2	Microparticles	Electrons		Muriel [14]
Au-198 colloid	Au-198	64.8	Microparticles	Electrons	Gamma camera	Metz [15]
Specific Radiolabeled MoAb:						
HMFG1/2, UJ181.4, F811.13, FD32	I-131	193.7	Protein	Electrons, photons	Gamma camera	Lashford [16]
I-131 Mel 14	I-131	193.7	Protein	Electrons, photons	Gamma camera	Bigner [17]
I-131 81C6	I-131	193.7	Protein	Electrons, photons	Gamma camera	Bigner [17]
I-131 3F8	I-131	193.7	Protein	Electrons, photons	Gamma camera	Kramer [34]
I-124 3F8	I-124	100.8	Protein	Positrons, photons	PET	Kramer [34]
I-131 Omburtamab	I-131	193.7	Protein	Electrons, photons	Gamma camera	Pandit-Taska [19]
I-124 Omburtamab	I-124	100.8	protein	Positron, photons	PET	Pandit-Taska [19]
Lu-177 DTPA-Omburtamab	Lu-177	159.6	protein	Electrons, photons	Gamma camera/SPECT	Wong (2022) (this chapter)

P-32 Chromic Phosphate Colloids

An earlier trial was reported from Argentina using P-32 chromic phosphate colloids (3 mCi/dose) injected intrathecally via lumbar puncture for prophylaxis of 16 patients with leukemia [14]. These patients had achieved CSF remission (CSF cytology conversion to negative) from prior treatment. Comparison was made with 16 patients receiving methotrexate and dexamethasone preventive treatment and with historical control without preventive treatment. Repeated intrathecal doses in 2 weeks, then 4 weeks, and then every 6 weeks were administered (Table 8.2). The resulting median progression free survival (CSF cytology positive from malignant cell) was comparable (360, 550, and 102 days, respectively) for those treated with P-32 and those treated with methotrexate plus dexamethasone versus the historic control without preventive treatment (Table 8.3). Severe unexpected adverse effects of cauda equina syndrome in 3/16 patients, headache, back pain, and bacterial meningitis were reported.

There were other earlier P-32 studies in abstracts reporting observations of low acute or chronic toxicities and adherence of the colloids in the spinal and posterior fossa [20]. Phase 2 studies using P-32 colloids reported temporary shrinkage of tumor after intratumoral injection into solid tumors but there was no persistent tumor control [21]. P-32 chromic phosphate was removed from the US market in 2009 but is available for compounding in colloid/microaggregate suspensions and was used in US locoregional cancer therapy trials [22].

Table 8.2 Published intrathecal radiopharmaceutical therapy trials

Intrathecal radiopharmaceuticals	Primary target	Goal	Cancer	Max mCi	Mass (mg)	Interval (weeks)	Cycles	Source
Nonspecific Colloids:								
P-32 chromic phosphate	CSF + meninges	Prophylaxis	Leukemia	3	0.30[a]	2, 4 then 6	4 – 8	Muriel [14]
Au-198 colloid	CSF + meninges	Prophylaxis	Leukemia	1.5–5.4	0.015 – 0.05[b]	Single-dose	1	Metz [15]
Small molecules:								
I-125 iododeoxyuridine (IUDR)	Thymidine kinase	Treatment	Pancreatic	50	0.0088[c]	Single-dose	1	Rebischung [7]
Specific radiolabeled MoAb:								
I-131 HMFG1/2, UJ181.4, F811.13	Mucin/brain	Treatment	Multiple#	11 – 45	2.5 – 10.0	Single-dose	1	Lashford [16]
I-131 Mel 14	Melanoma	Treatment	Melanoma+	42 – 80	10.5 – 20.0	Single-dose	1	Bigner [17]
I-131 81C6	Tenascin	Treatment	Glioma+	20 –100	4.0 – 20.0	Single-dose	1	Bigner [17]
I-131 3F8	GD2	Treatment	Medulloblastoma	10	2.0	1	4	Kramer [34]
I-124 3F8	GD2	Dosimetry	Medulloblastoma	2.0	2.0	Single-dose	1	Kramer [34]
I-131 Omburtamab (8H9)	B7-H3	Treatment	Neuroblastoma	34 – 80	1.0 – 1.6	Single-dose	1	Pandit-Taska [19]
I-124 Omburtamab (8H9)	B7-H3	Dosimetry	Neuroblastoma	2.0	1.0	Single-dose	1	Pandit-Taska [19]
Lu-177 -DTPA-Omburtamab	B7-H3	Dosimetry + RX	Medulloblastoma	10.0 – 85.0	1.0 – 8.0	5	2 – 5	Wong (2022) (this chapter)

[a]Based on 10 mCi/mg (Ingrand J 1973)

[b]Based on 100 mCi/mg of MURR supply (Black K 2014)

[c]Based on 74 TBq/mmole of Amersham supply of (Mairs R 2000)

Multiple# tumors: pineablastoma, lymphoma, teratoma, neuroendorcine tumor, Melanoma and ependymoma

GBM+ other glioma, ependymoma and medulloblastoma in children

Table 8.3 Intrathecal radiopharmaceutical trial results

Radiopharmaceutical	*N* (subjects)	Route	Dose (mCi)	Cycles	Clin response*	Median PFS (weeks)	Hematotoxicity	Other toxicity	Source
Nonspecific colloids:									
P-32 chromic phosphate	16	Lumbar	3	4–8	Prophylaxis	51 vs 15 (no rx)	No	archnoditis	Muriel [14]
Au-198 colloid	73	Lumbar	1.5–5.4	1	Prophylaxis	6.8% relapse/8 years	No	3 cauda equina sx	Metz [15]
Small molecules:									
I-125 iododeoxyuridine (IUDR)	1	Ventricular	50	1	1/1	26	No	No	Rebischung [7]
Specific radiolabeled MoAb:									
I-131 HMFG1/2, UJ181.4, F811.13	1 each (5)	Lumbar	11–45	1	4/5	Not recorded	Yes	2/5 pyrexia	Lashford [16]
I-131 Mel 14	10	Ventricular	42–80	1	3/8 CSF	Not recorded	Yes	None	Bigner [17]
I-131 81C6	23	Ventricular	20–100	1	20/28 stable	Not recorded	Yes	None	Bigner [17]
I-131 3F8	42	Ventricular	10	4	10/22 stable	45	No	Chemical menigitis	Kramer [34]
I–124 3F8	42	Ventricular	2.0	1	Dosimetry				Kramer [34]
I-131 Omburtamab	42	Ventricular	34–80	1	Pending analysis	Pending analysis	Pending analysis	Pending analysis	Pandit–Taska [19]
I-124 Omburtamab	42	Ventricular	2.0	1	Dosimetry				Pandit–Taska [19]
Lu-177-DTPA-Omburtamab	2	Ventricular	10.0	2	Pending analysis	Pending analysis	Pending analysis	Pending analysis	This chapter

Au-198 Gold Colloids

A study over 10 years in LM prophylaxis in pediatric leukemia of 73 children in Germany was reported by Metz [15] using injected doses from 1.2 to 4.8 mCi Au-198 colloids (Behringwerke FRG) in volumes of 12–15 mL/m^2 body surface area. The patients were placed in a head low position for 30 min after injection to facilitate transport to the head. The duration to first relapse was not reported but the overall survival (with additional other therapy) was 5 years. For a 3 mCi injection, the CSF dosimetry was estimated at 35 Gy. This Au-198 study did not report severe neurologic adverse reactions although earlier case series using intrathecal Au-198 in similar radioactivity and volume to treat medulloblastoma reported 5/5 cauda equina syndrome [23] and the intrathecal P-32 colloid prophylaxis of LM in leukemia also reported that adverse effect in 3/16 patients [14].

Another study of 77 children with acute leukemia treated with 81 intrathecal injections of Au-198 colloid was conducted in Germany with evaluation of Au-198 retention, radiation dosimetry as well as efficacy for prophylaxis of leptomeningeal metastasis [15]. In another study of 77 pediatric patients with leukemia, Au-198 colloid was injected via lumbar puncture at doses of 1.5–5.4 mCi in volumes of 12–15 mL/m^2 body surface area for prophylaxis after initial CSF remission. Scintigraphic imaging was incorporated to delineate subarachnoid spaces in the cerebrum, cerebellum, and spine areas to report dosimetry [24]. After distribution for 20 h after injection, 36/73 patients with normal distribution of Au-198 demonstrated 52% and 26% of injection dose in the intracranial subarachnoid space (ISS) and spinal subarachnoid space (SSS), respectively. The radiation absorbed doses from intrathecal Au-198 to the ISS and SSS meninges were 1.6 Gy/mCi and 7.0 Gy/mCi, respectively. It was thus estimated that 400 MBq (10.8 mCi) would be required to ablate the SSS meninges with 18 Gy and SSS with 76 Gy, respectively [24]. The outcome data from radionuclide therapy alone was not reported, partly because of other concurrent therapy including methotrexate and dexamethasone. Furthermore, with the reported cauda equina syndromes and the high radiation doses to the spinal subarachnoid space, this approach has not been expanded to the mainstream of LM treatment.

I-125 Iododeoxyuridine (IUDR)

The use of nucleoside carrying a lethal radionuclide incorporated into the DNA of reproducing cell is an attractive means to treat neoplastic disease. A DNA-targeting radiopharmaceutical 5-Iodo-2′-deoxyuridine (IUDR) is a thymidine analog that is efficiently incorporated into the DNA of cycling cells to effect ablation. Upon labeling with I-125 which emits multiple low-energy short-range electrons, I-125 IUDR can deliver lethal radiation for cell killing. However, IUDR is rapidly metabolized in vivo as exemplified by its short effective half-life of 1.6 min in serum for I-131 IUDR [25]. Radiolabeled IUDR is expected to be more effective in treating tumors when delivered locoregionally, such as via intratumoral injection or intrathecal injection. Intratumoral (glioma) injection of I-124 IUDR has found variable extents of pharmacokinetics and metabolism of I-124 IUDR [26]. IUDR also has a fast intrathecal half-life of 28 min [27]. Combination schemes have been designed to use I-125 IUDR together with methotrexate (MTX) which also inhibits IUDR intrathecal metabolism [28].

A single patient case study has been reported with intrathecal injection of I-125 IUDR [7]. This was a patient with pancreatic cancer and brain metastasis treated with systemic therapy, intrathecal methotrexate, and whole brain irradiation who subsequently developed refractory LM by cytology.

After the patient underwent implantation of ventricular catheter (Rickham reservoir) and lumbar catheter and pretreated with thyroid blockade and intrathecal MTX, she received 50 mCi of I-125 IUDR into the Rickham reservoir. No toxicity was reported but she required radiation therapy to the lumbar spine at 26th day after injection of I-125 IUDR effectively rendering a PFS of 26 days (nadir of CA 19.9

level in CSF). CSF relapse was confirmed by CSF cytology on day 152. Multiple therapies before I-125 IUDR injection (including intrathecal MTX) and multiple therapies soon after I-125 IUDR injection including radiation therapy make it difficult to delineate efficacy of the single case study.

Radiolabeled Monoclonal Antibodies

Radiolabeled monoclonal antibodies have been produced against multiple surface antigens on tumor cells since 1980s. Their obvious advantage is the high sensitivity and specificity to target specific tumor antigens. Radiolabeled monoclonal antibodies have been FDA-approved for intravenous injection for cancer diagnosis (for instance, In111-labeled Oncoscint to detect CEA on colorectal cancer [29]) and for cancer therapy (for instance, yttrium-90 Zevalin [30] and I-131 Bexxar [31], both of which target CD 20 on lymphomas). Multiple clinical trials have been conducted with intrathecal injection of radiolabeled monoclonal antibodies to ablate tumor cells in leptomeningeal metastasis. The added advantage of intrathecal injection is that the radiopharmaceutical is in direct contact with tumor cells bathed by the CSF with fewer barriers (compared to iv injection) to harness markedly enhanced payloads with high sensitivity and specificity of monoclonal antibodies.

I-131 MoAb (HMGF1, HMFG2, UJ181.4, F811.13, FD32)

Intrathecal application of radiolabeled monoclonal antibodies has been reported from Bristol, UK with publications reporting clinical findings from collections of single patient study treated with monoclonal antibodies of different specificities, labeled with I-131 [16, 32]. These studies involve intrathecal injection via lumbar puncture. Attempts were made to derive radiation dosimetry from intralumbar injection of I-131 labeled monoclonal antibodies [33]. Among these different radiolabeled monoclonal antibodies, 81C6 (against tenascin in glioma basement membrane) and Mel 14 (against melanoma) have undergone additional development to transition to intraventricular injection. They have been studied in more formal clinical trials in the USA.

I-131 Mel 14 F $(ab')_2$

Radioiodide (I-131)-labeled monoclonal antibody fragment Mel 14 F$(ab')_2$ binds is designed to bind avidly to melanoma and glioma proteoglycan chondroitin sulfate associated proteins. It has less hematotoxicity compared with the whole antibody I-131 Mel 14 [16]. A Phase I study was reported [17] along with intracavitary application on postsurgical cavities to treat melanoma and gliomas.

I-131 81C6

Radioiodide (I-131)-labeled murine monoclonal antibody 81C6 targets polymorphic glycoprotein tenascin that is commonly found in glioma base membrane. Several Phase I studies were conducted to study gliomas by different routes of administration. Along with the intracavitary administration, intraventricular injection was reported [17] with clinical responses but hematotoxicity is the dose-limiting toxicity at doses above 80 mCi.

I-124 and I-131 3F8

A Phase II study of intraventricular I-131-labeled 3F8 has been reported for dosimetry and LM therapy of medulloblastoma patients. This murine antibody targets disaloganglioside GD2, a tumor antigen homogenously distributed on the surface of solid tumors of neuroectodermal origin including medulloblastoma. Dosimetry was derived from I-124 3F8 PET and I-131 3F8 SPECT, radioactivity counting of CSF and of blood sampling [34].

I-124 and I-131 Omburtamab

The same team that conducted the I-124/I-131 3F8 studies also conducts a similar dosimetry/therapy study using I-124 labeled Omburtamab (8H9) for dosimetry and 131 labeled 8H9 for neuroblastoma therapy [19]. The radiolabeled murine antibodies of 8H9 avidly target B7-H3 on cell membranes expressed in selected human solid tumor including neuroblastoma.

Lu-177 DTPA-Omburtamab

A more recent study involves the radionuclide Lu-177 which has favorable diagnostic and characteristic potentials (modest half-life and abundant emissions at medium energy ranges for diagnosis and therapy). There are obvious advantages of using the same radiopharmaceutical at lower dose to perform pretherapy imaging for treatment planning and at high dose for therapy. This first in human scan of Lu-177 DTPA Omburtamab in our institution was acquired over 7 days following intraventricular injection of 5 mCi of Lu-177 DTPA-Omburtamab. Expected biodistribution of the tracer is confirmed, while serial radioactivity counting of regions of interest from outlined area allows calculation of whole-body and organ dosimetry, in imaging schemes similar to those described in Chap. 10. Following confirmation of biodistribution, the therapy was conducted at 10 mCi as the starting dose which would be escalated stepwise to 85 mCi pe protocol (Table 8.1).

Intrathecal Radionuclide Therapy Dosing Scheme (Table 8.2)

Therapeutic radionuclide LM trials since the 1990s mostly use the intraventricular approach, likely because of availability of the Ommaya reservoir and the acceptance of the notion that intraventricular approach provides more comprehensive coverage of the CSF space.

Earlier studies with nonspecific radiocolloids were designed to accomplish prophylaxis after LM was controlled. Relatively low radioactivities and physical mass are required because of high specific activities as in the case of P-32 colloids at 10 mCi/mg [35] and Au-198 colloids at 100 mCi/mg [36]. When specific targets are identified and specific ligands are available, tumor-specific treatment of LM can be also accomplished.

The use of I-125 IUDR also involves high specific activity at 74 TBq/mmol [37]. Although high I-125 radioactivity at 50 mCi was used, the physical mass was 8.8 μg. The higher radioactivity was required based on preclinical studies and likely related to rapid catabolism of IUDR in the spinal fluid and in the general circulation. Most recent radiopharmaceuticals are radiolabeled monoclonal antibodies, which are macromolecules that require high physical mass that could lead to undesirable adverse effects. With better radiochemistry techniques and high radiolabeling yields, lower physical mass is needed in recent trials.

Repeating radiopharmaceutical treatments in cycles following cancer therapeutic schemes allows recovery of vital organs (bone marrow) to achieve higher efficacy.

Efficacy and Toxicity of Intrathecal Radionuclide Therapy (Table 8.3)

Efficacy is difficult to compare for prophylaxis versus treatment. Nevertheless, CSF conversion is a good indicator of treatment, while clinical response could be more subjective and imaging improvement may be less sensitive. Most LM therapeutic trials had some transient improvement but relapse is the rule. CSF conversion is a specific indicator of efficacy but is not sensitive to proof effectiveness. Both efficacy and toxicity are difficult to evaluate in patients with LM because of difficulty to distinguish treatment effects from intervening neurological deterioration versus neurotoxicity. The recent proposal of RANO criteria for LM may be a good starting point for evaluation of LM.

Arachnoiditis and cauda equina syndrome were common toxicity with radiocolloids injections, likely related to pooling of radiocolloid in the thecal sac. Large volume of injectate (up to 15 mL) was required for lumbar injection which has been laterally replaced with intraventricular injection via Ommaya reservoirs. Hematotoxicity is often encountered with radiolabeled monoclonal antibodies, likely related to the prolonged circulation in the general circulation after it leaves the CSF. Such problems can be partly overcome by using smaller physical mass of the protein or overcome by bone marrow stimulating trophic factors.

Radiation Dosimetry as Potential Guidance (Table 8.4)

Recent technologic advances have allowed precise measurement of radioactivity from imaging and therefore translating into radiation absorbed doses. There have been established dosimetry schemes to account for radiation exposure of each organ

Table 8.4 Intrathecal radiopharmaceutical dosimetry results

Median cGy/mCi	I-124 3F8	I-131 3F8	Omburtamab	Omburtamab
Organ/radionuclide	I-124	I-131	I-124	I-131
Adrenals			1.480	
Brain			3.737	
Breasts				
Eyes				
Lens of eyes				
Gallbladder wall			1.702	
LLIWall			1.258	
Small intestine			1.406	
Stomach			2.627	
ULI wall			1.443	
Heart wall			1.369	
Kidneys			1.406	
Liver			5.994	
Lungs			1.258	
Muscle			1.147	
Ovaries				
Pancreas			1.628	
Red marrow			1.110	
Bone surfaces			2.183	
Skin			0.999	
Spleen			2.035	
Testes				
Thymus			1.184	
Thyroid			1.480	
Urin bladder wall			1.258	
Uterus				
Total Body			1.665	
ED			1.739	
EDE			1.961	
Ventricle CSF	31.100	89.200	2.294	1.930
C-Spine CSF			1.665	1.432
T-spine CSF	17.200	19.600		1.635
L-Spine CSF			2.072	2.042
CSF from CSF I-124 count				5.339
CSF from CSF I-131 count		47.900		4.070
CSF by imaging				
Blood from blood I-124 count				0.144
Blood from blood I-131 count		1.600		0.255

from all radioactive sources in order to arrive at accurate and repeatable dosimetry measures such as with the OLINDA 2.0 software. However, radiation sources from the CSF have been less studied than from systemic administration of radionuclides. Such difficulty can be illustrated by the recent studies of intraventricular 3F8 and Omburtamab that are labeled with I-124 and with I-131. Both studies report the median radiation dosimetry as the main parameter. Radiation dosimetry from intrathecal injection was only reported in the CSF and in the blood from dose to radionuclides in 3F8 [34]. Subsequent study of Omburtamab labeled with I-124 and I-131 managed to report on radiation dosimetry of whole-body organs as well as on CSF in the cervical, thoracic, and lumbar spine [19]. This study also compared dosimetry measurement from imaging with those from direct CSF sampling and radioactivity counting of blood and CSF. The conclusion is that imaging can provide a more reliable radiation dosimetry because technical variations in sampling and counting may result in larger standard deviations.

With more precise and perhaps accurate radiation dosimetry estimates, both the efficacy and toxicity may be correlated to serve as reliable indication to contrast and compare different therapy schemes to choose the optimal treatment of LM, the deadly cancer complication.

Conclusions

A review of the published radionuclide LM therapeutic trials has shown trends of favoring the intraventricular approach of injection, unrelenting LM relapse, use of radiopharmaceuticals with and without tumor specificity as well as increasing use of radiation dosimetry for correlation. Advances have been made in each of these areas. Continuing efforts are needed for better radiopharmaceuticals design, imaging scheme, more effective treatment cycles, and more accurate radiation dosimetry.

Acknowledgments The author is a co-principal investigator of MD Anderson Cancer Center protocol 2020-0595 using Lu-177 DTPA-Omburtamab. Sponsoring of Protocol 2020-0595 by Y mabs Inc. for the Lu-177 DTPA-Omburtamab trial (301 trial) is greatly appreciated. The author also thanks Dr. Zsilla Sadighi from MDACC pediatric neurology, the protocol principal investigator for making this protocol possible.

References

1. Iacoangeli M, et al. Intrathecal chemotherapy for treatment of overt meningeal leukemia: comparison between intraventricular and traditional intralumbar route. Ann Oncol. 1995;6(4):377–82.
2. Grossman SA, et al. Cerebrospinal fluid flow abnormalities in patients with neoplastic meningitis. An evaluation using 111indium-DTPA ventriculography. Am J Med. 1982;73(5):641–7.
3. Goodwin DA, et al. Preparation, physiology, and dosimetry of 111 In-labeled radiopharmaceuticals for cisternography. Radiology. 1973;108(1):91–8.

4. Lette J, et al. A reproducible radionuclide procedure for measurement of cerebrospinal fluid shunt flow. Eur J Nucl Med. 1986;12(5–6):240–3.
5. Hosain F, Reba RC, Wagner HN Jr. Ytterbium-169 diethylenetriaminepentaacetic acid complex. A new radiopharmaceutical for brain scanning. Radiology. 1968;91(6):1294. passim.
6. Larson SM, et al. The radionuclide ventriculogram. JAMA. 1973;224(6):853–7.
7. Rebischung C, et al. First human treatment of resistant neoplastic meningitis by intrathecal administration of MTX plus (125)IUdR. Int J Radiat Biol. 2008;84(12):1123–9.
8. de Rougemont J, et al. [Outflow in ventricular peritoneal derivations. Its determination with Na 131-I]. Neurochirurgie. 1970;16(4):307–18.
9. Wong FC, Groves M, Papadopulos N, Conrad C, Meyers C, Kim S, Puduvali V, Hsu S, Kim EE. Toxicity and efficacy profiles of intrathecal injection of I-131 NaI via intraventricular (IVent) or intralumbar (Ilumb) route for leptomeningeal metastases (LM) therapy. J Clin Oncol. 2006;24(18S):70s.
10. Dichiro G, Reames PM, Matthews WB Jr. Risa-ventriculography and risa-cisternography. Neurology. 1964;14:185–91.
11. Bergstrand G, et al. Positron emission tomography with 68Ga-EDTA in the diagnosis and localization of CSF fistulas. J Comput Assist Tomogr. 1982;6(2):320–4.
12. Maziere B, et al. [55Co]- and [64Cu]DTPA: new radiopharmaceuticals for quantitative tomocisternography. Int J Appl Radiat Isot. 1983;34(3):595–601.
13. Freesmeyer M, et al. High-resolution PET cisternography with 64Cu-DOTA for CSF leak detection. Clin Nucl Med. 2019;44(9):735–7.
14. Muriel FS, et al. Remission maintenance therapy for meningeal leukaemia: intrathecal methotrexate and dexamethasone versus intrathecal craniospinal irradiation with a radiocolloid. Br J Haematol. 1976;34(1):119–27.
15. Metz O, Stoll W, Plenert W. Meningosis prophylaxis with intrathecal 198Au-colloid and methotrexate in childhood acute lymphocytic leukemia. Cancer. 1982;49(2):224–8.
16. Lashford LS, et al. A pilot study of 131I monoclonal antibodies in the therapy of leptomeningeal tumors. Cancer. 1988;61(5):857–68.
17. Bigner DD, Brown M, Coleman RE. Phase I studies of treatment of malignant gliomas and neoplastic meningitis with 131I-radiolabeled monoclonal antibodies anti-tenascin 81C6 and anti-chondroitin proteoglycan sulfate Me1-14 F (ab')2–a preliminary report. J Neurooncol. 1995;24(1):109–22.
18. Kramer K, Humm JL, Souweidane MM. Phase I study of targeted radioimmunotherapy for leptomeningeal cancers using intra-Ommaya 131-I-3F8. J Clin Oncol. 2007;25(34):5465–70.
19. Pandit-Taskar N, et al. Biodistribution and dosimetry of intraventricularly administered (124)I-omburtamab in patients with metastatic leptomeningeal tumors. J Nucl Med. 2019;60(12):1794–801.
20. Harbert JC. Intrathecal radiocolloids in meningeal leukemia. In: Harbert JC, Eckelman WC, Neumann RD, editors. Nuclear medicine: diagnosis and therapy. Thieme; 1996. p. 1157–61.
21. Firusian N, Dempke W. An early phase II study of intratumoral P-32 chromic phosphate injection therapy for patients with refractory solid tumors and solitary metastases. Cancer. 1999;85(4):980–7.
22. Halperin E, Fallat M, Bond S, Crew J, et al. Role of 32P-chromic phosphate colloids in the treatment of Askin tumors, Ewing's sarcoma. J Nucl Med. 2012;53:1079.
23. Gold LH, et al. Current status of intrathecal radiogold in the treatment of medulloblastoma. Acta Radiol Ther Phys Biol. 1972;11(4):329–40.
24. Doge H, Hliscs R. Intrathecal therapy with 198Au-colloid for meningosis prophylaxis. Eur J Nucl Med. 1984;9(3):125–8.
25. Tjuvajev JG, et al. Imaging of brain tumor proliferative activity with iodine-131-iododeoxyuridine. J Nucl Med. 1994;35(9):1407–17.
26. Roelcke U, et al. PET imaging drug distribution after intratumoral injection: the case for (124) I-iododeoxyuridine in malignant gliomas. J Nucl Med. 2002;43(11):1444–51.

27. Gutin PH, et al. Perfusion and molecular modification of idoxuridine to alter its cerebrospinal fluid metabolism. J Pharm Sci. 1977;66(9):1338–40.
28. Kassis AI, Dahman BA, Adelstein SJ. In vivo therapy of neoplastic meningitis with methotrexate and 5. Acta Oncol. 2000;39(6):731–7.
29. Abdel-Nabi HH, Doerr RJ. Multicenter clinical trials of monoclonal antibody B72.3-GYK-DTPA 111In (111In-CYT-103; OncoScint CR103) in patients with colorectal carcinoma. Target Diagn Ther. 1992;6:73–88.
30. Wiseman GA, et al. Biodistribution and dosimetry results from a phase III prospectively randomized controlled trial of Zevalin radioimmunotherapy for low-grade, follicular, or transformed B-cell non-Hodgkin's lymphoma. Crit Rev Oncol Hematol. 2001;39(1–2):181–94.
31. Rutar FJ, et al. Feasibility and safety of outpatient Bexxar therapy (tositumomab and iodine I 131 tositumomab) for non-Hodgkin's lymphoma based on radiation doses to family members. Clin Lymphoma. 2001;2(3):164–72.
32. Moseley RP, et al. Carcinomatous meningitis: antibody-guided therapy with I-131 HMFG1. J Neurol Neurosurg Psychiatry. 1991;54(3):260–5.
33. Richardson RB, et al. Dosimetry of intrathecal iodine131 monoclonal antibody in cases of neoplastic meningitis. Eur J Nucl Med. 1990;17(1–2):42–8.
34. Kramer K, et al. A phase II study of radioimmunotherapy with intraventricular (131) I-3F8 for medulloblastoma. Pediatr Blood Cancer. 2018;65(1):e26754.
35. Ingrand J. Characteristics of radio-isotopes for intra-articular therapy. Ann Rheum Dis. 1973;32 Suppl 6(Suppl):3–9.
36. Black KC, et al. Radioactive 198Au-doped nanostructures with different shapes for in vivo analyses of their biodistribution, tumor uptake, and intratumoral distribution. ACS Nano. 2014;8(5):4385–94.
37. Mairs RJ, et al. Comparison of different methods of intracerebral administration of radioiododeoxyuridine for glioma therapy using a rat model. Br J Cancer. 2000;82(1):74–80.

Chapter 9
Simulated Radiation Dosimetry Models After Intraventricular and Intralumbar Injection of Radiopharmaceuticals

Franklin C. L. Wong and Richard B. Sparks

Introduction

Recent advances in nuclear medicine have provided many radiopharmaceuticals for diagnosis and therapy of cancers. Advantages of radiopharmaceuticals include low mass doses and visualization of active drug action, as well as ready customization for various biologic pathways. Increasing number of radiopharmaceuticals are becoming commercially available to diagnose and treat human cancers. The evaluation of both potential efficacy and toxicity of these agents can be enhanced by the determination of the radiation absorbed dose (RAD). After biologic tissues are exposed to a radionuclide emitting alpha, beta, and/or gamma radiations, RAD is defined as the total energy deposited per unit mass from all emissions during the exposure time, which is governed by specific biodistribution, emissions, radiation transport, and the physical half-life of the radionuclide. The standard dosimetric methodologies break the determination of radiation dosimetry into two components: (1) determination of the number of radioactive decays (residence times) that occur in all relevant organs, tissues, and spaces (source organs) and (2) the amount of each emission's energy that is deposited in any organ/tissue/space of interest (target organs). The residence times in any source organ can be estimated by theoretical simulation using assumed biokinetic models to predict the biodistribution (this chapter) or by empirical image-based measurement of radionuclide

F. C. L. Wong (✉)
Department of Nuclear Medicine, University of Texas M. D. Anderson Cancer Center, Houston, TX, USA
e-mail: fwong@mdanderson.org

R. B. Sparks
CDE Dosimetry Service, Inc., Knoxville, TN, USA
e-mail: rsparks@creativedevelopment.com

F. C. L. Wong (ed.), *Radiopharmaceuticals in the Management of Leptomeningeal Metastasis*, https://doi.org/10.1007/978-3-031-14291-8_9

biodistribution over time (Chap. 10). The simulation approach has the inherent limitation of oversimplification and gross approximation of compartments of radionuclide deposition, but can be performed for scenarios where no empirical data are available for a first approximation of radiation exposure. The empirical imaging approach is limited by the spatial resolution of clinical scanners and the temporal limitations of practical clinical data collection. These approaches can be utilized together to obtain a better understanding of absorbed dose in various scenarios.

Dosimetry of some tissues or spaces can be determined using a simplified empirical data collection scheme. For example, absorbed dose estimates within the CSF compartments themselves, utilized for efficacy evaluations, may be estimated using serial CSF sampling alone. Concordance of dosimetry estimates from different approaches would strengthen the confidence of the evaluation and potentially allow for more precise correlations with outcome of LM therapy.

Human cerebrospinal fluid is mostly produced from the choroid plexus in the roof of lateral ventricles. It passes through the third and fourth ventricles to reach the subarachnoid space of the brain and spinal cord and then returns to the systemic circulation through the cristae villi along the parasagittal sinuses [1]. The flow of CSF in the cervical spinal canal consists primarily of bulk flow which is likely propelled by respiration [2] and also through pulsatile flow driven by vascular pulsation during the cardiac cycle [3]. The combination of respiratory and vascular pulsation results in opposite CSF flows in the anterior (cephalic) versus the posterior (caudal) spinal subarachnoid space across the dentate ligament partition [4]. CSF in the cephalid flow joins the rest of the CSF distributed to the convexity to be returned to the general circulation. Small amounts of CSF also directly return to the general circulation from each compartment.

This chapter examines simulation of CSF biokinetics using compartmental models, along with anthropomorphic radiation transport models of the CSF spaces and normal organs, and published dosimetry models for activity reaching the systemic circulation to estimate radiation dosimetry of CSF compartments and vital organs from intrathecal application of radiopharmaceuticals via intraventricular or intralumbar injection. Using a common set of 5-compartment models of CSF compartments with considerations of outflow from the spinal canal to the convexity, along with anthropomorphic radiation transport models, the absorbed doses for the ventricles, spinal cord, and cerebral convexity CSF spaces and the absorbed dose vs. depth for the tissues immediately adjacent to these CSF spaces are determined. Normal organ absorbed dose estimates are determined using radiation transport results from the CSF modeling and biokinetic models for systemic activity from the literature. Results from the 5-compartment model are compared with those of a 4-compartment ICRP-53 model [5, 6] where the spinal CSF is considered as one compartment.

The hypothesis is that biokinetic models will allow for comparison of intrathecal radiopharmaceuticals in terms of their potential efficacy (by evaluation of CSF spaces absorbed doses) as well as potential risk in critical organs including the bone marrow (by evaluation of the normal organ absorbed doses).

Methodology

Radionuclides and Radiopharmaceuticals

A plethora of novel radiopharmaceuticals have been developed for diagnosis and treatment of human cancer. Many are designed for specific biologic pathways such as antigen localization on cancers, while others are used to diagnose blood flow, lymphatic flow, urine flow, or CSF flows. This study examines 14 commercially available radiopharmaceuticals (see Table 9.1) with respect to radiation absorbed doses to normal organs, CSF compartments, and neural tissue immediately surrounding CSF compartments to assess their potential use to treat LM.

It should be noted that most of these radionuclides have photon emissions that can be imaged by PET or SPECT to evaluate the distribution of activity in the body over time. The beta emitter Y-90 can also be detected by SPECT using Bremsstrahlung produced photon emissions or by PET using photons produced via internal pair production. Thus, patient image data could be utilized as a complimentary analysis to refine the theoretic biokinetic models used in this analysis.

Table 9.1 Available radiopharmaceuticals with potential to ablate leptomeningeal metastasis

Radiopharmaceutical	Systemic organ dosimetry source	Radiation emission	Possible detection method
Sm-153 EDTMP	Eary JNM 1993 [8]	Electrons, photons	Gamma camera, SPECT
Ga-66 citrate	ICRP-53 [5, 6]	Positrons, photons	PET
Ga-67 citrate	ICRP-53 [5, 6]	Electrons, photons	Gamma camera, SPECT
Ga-68 citrate	ICRP-53 [5, 6]	Positrons, photons	PET
In-111pentetreotide	Stabin JNM 1997 [9]	Electrons, photons	Gamma camera, SPECT
Tl-201 chloride	ICRP-53 [5, 6]	Electrons, photons	Gamma camera, SPECT
I-123 NaI + thyroid block	ICRP-53 [5, 6]	Electrons, photons	Gamma camera, SPECT
I-124 NaI + thyroid block	ICRP-53 [5, 6]	Positrons, photons	PET
I-125 NaI + thyroid block	ICRP-53 [5, 6]	Electrons, photons	Gamma camera, SPECT
I-131 NaI + thyroid block	ICRP-53 [5, 6]	Electrons, photons	Gamma camera, SPECT
F-18 fluorodeoxyglucose FDG	Hays JNM 2002 [10]	Positrons, photons	PET
Y-90 chloride	ICRP-30 [11]	Electrons	SPECT, PET
Y-90 DTPA	ICRP-53 [5, 6] In111-DTPA	Electrons	SPECT, PET
Y-90 zevalin (Aby)	Zevalin Package Insert 2002 [12]	Electrons	SPECT, PET

Biokinetic Models of CSF and Flow

Residence time estimates in the cranial and spinal CSF spaces are determined using modified kinetics models (5-compartment) for the CSF from ICRP-53 to include cephalid outflow to the convexity as the biokinetic model in illustrated in Fig. 9.1 for intraventricular injection with and without stasis. An alternative model is also investigated using a 4-compartment ICRP-53 scheme as shown in Fig. 9.2. The biokinetic model for intralumbar injection with and without stasis is illustrated in Fig. 9.3. Simulation of stasis is made with increasing CSF outflow biologic half-life to 90 h in ventricular stasis or VS (from compartment V in Fig. 9.3) and in lumbar stasis or LS (from compartment A in Fig. 9.5).

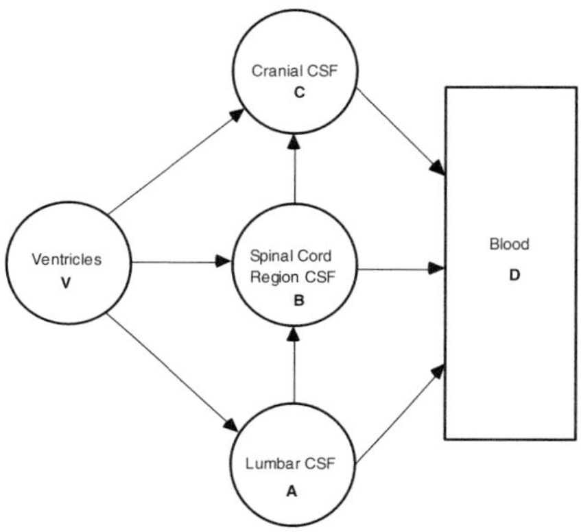

Flow	Fraction of Dose	Biologic Half Time	Associated Fraction
A→B	0.4	20 minutes 8 hours	0.25 0.75
A→D	0.4	8 hours 30 days	0.97 0.03
B→C	0.25	18 hours	1.0
B→D	0.25	18 hours 30 days	0.97 0.03
C→D	0.35	18 hours 30 days	0.97 0.03
V→A	0.8	1 hr	1
V→B	0.1	1 hr	1
V→C	0.1	1 hr	1

Flow in VS	Fractionof Dose	Biologic Half Time	Associated Fraction
A→B	0.5	20 minutes 8 hours	0.25 0.75
A→D	0.5	8 hours 30 days	0.97 0.03
B→C	0.25	18 hours	1.0
B→D	0.25	18 hours 30 days	0.97 0.03
C→D	0.25	18 hours 30 days	0.97 0.03
V→A	0.8	**90 hr**	1
V→B	0.1	**90 hr**	1
V→C	0.1	**90 hr**	1

Fig. 9.1 5-Compartment model for CSF flow of intraventricular injection with and without ventricular stasis (VS)

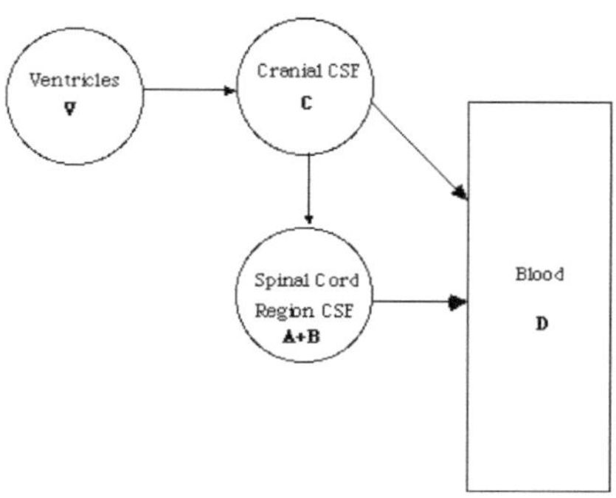

ICRP53 Flow	Fraction of Dose	Biologic Half Time	Associated Fraction
V→C	1.0	1 hour	1.0
C→(A+B)	0.5	18 hours	1.0
C→D	0.5	18 hours 30 days	0.97 0.03
(A+B)→D	1.0	18 hours 30 days	0.97 0.03

Fig. 9.2 4-Compartment ICRP53 CSF flow model after intraventricular injection

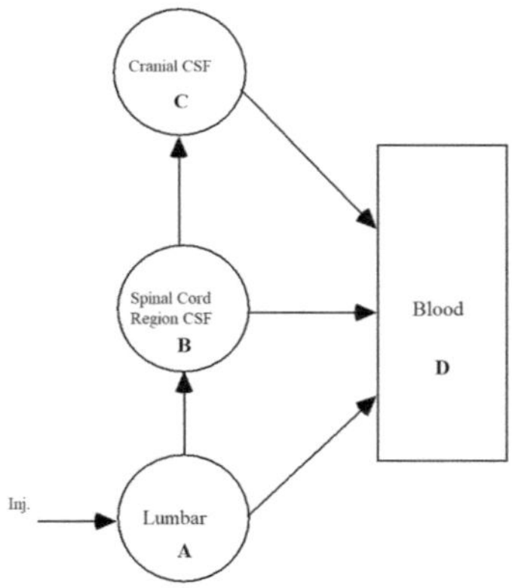

Flow	Fraction of Dose	Biologic Half Time	Associated Fraction
A→B	0.5	20 minutes 8 hours	0.25 0.75
A→D	0.5	8 hours 30 days	0.97 0.03
B→C	0.25	18 hours	1.0
B→D	0.25	18 hours 30 days	0.97 0.03
C→D	0.25	18 hours 30 days	0.97 0.03

Flow in LS	Fraction of Dose	Biologic Half Time	Associated Fraction
A→B	0.5	**90 hours**	1.0
A→D	0.5	**90 hours** 30 days	0.97 0.03
B→C	0.25	18 hours	1.0
B→D	0.25	18 hours 30 days	0.97 0.03
C→D	0.25	18 hours 30 days	0.97 0.03

Fig. 9.3 Biokinetic model of CSF flow after intralumbar injection with and without lumbar stasis (LS)

Radiation Dosimetry from Activity Absorbed into the Systemic Circulation

Since some of the radiopharmaceuticals injected into the CSF could be resorbed into the systemic circulation, absorbed dose from this component must also be evaluated and summed with the absorbed doses caused by activity in the CSF. Residence times estimates for all organs from a bolus introduction into the ventricle are determined by coupling [7] the CSF transport to the blood with models of I.V. injection of the radiopharmaceutical in published literature (systemic organ dosimetry model sources are listed in Table 9.1). All model sources are from ICRP-53 except for Sm-153 EDTMP [8], In-111 Pentetreotide [9], F-18 FDG [10], Y-90 chloride [11], and Y-90 Zevalin [12]. The simulation of intrathecal radioiodides assumes successful pretreatment thyroid blocking to achieve thyroidal radioiodide uptake below 0.1%. MIRDose3.1 is used to determine the absorbed dose estimates from the activity reaching the systemic circulation.

MCNP Monte Carlo Radiation Transport Simulations

Anthropomorphic models for the radiation transport analysis are illustrated in Fig. 9.4. MCNP 4b [13] is used to calculate the absorbed fractions from cranial CSF to brain margins, from spinal CSF to spinal cord margins, for photon dose from the ventricles to the brain, and for depth dose profiles around the ventricles. Between 6 and 15 million particle histories are run in four geometry setups. Emission energies and yields are derived from Weber et al. [14]. For all the simulations sufficient

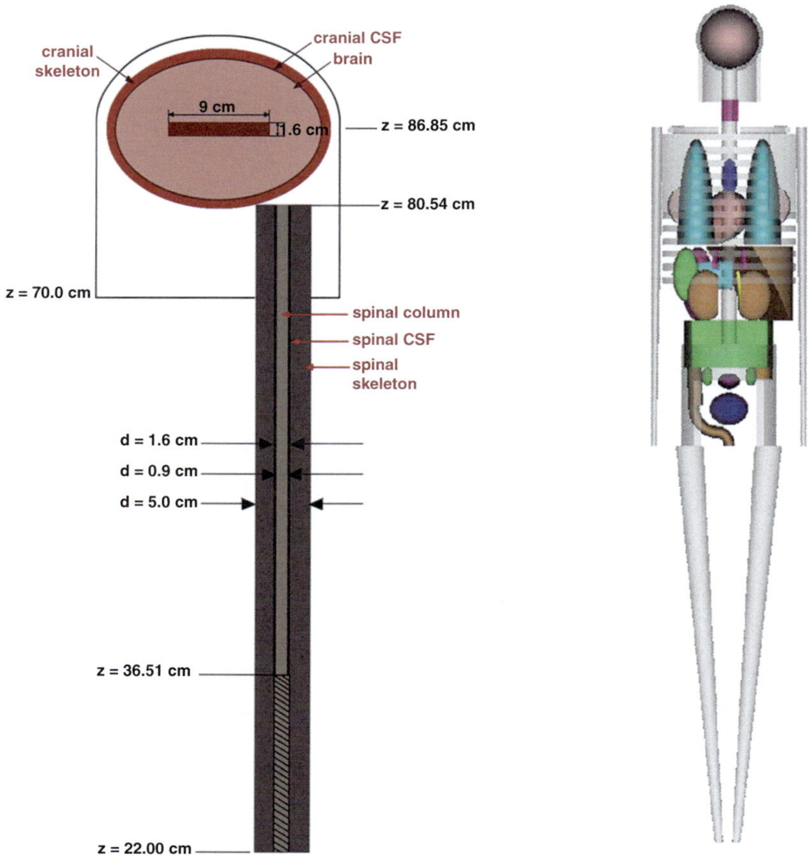

Fig. 9.4 Anthropomorphic models of spinal fluids and vital organs

numbers of histories are run such that the relative errors are less than 8% for all shells. MCNP results with errors less than 10% are generally considered reliable [13]. Equations describing the assumed anatomy for the radiation transport models are listed in Appendix. An example of the energies and abundance of radiation emissions used for simulation is illustrated for I-131 in Fig. 9.5a, b.

The tally results from the MCNP simulations are converted to absorbed fractions. These absorbed fractions are used with calculated masses of the target margins, and delta values are taken from Weber et al. [14] to determine S-values using the standard MIRD methodology [15].

Radiation transport results for normal organs and tissues such as kidneys, liver, and red marrow from activity in CSF sources are determined by using the absorbed fractions taken from Evans et al. [16] and the standard MIRD methodology. The Evans model consisted of the spinal cord, the spinal CSF, the surrounding bone all contained in a soft tissue trunk as defined in the Cristy–Eckerman phantom [17].

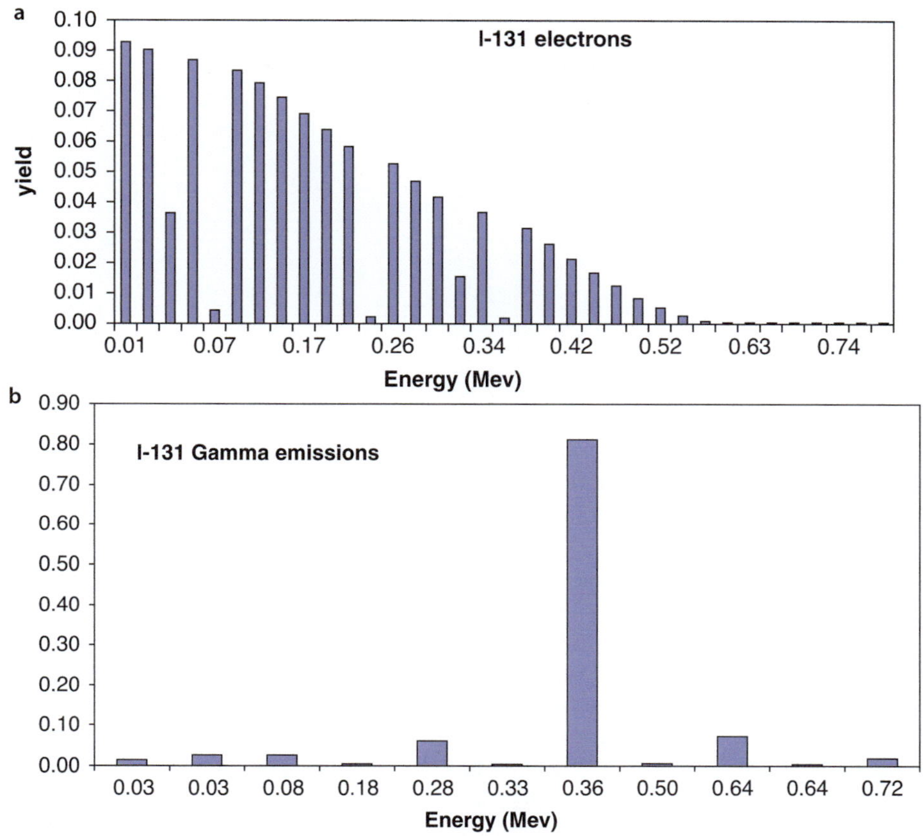

Fig. 9.5 (**a**) Multiple beta emissions (electrons) from I-131. (**b**) Multiple gamma emissions (photons) from I-131

Final Dosimetry Estimates

Residence times and S-values are combined to form absorbed dose contributions to the CSF spaces, tissues immediately adjacent to the CSF spaces, and normal organs and tissues using the standard MIRD methodology [15]. ED and EDE are determined using the standard ICRP methodology [18].

Results from Intraventricular Injections [19]

CSF and Organ Dosimetry

Residence times in CSF as determined using the theoretical biokinetic models described herein are listed in Table 9.2. Also listed are residence times of normal source organs and tissues for systemic administration from the literature references

Table 9.2 Residence times of CSF compartments and source organs for intraventricular injection models

Residence time (h) Source organ	Physical T1/2	Ventricle	Lower CSF	Upper CSF	Cranial CSF	Adrenals	Brain	LL bowel	Sm bowel	UL bowel	Heart	Kidneys	Liver	Red marrow	Cort bone	Trab bone	Spleen	Lungs	Thyroids	Urin bladder	Remainder
Sm-153 EDTMP	46.7	1.27	7.43	8.66	5.2							0.0190	0.0140		3.4000	3.4000		0.0130		1.7000	0.4900
Sm-153 EDTMP VS	46.7	39.9	2.6	3	1.8																
Ga-66 citrate	9.49	1.31	4.09	2.94	1.33	0.0020		0.0907	0.0819	0.1360		0.0319	0.1890	0.2040	0.1880	0.3040	0.0280			0.0240	2.8200
Ga-66 citrate ICRP M	9.49	1.31	0.46	0.96	8.17	0.0014		0.0630	0.0568	0.0942		0.0221	0.1310	0.1410	0.1300	0.2110	0.0194			0.0167	1.9600
Ga-67 citrate	78.3	1.28	8.37	10.4	6.78	0.0360		1.2000	2.7000	0.7700		0.5700	3.4000	3.6000	7.0000	1.8000	0.5100			0.2600	51.0000
Ga-67 citrate VS	78.3	54.4	3.94	4.9	3.2																
Ga-67 citrate ICRP M	78.3	1.42	3.08	6.37	22.05	0.0354		1.0900	0.2480	0.7160		0.5240	3.1300	3.3900	6.5200	1.6300	0.4680			0.2480	47.0000
Ga-68 citrate	1.1	0.69	0.55	0.18	0.09	0.0000		0.0001	0.0033	0.0012		0.0004	0.0026	0.0028	0.0054	0.0014	0.0038			0.0002	0.0390
Ga-68 citrate VS	1.1	1.45	0.01	0	0																
In-111 Pentetreotide	67.9	1.28	8.11	9.95	6.35			0.2800	0.0660	0.1800		2.6000	0.9400				0.9400			2.1000	7.2000
In-111 Pentetreotide VS	67.9	50.3	3.5	4.34	2.8																
Tl-201 Chloride	73.1	1.42	8.24	10.18	6.57		1.3900	2.0200	8.2400	2.7000	1.9000	3.0100	2.7100					0.6000	0.3200	0.0100	38.6000
I-123 sodium iodide	13.2	1.2	4.85	3.97	1.89							0.3100							0.0043	0.4000	2.6000
I-124 sodium iodide	100.32	1.29	8.84	11.16	7.54							0.1000							0.1000	1.4000	8.4000
I-125 sodium iodide	1443.36	1.3	16.25	17.76	15.8							0.1300							0.1000	1.8000	9.4000
I-131 sodium iodide	193	1.29	10.26	12.96	9.53							1.1000							0.2100	1.4000	9.4000
I-131 sodium iodide VS	193	79.7	7.03	8.9	6.5																
I-131 sodium iodide ICRP M	193	1.44	4.39	9.09	26.56							0.0936							0.1790	1.2800	8.0000
F-18 flurodeoyglucose FDG	1.83	0.93	1	0.37	0.17		0.0320				0.0072	0.0018	0.0084				0.0006	0.0036		0.0078	0.1000
F-18 FDG ICRP M	1.83	0.93	0.02	0.05	1.55		0.0070				0.0038	0.0009	0.0044				0.0003	0.0019		0.0041	0.0526
Y-90 chloride	64	1.42	8	9.75	6.16								10.0900		12.7700	20.7500				0.6200	6.7100
Y-90 DTPA	64	1.42	8	9.75	6.16																
Y-90 DTPA ICRP M	64	1.42	2.78	5.76	20.91							0.0537								1.3800	1.9300
Y-90 Zevalin	64	1.42	8	9.75	6.16																

noted in Table 9.1. Residence times are potential parameters for reconciliation between theoretic biokinetic models and empirical imaging finding results. They may also provide a basis for choice of biokinetic models, using the image-based residence times for arbitration.

As expected, the ratios of the absorbed doses to the CSF spaces vs to the normal organs are quite large [19]. The absorbed doses to the CSF spaces and normal organs, as well as the dose ratio of CSF to active (red) marrow are listed in Table 9.3 and illustrated in Fig. 9.6. Higher radiation absorbed doses in the CSF compartments are noted with Sm-153, I-131, Ga-66, and Y-90 compounds. Radiopharmaceuticals with the same chemical properties can be compared when different radionuclides are attached. For example, I-123, I-124, I-125, and I-131 sodium iodide absorbed doses are shown in Fig. 9.7 which indicates that I-131 would provide the highest payload to the CSF compartments. When comparison of CSF dosimetry is made with red marrow, wide therapeutic windows indicate potential safety. Similarly, results from the 4-compartment ICRP-53 models for 5 radiopharmaceuticals are listed in Table 9.4. In general, increased radiation doses in the convexity and decreased doses in the upper and lower spine are noted with the 4-compartment ICRP-53 model. Both models confirm that I-131 NaI, Y90-DTPA, and Ga-66 citrate would provide large radiation absorbed doses to the CSF compartments while maintaining wide therapeutic windows.

Absorbed Dose as a Function of Depth Surrounding CSF Spaces

Radiation absorbed doses in brain tissue immediately surrounding the ventricles within 4.3 cm from the interface of the CSF are listed in Table 9.5 and illustrated in Fig. 9.8. Absorbed dose vs. depth over the cerebral convexity is the list in Table 9.6 and illustrated in Fig. 9.9. Absorbed dose vs. depth for the cervical spine level is shown in Table 9.7 and illustrated in Fig. 9.10.

The half-dose ranges are reported as the distances of the shell from CSF interface where radiation absorbed doses decrease to less than 50%. This most commonly occurs at the shell that is 0.10 cm from the ventricular CSF interface (Table 9.5 and Fig. 9.8). Shorter half-dose ranges are noted in the cerebral convexity with half-dose

Table 9.3 Simulated radiation dosimetry to organs and CSF from intraventricular injection of 14 radiopharmaceuticals

cGy/mCi														
Organ	Sm-153	Ga-67	Ga-68	In-111	Tl-201	I-123	I-124	I-125	I-131	Y-90 CI	Y-90 DTPA	Y-90 Aby	F-18 FDG	Ga-66
Adrenals	0.072	0.540	0.049	0.600	0.310	0.099	1.500	0.069	0.670	0.200	0.057	0.810	0.096	1.200
Brain	0.120	0.420	0.200	0.690	0.370	0.160	2.700	0.380	0.850	3.800	3.600	4.400	0.330	2.900
Breasts	0.009	0.150	0.005	0.065	0.094	0.011	0.220	0.013	0.120	0.200	0.057	0.810	0.009	0.230
Eyes	0.046	0.250	0.038	0.250	0.230	0.043	0.580	0.077	0.320				0.059	0.410
Lens of eyes	0.033	0.220	0.030	0.200	0.210	0.031	0.480	0.041	0.270				0.046	0.360
Gallbladder wall	0.007	0.240	0.002	0.140	0.270	0.025	0.420	0.018	0.110	0.200	0.057	0.810	0.021	0.400
LLI wall	0.018	0.590	0.004	0.250	0.850	0.017	0.310	0.021	0.160	0.200	0.057	13.000	0.008	0.940
Small intestine	0.023	0.270	0.018	0.220	1.100	0.032	0.500	0.023	0.250	0.200	0.057	3.800	0.024	0.600
Stomach	0.015	0.230	0.010	0.190	0.490	0.024	0.390	0.017	0.200	0.200	0.057	0.810	0.019	0.350
ULI wall	0.019	0.380	0.014	0.230	0.860	0.026	0.420	0.019	0.210	0.200	0.057	9.700	0.019	1.000
Heart wall	0.022	0.250	0.014	0.190	0.720	0.032	0.520	0.020	0.250	0.200	0.057	7.500	0.042	0.420
Kidneys	0.077	0.430	0.030	1.700	1.200	0.069	1.100	0.062	0.550	0.200	0.390	0.270	0.060	0.850
Liver	0.017	0.360	0.012	0.260	0.270	0.025	0.420	0.018	0.210	10.000	0.057	13.000	0.023	0.510
Lungs	0.026	0.230	0.014	0.180	0.160	0.031	0.490	0.024	0.240	0.200	0.057	5.400	0.029	0.400
Muscle	0.018	0.200	0.010	0.140	0.140	0.022	0.370	0.022	0.190	0.200	0.057	0.810	0.018	0.320
Ovaries	0.019	0.260	0.006	0.170	0.270	0.021	0.350	0.020	0.180	0.200	0.057	1.100	0.011	0.330
Pancreas	0.036	0.320	0.022	0.380	0.250	0.052	0.780	0.029	0.370	0.200	0.057	0.810	0.047	0.600
Red marrow	0.750	0.520	0.170	0.590	0.290	0.120	1.900	0.160	0.950	12.000	1.500	4.900	0.120	2.400
Bone surfaces	2.700	1.000	0.048	0.530	0.510	0.150	1.100	0.490	0.510	12.000	0.057	2.400	0.078	1.800
Skin	0.011	0.140	0.008	0.077	0.094	0.013	0.260	0.014	0.130	0.200	0.057	0.810	0.014	0.240
Spleen	0.018	0.440	0.014	1.000	0.180	0.027	0.440	0.019	0.220	0.200	0.057	25.000	0.024	0.639
Testes	0.011	0.160	0.002	0.076	2.000	0.010	0.190	0.016	0.110	0.200	0.057	24.000	0.003	0.180
Thymus	0.013	0.200	0.009	0.110	0.140	0.020	0.350	0.016	0.180	0.200	0.057	0.810	0.017	0.311
Thyroid	0.020	0.220	0.019	0.160	1.600	0.042	2.800	3.200	4.600	0.200	0.057	0.810	0.034	0.396
Urin bladder wall	2.400	0.240	0.004	0.980	0.130	0.120	2.300	0.350	1.900	3.000	7.100	2.400	0.018	0.317
Uterus	0.029	0.240	0.006	0.210	0.230	0.026	0.430	0.033	0.220	0.200	0.057	1.100	0.011	0.300
Total body	0.091	0.240	0.016	0.200	0.200	0.036	0.490	0.075	0.240	1.400	0.066	1.300	0.047	0.668
ED	0.340	0.360	0.080	0.460	0.800	0.045	0.700	0.260	0.620	2.500	0.430	8.600	0.039	0.752
EDE	0.250	0.330	0.030	0.290	0.920	0.060	1.000	0.190	0.600	3.000	0.890	12.000	0.060	0.930
Ventricle CSF	**22.000**	**3.500**	**30.000**	**4.200**	**4.000**	**2.900**	**16.000**	**2.200**	**17.000**	**63.000**	**63.000**	**63.000**	**15.000**	**52.000**
C-Spine CSF	**74.000**	**14.000**	**3.400**	**16.000**	**16.000**	**4.600**	**62.000**	**15.000**	**83.000**	**200.000**	**200.000**	**200.000**	**3.300**	**49.000**
L-Spine CSF	**140.000**	**25.000**	**25.000**	**29.000**	**28.000**	**12.000**	**130.000**	**31.000**	**140.000**	**440.000**	**440.000**	**440.000**	**19.000**	**200.000**
Convexity CSF	**41.000**	**9.600**	**0.900**	**8.750**	**11.000**	**2.100**	**23.000**	**13.000**	**56.000**	**67.000**	**67.000**	**67.000**	**1.300**	**9.800**
Skull	0.740	0.310	0.093	0.878	0.330	0.160	3.500	1.160	1.500	6.700	6.700	6.700	0.350	1.800
Vertebra	0.940	0.710	0.260	2.100	0.760	0.640	5.800	2.100	2.100	7.000	7.000	7.000	0.310	7.600
Red marrow	0.750	0.520	0.170	0.590	0.290	0.120	1.900	0.160	0.950	12.000	1.500	4.900	0.120	2.400
Ratios (Therapeutic windows)														
Ventricle CSF to marrow	**29.3**	**6.7**	**176.5**	**7.1**	**13.8**	**24.2**	**8.4**	**13.8**	**17.9**	**5.3**	**42.0**	**12.9**	**125.0**	**21.7**
C-Spine CSF to marrow	**98.7**	**26.9**	**20.0**	**27.1**	**55.2**	**38.3**	**32.6**	**93.8**	**87.4**	**16.7**	**133.3**	**40.8**	**27.5**	**20.4**
L-Spine CSF to marrow	**186.7**	**48.1**	**147.1**	**49.2**	**96.6**	**100.0**	**68.4**	**193.8**	**147.4**	**36.7**	**293.3**	**89.8**	**158.3**	**83.3**
Convex CSF to marrow	**54.7**	**18.5**	**5.3**	**14.8**	**37.9**	**17.5**	**12.1**	**81.3**	**58.9**	**5.6**	**44.7**	**13.7**	**10.8**	**4.1**

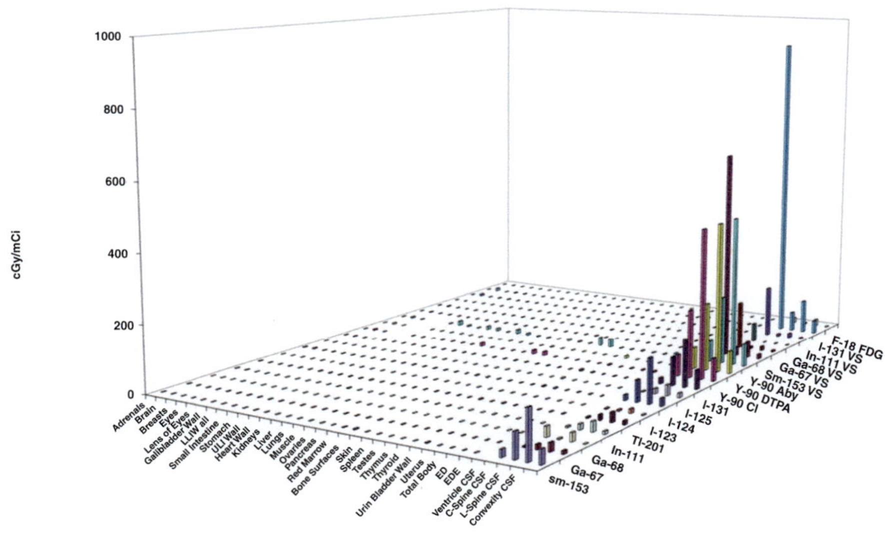

Fig. 9.6 Simulated radiation dosimetry in the CSF Spaces and vital organs after intraventricular injection of 14 radiopharmaceuticals and 5 radiopharmaceuticals with ventricular stasis

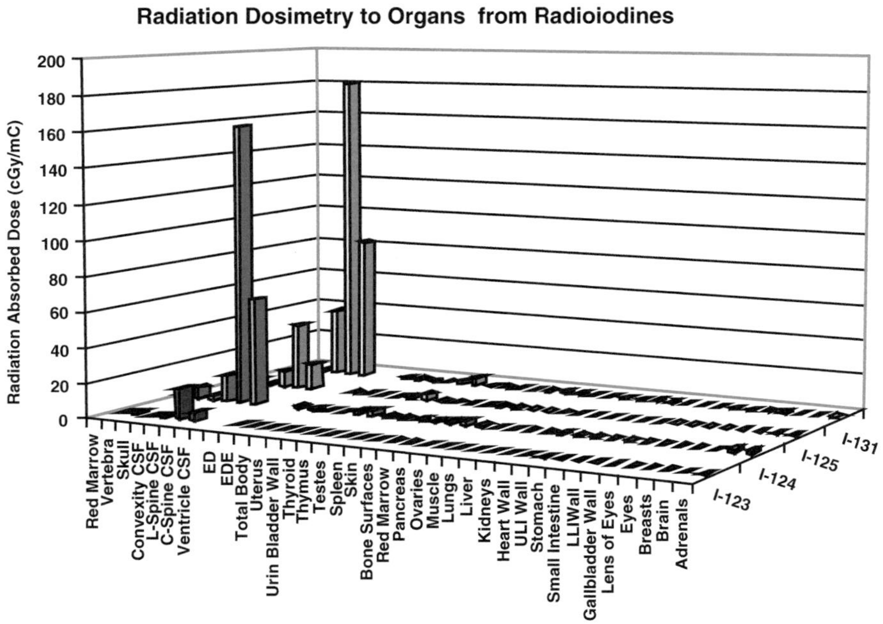

Fig. 9.7 Simulated radiation dosimetry of I-123, I-124, I-125, and I-131 from intraventricular Injection

ranges typically occurring at the shells that are at distances of 0.05–0.15 cm (Table 9.6). These dosimetry models allow comparison of absorbed dose vs depth of radiopharmaceuticals with identical chemical properties, but different isotopes as illustrated by Ga-66, Ga-67, and Ga-68 as gallium citrate (Fig. 9.9). Except for Ga-66, the half-dose ranges occur at 0.01–0.09 cm in the cervical spine (Table 9.7 and Fig. 9.10). The high half-dose range of Ga-66 in the spinal cord may be less desirable because of potential adverse effects to excessively irradiating underlying neural tissues.

Another measure of potential efficacy and toxicity is the 90% total dose range, i.e., the distance the shell from the CSF interface that receives more than 90% of total radiation deposition. This parameter varies from 0.10 to 1.1 cm in the periventricular tissues (Table 9.5), from 0.05 to 2.35 cm in the convexity (Table 9.6), and from 0.06 to 0.36 cm in the spinal cord (Table 9.7). This parameter of range may provide another guidance for safety and efficacy for the design of radiopharmaceutical therapy against LM.

Ventricular Stasis (VS)

The absorbed doses in the CSF spaces and the normal organs and tissues using the same methods as described above but with the assumption of ventricular stasis in five selected radiopharmaceuticals are shown in Table 9.8. Absorbed dose vs. depth

Table 9.4 Comparison of simulated radiation dosimetry of an alternative CSF flow intraventricular model (ICRP-53 M) of 5 radiopharmaceuticals

cGy/mCi	Ivent	Ivent	Ivent	IVent	Ivent	ICRP53 M	ICRP53 M	ICRP53 M	ICRP53 M	ICRP53 M
Organ	Ga-67	I-131	Y-90 DTPA	F-18 FDG	Ga-66	Ga-66	Ga-67	F-18 FDG	I-131	Y90 DTPA
Adrenals	0.540	0.670	0.057	0.096	1.200	0.440	0.430	0.007	0.420	0.053
Brain	0.420	0.850	3.600	0.330	2.900	9.000	4.600	0.610	2.500	11.000
Breasts	0.150	0.120	0.057	0.009	0.230	0.140	0.130	0.003	0.094	0.053
Eyes	0.250	0.320		0.059	0.410	0.830	0.360	0.120	0.610	0.053
Lens of eyes	0.220	0.270		0.046	0.360	0.690	0.310	0.093	0.490	0.053
Gallbladder wall	0.240	0.110	0.057	0.021	0.400	0.200	0.240	0.003	0.160	0.053
LLI wall	0.590	0.160	0.057	0.008	0.940	0.630	0.540	0.002	0.130	0.053
Small intestine	0.270	0.250	0.057	0.024	0.600	0.320	0.230	0.003	0.170	0.053
Stomach	0.230	0.200	0.057	0.019	0.350	0.180	0.200	0.003	0.140	0.053
ULI wall	0.380	0.210	0.057	0.019	1.000	0.630	0.340	0.002	0.150	0.053
Heart wall	0.250	0.250	0.057	0.042	0.420	0.200	0.210	0.012	0.180	0.053
Kidneys	0.430	0.550	0.390	0.060	0.850	0.350	0.350	0.006	0.370	0.360
Liver	0.360	0.210	0.057	0.023	0.510	0.280	0.320	0.004	0.150	0.053
Lungs	0.230	0.240	0.057	0.029	0.400	0.200	0.190	0.007	0.170	0.053
Muscle	0.200	0.190	0.057	0.018	0.320	0.200	0.180	0.009	0.160	0.053
Ovaries	0.260	0.180	0.057	0.011	0.330	0.190	0.230	0.002	0.140	0.053
Pancreas	0.320	0.370	0.057	0.047	0.600	0.230	0.260	0.005	0.240	0.053
Red marrow	0.520	0.950	1.500	0.120	2.400	1.800	0.440	0.073	0.670	1.800
Bone surfaces	1.000	0.510	0.057	0.078	1.800	1.800	0.970	0.090	0.620	1.800
Skin	0.140	0.130	0.057	0.014	0.240	0.220	0.140	0.015	0.140	0.053
Spleen	0.440	0.220	0.057	0.024	0.639	0.360	0.400	0.004	0.160	0.053
Testes	0.160	0.110	0.057	0.003	0.180	0.120	0.150	0.001	0.095	0.053
Thymus	0.200	0.180	0.057	0.017	0.311	0.180	0.180	0.006	0.140	0.053
Thyroid	0.220	4.600	0.057	0.034	0.396	0.420	0.220	0.039	4.000	0.053
Urin bladder wall	0.240	1.900	7.100	0.018	0.317	0.210	0.220	0.009	1.500	6.500
Uterus	0.240	0.220	0.057	0.011	0.300	0.170	0.220	0.002	0.170	0.053
Total body	0.240	0.240	0.066	0.047	0.668	0.670	0.270	0.047	0.480	0.920
ED	0.360	0.620	0.430	0.039	0.752	0.680	0.400	0.030	0.490	0.890
EDE	0.330	0.600	0.890	0.060	0.930	1.000	0.570	0.054	0.590	1.400
Ventricle CSF	3.50	17.00	63.00	15.00	52.00	52.00	2.50	15.00	16.00	63.00
C-Spine CSF	14.00	83.00	200.00	3.30	49.00	16.00	1.60	0.42	56.00	120.00
L-Spine CSF	25.00	140.00	440.00	19.00	200.00	23.00	1.80	0.45	59.00	150.00
Convexity CSF	9.60	56.00	67.00	1.30	9.80	60.00	20.00	11.00	150.00	230.00
Skull	0.31	1.50	6.70	0.35	1.80	15.00	1.10	0.55	3.00	17.00
Vertebra	0.71	2.10	7.00	0.31	7.60	1.60	0.10	0.02	0.94	2.60
Red marrow	0.52	0.95	1.500	0.12	2.400	1.800	0.440	0.073	0.670	1.800
Ratios (Therapeutic windows)										
Ventricle CSF to BM	6.7	17.9	42.0	125.0	21.7	28.9	5.7	205.5	23.9	35.0
C-Spine CSF to BM	26.9	87.4	133.3	27.5	20.4	8.9	3.6	5.8	83.6	66.7
L-Spine CSF to BM	48.1	147.4	293.3	158.3	83.3	12.8	4.1	6.2	88.1	83.3
Convex CSF to BM	18.5	58.9	44.7	10.8	4.1	33.3	45.5	150.7	223.9	127.8

in neural tissues adjacent to the CSF spaces are shown in Tables 9.5, 9.6, and 9.7. Ventricular stasis results in significantly higher radiation absorbed doses in the ventricle (Table 9.8), while the therapeutic window markedly increased, as expected because there is less available radionuclide to reach the bone marrow. Although absolute values of radiation absorbed doses increase in the ventricle with stasis, the half-dose range at the shell that is 0.01 cm in the spinal cord (Table 9.7), 0.05 cm in the cerebral convexity (Table 9.6) and 0.1 cm in the ventricle (Table 9.7) indicating likely low collateral damage to neural tissue beyond the spinal fluid. The 90% total dose ranges are relatively stable with and without stasis, except for Sm-153 in spinal cord (Table 9.7). Numerical values of the effects of ventricular stasis in the CSF and in the surrounding tissues may provide valuable guidance to manage LM treatment strategies when stasis is encountered.

Table 9.5 Periventricular absorbed dose vs. depth after intraventricular injection of 14 radiopharmaceuticals plus 5 with ventricular stasis (vs). Range parameters include distance (cm) of the shell that receives less than 50% of CSF radiation dose and distance of the shell that receives more than 90% of total radiation dose including CSF

cGy/mCi	Ivent	Ivent	Ivent	Ivent	Ivent	Ivent	Ivent	Ivent	Ivent	Ivent
Distance (cm)	Sm-153	Ga-67	Ga-68	In-111	Tl-201	I-123	I-124	I-125	I-131	Y-90 CI
0.00	22.00	3.50	30.00	4.20	4.00	2.90	16.00	2.20	17.00	63.00
0.10	2.20	0.32	10.00	0.91	0.26	0.44	6.10	0.34	2.00	23.00
0.20	0.16	0.20	4.30	0.66	0.15	0.32	3.20	0.27	0.52	11.00
0.30	0.10	0.16	1.90	0.54	0.12	0.27	1.90	0.23	0.44	5.40
0.40	0.09	0.15	0.93	0.50	0.10	0.24	1.30	0.19	0.38	2.50
0.50	0.08	0.12	0.55	0.42	0.09	0.21	1.00	0.17	0.33	1.10
0.60	0.07	0.11	0.41	0.38	0.08	0.19	0.86	0.15	0.30	0.40
0.70	0.06	0.10	0.37	0.34	0.07	0.17	0.74	0.13	0.26	0.12
0.80	0.06	0.09	0.33	0.31	0.06	0.15	0.68	0.12	0.25	0.03
0.90	0.06	0.08	0.30	0.28	0.06	0.14	0.60	0.11	0.22	0.01
1.00	0.05	0.07	0.28	0.26	0.05	0.13	0.56	0.10	0.21	0.00
1.10	0.05	0.07	0.25	0.24	0.05	0.11	0.52	0.09	0.19	0.00
1.20	0.04	0.06	0.24	0.22	0.04	0.11	0.49	0.08	0.17	0.00
1.30	0.04	0.06	0.22	0.20	0.04	0.10	0.44	0.08	0.17	0.00
1.80	0.03	0.05	0.18	0.16	0.03	0.08	0.36	0.06	0.13	0.00
2.30	0.02	0.04	0.13	0.11	0.03	0.06	0.27	0.04	0.10	0.00
2.80	0.02	0.03	0.10	0.09	0.02	0.04	0.21	0.03	0.08	0.00
3.30	0.01	0.02	0.08	0.07	0.02	0.03	0.16	0.02	0.06	0.00
3.80	0.01	0.02	0.07	0.05	0.01	0.02	0.13	0.01	0.05	0.00
4.30	0.01	0.01	0.05	0.04	0.01	0.02	0.11	0.01	0.04	0.00
Ventricles	22.00	3.50	30.00	4.20	4.00	2.90	16.00	2.20	17.00	63.00
CSF % of Total	87.47	66.57	59.18	42.11	75.86	50.63	44.91	49.86	74.26	59.11
Range (cm)										
50% Dose	0.10	0.10	0.10	0.10	0.10	0.10	0.10	0.10	0.10	0.10
90% Total dose	0.10	0.80	0.30	1.10	0.60	1.00	0.90	1.00	0.90	0.20
Dose ratios										
Red marrow	0.750	0.520	0.170	0.590	0.290	0.120	1.900	0.160	0.950	12.000
CSF to marrow	29.33	6.73	176.47	7.12	13.79	24.17	8.42	13.75	17.89	5.25

cGy/mCi	Ivent	Ivent	Ivent	Ivent	Ivent	Ivent	Ivent	IVent	Ivent
Distance (cm)	Y-90 DTPA	Y-90 Aby	Sm-153 VS	Ga-67 VS	Ga-68 VS	In-111 VS	I-131 VS	F-18 FDG	Ga-66
0.00	63.00	63.00	610.00	140.00	56.00	150.00	920.00	15.00	52.00
0.10	23.00	23.00	62.00	12.00	19.00	32.00	110.00	2.60	25.00
0.20	11.00	11.00	4.40	7.70	8.00	23.00	29.00	0.90	17.00
0.30	5.40	5.40	2.80	6.20	3.60	19.00	24.00	0.76	12.00
0.40	2.50	2.50	2.40	5.60	1.70	18.00	21.00	0.68	8.90
0.50	1.10	1.10	2.20	4.50	1.00	15.00	18.00	0.59	6.50
0.60	0.40	0.40	2.00	4.20	0.77	13.00	16.00	0.51	4.70
0.70	0.12	0.12	1.80	3.70	0.69	12.00	15.00	0.47	3.50
0.80	0.03	0.03	1.60	3.40	0.63	11.00	14.00	0.43	2.50
0.90	0.01	0.01	1.60	3.00	0.56	10.00	12.00	0.38	1.90
1.00	0.00	0.00	1.30	2.80	0.53	9.10	11.00	0.36	1.50
1.10	0.00	0.00	1.30	2.60	0.48	8.30	10.00	0.33	1.20
1.20	0.00	0.00	1.20	2.50	0.46	7.70	9.70	0.31	1.00
1.30	0.00	0.00	1.10	2.40	0.41	7.20	9.30	0.29	0.88
1.80	0.00	0.00	0.91	1.90	0.34	5.70	7.50	0.24	0.67
2.30	0.00	0.00	0.67	1.40	0.25	4.00	5.40	0.17	0.49
2.80	0.00	0.00	0.50	1.10	0.20	3.00	4.20	0.13	0.38
3.30	0.00	0.00	0.39	0.85	0.15	2.30	3.30	0.11	0.31
3.80	0.00	0.00	0.30	0.66	0.12	1.90	2.70	0.09	0.25
4.30	0.00	0.00	0.23	0.52	0.10	1.40	2.10	0.07	0.20
Ventricles	63.00	63.00	610.00	140.00	56.00	150.00	920.00	15.00	52.00
CSF % of Total	59.11	59.11	87.30	67.62	58.95	42.42	73.94	61.43	36.91
Range (cm)									
50% Dose	0.10	0.10	0.10	0.10	0.10	0.10	0.10	0.10	0.10
90% Total dose	0.20	0.20	0.10	0.80	0.30	1.10	0.50	0.90	0.70
Dose ratios									
Red marrow	1.500	4.900	0.300	0.350	0.019	0.500	1.000	0.120	2.400
CSF to marrow	42.00	12.86	2033.33	400.00	2947.37	300.00	920.00	125.00	21.67

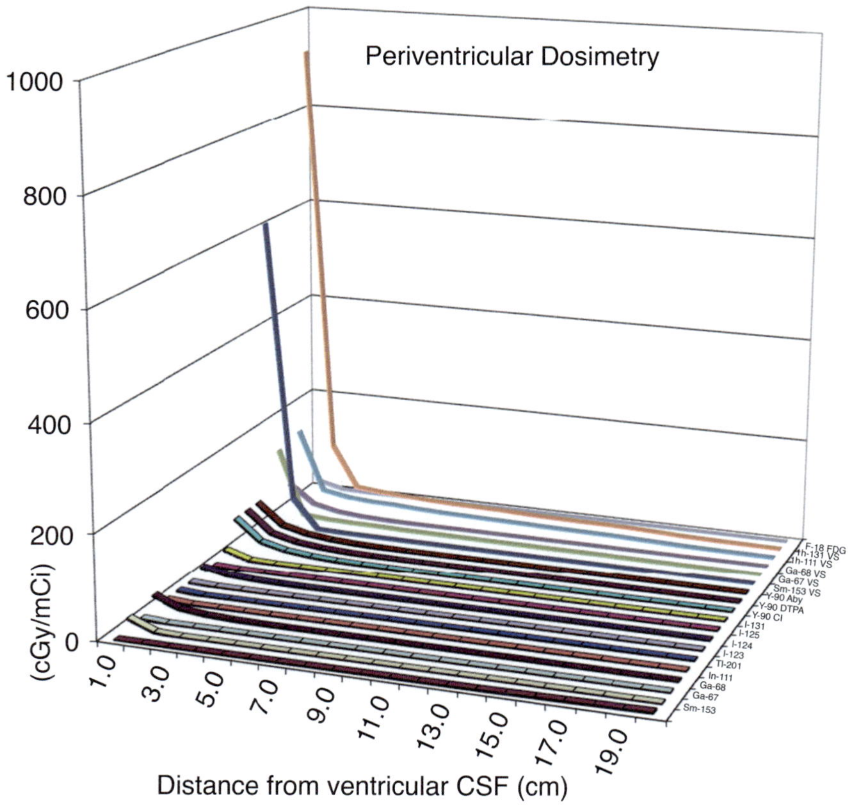

Fig. 9.8 Simulated depth radiation dosimetry in periventricular tissues from intraventricular injection of 14 radiopharmaceuticals

Table 9.6 Cerebral convexity absorbed dose vs. depth to 3 cm after intraventricular injection of 14 radiopharmaceuticals plus 5 radiopharmaceuticals with ventricular stasis (VS). Range parameters include distance (cm) to the shell that receives less than 50% of CSF radiation dose and distance to the shell that receives more than 90% of total radiation dose including CSF

cGy/mCi	Ivent	Ivent	Ivent	Ivent	Ivent	Ivent	Ivent	Ivent	Ivent
Distance (cm)	Sm-153	Ga-67	Ga-68	In-111	Tl-201	I-123	I-124	I-125	I-131
0.00	41.00	9.60	0.90	8.75	11.00	2.10	23.00	13.00	56.00
0.05	5.30	0.54	0.47	1.23	0.42	0.17	12.00	0.76	7.40
0.15	0.24	0.28	0.21	0.73	0.20	0.11	6.10	0.59	0.91
0.25	0.09	0.23	0.10	0.66	0.16	0.10	3.60	0.51	0.79
0.35	0.09	0.20	0.05	0.60	0.14	0.09	2.40	0.45	0.73
0.45	0.09	0.19	0.03	0.58	0.13	0.08	1.90	0.44	0.70
0.55	0.08	0.18	0.02	0.54	0.12	0.08	1.60	0.39	0.66
0.65	0.08	0.17	0.02	0.51	0.12	0.08	1.40	0.39	0.64
0.75	0.08	0.17	0.02	0.50	0.11	0.07	1.40	0.36	0.63
0.85	0.07	0.16	0.01	0.48	0.11	0.07	1.30	0.34	0.61
0.95	0.07	0.15	0.01	0.47	0.10	0.07	1.30	0.31	0.57
1.05	0.07	0.15	0.01	0.45	0.10	0.07	1.20	0.30	0.58
1.15	0.07	0.15	0.01	0.44	0.10	0.07	1.20	0.29	0.56
1.25	0.07	0.15	0.01	0.44	0.10	0.06	1.20	0.29	0.55
1.35	0.07	0.14	0.01	0.41	0.10	0.06	1.10	0.27	0.53
1.45	0.07	0.14	0.01	0.41	0.09	0.06	1.10	0.25	0.53
1.55	0.06	0.14	0.01	0.39	0.10	0.06	1.10	0.25	0.51
1.65	0.06	0.14	0.01	0.39	0.09	0.05	1.00	0.23	0.50
1.75	0.06	0.14	0.01	0.38	0.10	0.06	1.00	0.23	0.51
1.85	0.06	0.14	0.01	0.38	0.09	0.06	1.10	0.22	0.49
1.95	0.06	0.13	0.01	0.38	0.09	0.05	1.10	0.22	0.48
2.05	0.06	0.13	0.01	0.36	0.09	0.05	0.99	0.20	0.47
2.15	0.06	0.13	0.01	0.35	0.09	0.05	0.97	0.19	0.46
2.25	0.06	0.13	0.01	0.36	0.09	0.05	0.99	0.19	0.46
2.35	0.06	0.12	0.01	0.35	0.09	0.05	1.00	0.19	0.46
2.45	0.06	0.13	0.01	0.35	0.09	0.05	0.97	0.19	0.46
2.55	0.06	0.12	0.01	0.34	0.88	0.05	1.00	0.19	0.45
2.65	0.06	0.13	0.01	0.34	0.09	0.05	0.94	0.17	0.45
2.75	0.06	0.12	0.01	0.34	0.09	0.05	0.89	0.19	0.44
2.85	0.06	0.13	0.01	0.34	0.09	0.05	0.84	0.17	0.43
2.95	0.06	0.12	0.01	0.32	0.09	0.05	0.85	0.16	0.43
CSF % of Total	84.67	65.98	43.60	38.74	72.10	51.45	30.05	59.31	70.54
Range at layer (cm)									
50% dose	0.05	0.05	0.15	0.05	0.05	0.05	0.15	0.05	0.05
90% Total dose	0.05	1.85	1.15	2.35	2.15	2.15	2.15	1.85	1.35
Red marrow	0.750	0.520	0.170	0.590	0.290	0.120	1.900	0.160	0.950
CSF to marrovw	54.67	18.46	5.29	14.83	37.93	17.50	12.11	81.25	58.95

cGy/mCi	Ivent	Ivent	Ivent	Ivent	Ivent	Ivent	Ivent	Ivent	IVent	Ivent
Distance (cm)	Y-90 CI	Y-90 DTPA	Y-90 Aby	Sm-153 VS	Ga-67 VS	Ga-68 VS	In-111 VS	I-131 VS	F18 FDG	Ga-66
0.00	67.00	67.00	67.00	14.00	4.50	0.00	3.80	39.00	1.30	9.80
0.05	35.00	35.00	35.00	1.90	0.26	0.00	0.54	5.10	0.25	6.30
0.15	18.00	18.00	18.00	0.08	0.13	0.00	0.32	0.62	0.05	4.30
0.25	9.90	9.90	9.90	0.03	0.11	0.00	0.29	0.54	0.04	3.30
0.35	5.30	5.30	5.30	0.03	0.09	0.00	0.26	0.50	0.04	2.50
0.45	2.70	2.70	2.70	0.03	0.09	0.00	0.25	0.48	0.04	2.10
0.55	1.10	1.10	1.10	0.03	0.08	0.00	0.23	0.45	0.03	1.60
0.65	0.42	0.42	0.42	0.03	0.08	0.00	0.22	0.44	0.03	1.30
0.75	0.12	0.12	0.12	0.03	0.08	0.00	0.22	0.43	0.03	1.00
0.85	0.03	0.03	0.03	0.03	0.08	0.00	0.21	0.42	0.03	0.84
0.95	0.01	0.01	0.01	0.03	0.07	0.00	0.20	0.39	0.03	0.70
1.05	0.01	0.01	0.01	0.03	0.07	0.00	0.20	0.40	0.03	0.60
1.15	0.01	0.01	0.01	0.02	0.07	0.00	0.19	0.38	0.03	0.53
1.25	0.01	0.01	0.01	0.02	0.07	0.00	0.19	0.38	0.03	0.49
1.35	0.01	0.01	0.01	0.02	0.07	0.00	0.18	0.36	0.03	0.43
1.45	0.00	0.00	0.00	0.02	0.07	0.00	0.18	0.36	0.03	0.43
1.55	0.00	0.00	0.00	0.02	0.07	0.00	0.17	0.35	0.03	0.40
1.65	0.00	0.00	0.00	0.02	0.06	0.00	0.17	0.34	0.03	0.39
1.75	0.00	0.00	0.00	0.02	0.06	0.00	0.17	0.35	0.03	0.37
1.85	0.00	0.00	0.00	0.02	0.07	0.00	0.17	0.33	0.02	0.38
1.95	0.00	0.00	0.00	0.02	0.06	0.00	0.16	0.33	0.02	0.37
2.05	0.00	0.00	0.00	0.02	0.06	0.00	0.16	0.32	0.02	0.36
2.15	0.00	0.00	0.00	0.02	0.06	0.00	0.15	0.32	0.02	0.37
2.25	0.00	0.00	0.00	0.02	0.06	0.00	0.16	0.32	0.02	0.37
2.35	0.00	0.00	0.00	0.02	0.06	0.00	0.15	0.32	0.02	0.36
2.45	0.00	0.00	0.00	0.02	0.06	0.00	0.15	0.32	0.02	0.36
2.55	0.00	0.00	0.00	0.02	0.06	0.00	0.15	0.31	0.02	0.35
2.65	0.00	0.00	0.00	0.02	0.06	0.00	0.15	0.31	0.02	0.35
2.75	0.00	0.00	0.00	0.02	0.06	0.00	0.15	0.30	0.02	0.33
2.85	0.00	0.00	0.00	0.02	0.06	0.00	0.15	0.30	0.02	0.34
2.95	0.00	0.00	0.00	0.02	0.06	0.00	0.14	0.30	0.02	0.32
CSF % of Total	47.97	47.97	47.97	84.12	65.75		38.66	70.82	55.58	23.54
Range at layer (cm)										
50% dose	0.15	0.15	0.15	0.05	0.05		0.05	0.05	0.05	0.15
90% Total dose	0.25	0.25	0.25	0.05	1.85		2.35	1.35	1.95	1.85
Red marrow	12.000	1.500	4.900	0.300	0.350	0.019	0.500	1.000	0.120	2.400
CSF to marrovw	5.58	44.67	13.67	46.67	12.86	0.00	7.60	39.00	10.83	4.08

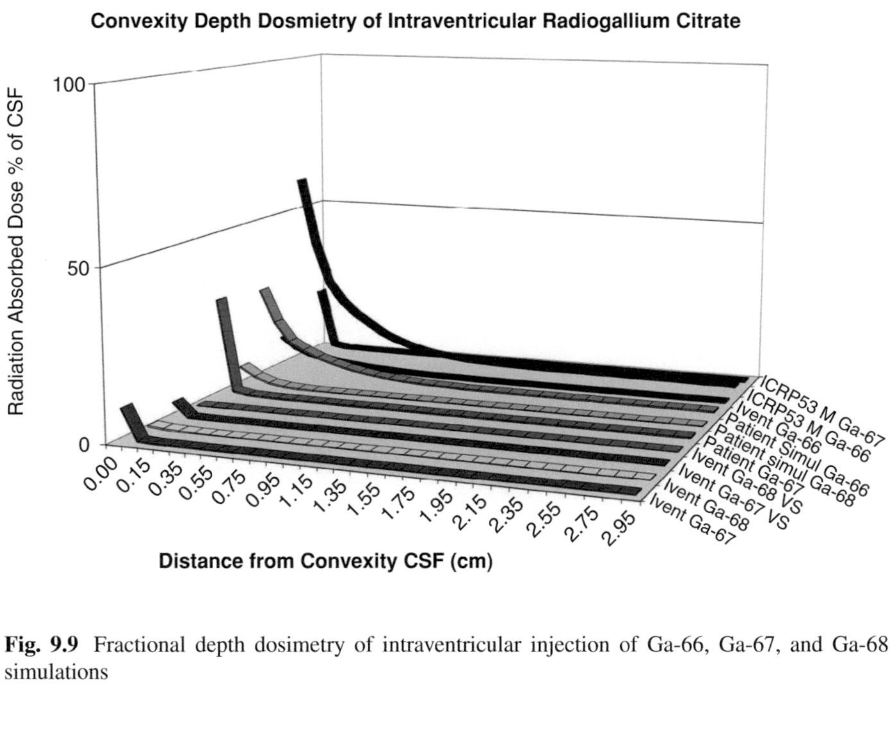

Fig. 9.9 Fractional depth dosimetry of intraventricular injection of Ga-66, Ga-67, and Ga-68 simulations

Table 9.7 Cervical spine absorbed dose vs. depth from CSF interface to 0.4 cm after intraventricular injection of 14 radiopharmaceuticals plus 5 radiopharmaceuticals with ventricular stasis (VS). Range parameters include distance (cm) to the shell that receives less than 50% of CSF radiation dose and distance to the shell that receives more than 90% of total radiation dose including CSF

cGy/mCi	Ivent	Ivent	Ivent	Ivent	Ivent	Ivent	Ivent	Ivent	Ivent	Ivent	Ivent	Ivent	Ivent	Ivent	Ivent	Ivent	Ivent	Ivent	Ivent
(cm)	Sm-153	Ga-67	Ga-68	In-111	Tl-201	I-123	I-124	I-125	I-131	Y-90 Cl	Y-90 DTPA	Y-90 Aby	Sm-153 VS	Ga-67 VS	Ga-68 VS	In-111 VS	I-131 VS	F18 FDG	Ga-66
0.00	74.00	14.00	3.40	16.00	16.00	4.60	62.00	15.00	83.00	200.00	200.00	200.00	26.00	6.80	0.00	6.80	57.00	3.30	49.00
0.01	21.00	2.30	2.20	5.70	2.00	1.20	43.00	3.10	25.00	140.00	140.00	140.00	7.20	1.10	0.00	2.50	17.00	1.30	45.00
0.04	8.50	1.60	1.80	3.90	1.10	0.80	36.00	2.90	11.00	120.00	120.00	120.00	3.00	0.73	0.00	1.70	7.30	0.69	42.00
0.06	4.00	1.40	1.50	3.60	1.00	0.79	32.00	2.80	5.80	110.00	110.00	110.00	1.40	0.65	0.00	1.60	4.00	0.46	40.00
0.09	1.90	1.30	1.30	3.60	0.96	0.75	28.00	2.70	4.00	95.00	95.00	95.00	0.65	0.59	0.00	1.60	2.70	0.35	38.00
0.11	1.10	1.20	1.10	3.50	0.93	0.74	24.00	2.70	3.40	84.00	84.00	84.00	0.37	0.55	0.00	1.50	2.40	0.30	36.00
0.14	0.78	1.10	0.97	3.40	0.88	0.73	22.00	2.60	3.20	75.00	75.00	75.00	0.27	0.53	0.00	1.50	2.20	0.29	35.00
0.16	0.62	1.10	0.83	3.60	0.85	0.72	20.00	2.60	3.30	68.00	68.00	68.00	0.22	0.52	0.00	1.60	2.20	0.28	34.00
0.19	0.55	1.00	0.72	3.50	0.80	0.71	18.00	2.50	3.20	61.00	61.00	61.00	0.19	0.49	0.00	1.50	2.20	0.29	33.00
0.21	0.53	1.00	0.62	3.30	0.80	0.71	16.00	2.50	3.20	55.00	55.00	55.00	0.18	0.47	0.00	1.40	2.20	0.28	32.00
0.24	0.52	0.95	0.54	3.40	0.77	0.69	15.00	2.40	3.00	50.00	50.00	50.00	0.18	0.45	0.00	1.50	2.10	0.27	32.00
0.26	0.53	1.00	0.48	3.30	0.75	0.69	14.00	2.40	3.20	45.00	45.00	45.00	0.18	0.48	0.00	1.40	2.20	0.28	31.00
0.29	0.50	0.96	0.41	3.10	0.75	0.68	13.00	2.40	3.10	41.00	41.00	41.00	0.17	0.45	0.00	1.40	2.10	0.26	31.00
0.31	0.49	0.92	0.36	3.30	0.72	0.68	13.00	2.40	3.00	38.00	38.00	38.00	0.17	0.44	0.00	1.40	2.00	0.27	30.00
0.34	0.52	0.91	0.31	3.20	0.71	0.68	12.00	2.40	3.10	35.00	35.00	35.00	0.18	0.43	0.00	1.40	2.10	0.27	29.00
0.36	0.49	0.89	0.29	3.30	0.74	0.69	11.00	2.40	3.10	33.00	33.00	33.00	0.17	0.42	0.00	1.40	2.10	0.26	29.00
0.39	0.49	1.00	0.27	3.30	0.76	0.70	11.00	2.40	3.00	32.00	32.00	32.00	0.17	0.48	0.00	1.50	2.10	0.27	29.00
0.41	0.54	1.00	0.26	3.30	0.72	0.67	11.00	2.40	3.00	31.00	31.00	31.00	0.19	0.48	0.00	1.40	2.10	0.28	29.00
0.44	0.51	0.92	0.25	3.30	0.74	0.71	11.00	2.40	2.90	30.00	30.00	30.00	0.18	0.43	0.00	1.40	2.00	0.29	29.00
Top CSF	74.00	14.00	3.40	16.00	16.00	4.60	62.00	15.00	83.00	200.00	200.00	200.00	26.00	6.80	0.00	6.80	57.00	3.30	49.00
Bottom CSF	140.00	25.00	25.00	29.00	28.00	12.00	130.00	31.00	140.00	440.00	440.00	440.00	48.00	12.00	0.46	13.00	98.00	19.00	200.00
CSF % of Total dose	62.94	40.52	19.31	20.10	50.03	25.64	15.05	24.59	48.12	14.89	14.89	14.89	63.31	41.24		19.71	48.31	33.03	7.50
Range (cm)																			
50% Dose	0.01	0.01	0.06	0.01	0.01	0.01	0.09	0.01	0.01	0.09	0.09	0.09	0.01	0.01		0.01	0.01	0.01	>0.44
90% Total dose	0.06	0.36	0.29	0.39	0.34	0.39	0.36	0.39	0.31	0.34	0.34	0.34	0.29	0.36		0.39	0.31	0.36	0.39
Red marrow	0.750	0.520	0.170	0.590	0.290	0.120	1.900	0.160	0.950	12.000	1.500	4.900	0.300	0.350	0.019	0.500	1.000	0.120	2.400
Top CSF to marrow	98.67	26.92	20.00	27.12	55.17	38.33	32.63	93.75	87.37	16.67	133.33	40.82	86.67	19.43	0.03	13.60	57.00	27.50	20.42

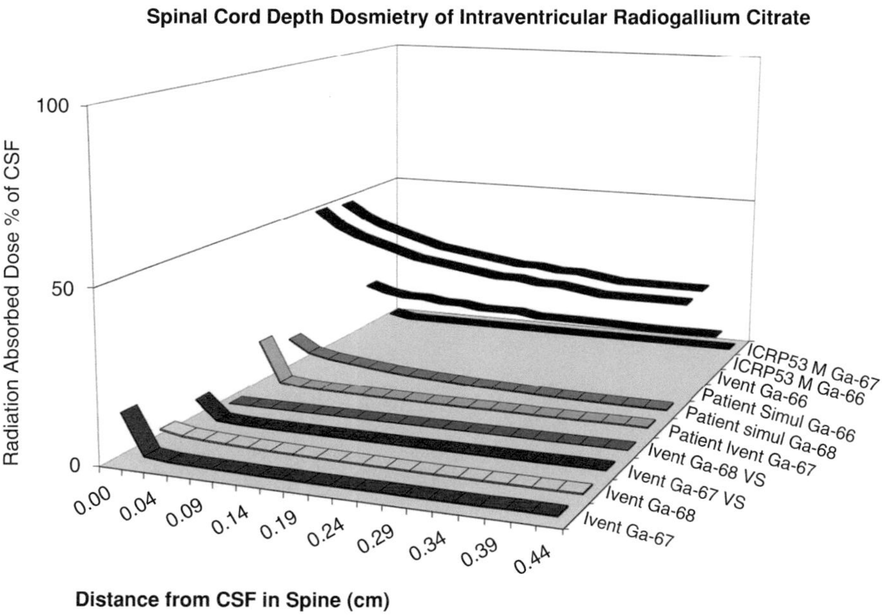

Fig. 9.10 Fractional dosimetry of intraventricular injection of Ga-66, Ga-67, and Ga-68

Table 9.8 Simulated radiation dosimetry of organs after intraventricular injection of 5 radiopharmaceuticals with and without ventricular stasis

cGy/mCi	Ivent	Ivent	Ivent	Ivent	Ivent	Ivent	Ivent	Ivent	Ivent	Ivent
Organ	Sm-153	Ga-67	Ga-68	In-111	I-131	Sm-153 VS	Ga-67 VS	Ga-68 VS	In-111 VS	I-131 VS
Adrenals	0.072	0.540	0.049	0.600	0.670	0.025	0.260	0.001	0.260	0.460
Brain	0.120	0.420	0.200	0.690	0.850	1.100	2.400	0.370	6.600	8.600
Breasts	0.009	0.150	0.005	0.065	0.120	0.003	0.072	0.001	0.035	0.097
Eyes	0.046	0.250	0.038	0.250	0.320	0.230	0.570	0.064	1.200	1.700
Lens of eyes	0.033	0.220	0.030	0.200	0.270	0.140	0.440	0.049	0.850	1.300
Gallbladder wall	0.007	0.240	0.002	0.140	0.110	0.002	0.110	0.000	0.063	0.073
LLI wall	0.018	0.590	0.004	0.250	0.160	0.006	0.280	0.000	0.110	0.110
Small intestine	0.023	0.270	0.018	0.220	0.250	0.008	0.130	0.000	0.098	0.170
Stomach	0.015	0.230	0.010	0.190	0.200	0.006	0.110	0.000	0.084	0.140
ULI wall	0.019	0.380	0.014	0.230	0.210	0.007	0.180	0.000	0.100	0.150
Heart wall	0.022	0.250	0.014	0.190	0.250	0.008	0.120	0.001	0.089	0.190
Kidneys	0.077	0.430	0.030	1.700	0.550	0.027	0.200	0.001	0.740	0.380
Liver	0.017	0.360	0.012	0.260	0.210	0.006	0.170	0.001	0.120	0.150
Lungs	0.026	0.230	0.014	0.180	0.240	0.010	0.110	0.002	0.096	0.200
Muscle	0.018	0.200	0.010	0.140	0.190	0.011	0.110	0.004	0.110	0.210
Ovaries	0.019	0.260	0.006	0.170	0.180	0.007	0.120	0.000	0.073	0.120
Pancreas	0.036	0.320	0.022	0.380	0.370	0.012	0.150	0.001	0.170	0.260
Red marrow	0.750	0.520	0.170	0.590	0.950	0.300	0.350	0.019	0.500	1.000
Bone surfaces	2.700	1.000	0.048	0.530	0.510	1.100	0.740	0.030	0.870	1.000
Skin	0.011	0.140	0.008	0.077	0.130	0.014	0.110	0.008	0.130	0.250
Spleen	0.018	0.440	0.014	1.000	0.220	0.006	0.210	0.001	0.450	0.160
Testes	0.011	0.160	0.002	0.076	0.110	0.004	0.076	0.000	0.033	0.077
Thymus	0.013	0.200	0.009	0.110	0.180	0.006	0.100	0.002	0.066	0.160
Thyroid	0.020	0.220	0.019	0.160	4.600	0.032	0.210	0.020	0.320	3.600
Urin bladder wall	2.400	0.240	0.004	0.980	1.900	0.830	0.110	0.000	0.430	1.300
Uterus	0.029	0.240	0.006	0.210	0.220	0.010	0.110	0.000	0.093	0.150
Total body	0.091	0.240	0.016	0.200	0.240	0.063	0.180	0.011	0.250	0.390
ED	0.340	0.360	0.080	0.460	0.620	0.200	0.320	0.031	0.640	0.990
EDE	0.250	0.330	0.030	0.290	0.600	0.100	0.190	0.006	0.210	0.530
Ventricle CSF	22.00	3.50	30.00	4.20	17.00	610.00	140.00	56.00	150.00	920.00
C-Spine CSF	74.00	14.00	3.40	16.00	83.00	26.00	6.80	0.00	6.80	57.00
L-Spine CSF	140.00	25.00	25.00	29.00	140.00	48.00	12.00	0.46	13.00	98.00
Convexity CSF	41.00	9.60	0.90	8.75	56.00	14.00	4.50	0.00	3.80	39.00
Skull	0.74	0.31	0.09	0.88	1.50	0.26	0.15	0.00	0.38	1.00
Vertebra	0.94	0.71	0.26	2.10	2.10	0.33	0.33	0.00	0.92	1.50
Red marrow	0.75	0.52	0.17	0.59	0.95	0.30	0.35	0.02	0.50	1.00
Ratios (Therapeutic windows)										
Ventricle CSF to BM	29.3	6.7	176.5	7.1	17.9	2033.3	400.0	2947.4	300.0	920.0
C-Spine CSF to BM	98.7	26.9	20.0	27.1	87.4	86.7	19.4	0.0	13.6	57.0
L-Spine CSF to BM	186.7	48.1	147.1	49.2	147.4	160.0	34.3	24.2	26.0	98.0
Convex CSF to BM	54.7	18.5	5.3	14.8	58.9	46.7	12.9	0.0	7.6	39.0

Results from Intralumbar Injections

CSF and Organ Dosimetry

Residence time estimates determined using the methodology described above for CSF spaces and all other organs from a bolus introduction into the lumbar CSF are shown in Table 9.9. Radiation absorbed doses to the normal organs and CSF compartments are listed in Table 9.10. High radiation absorbed dose to upper and lower spinal CSF compartments are noted with good therapeutic windows (i.e., high CSF to bone marrow ratios). Radiopharmaceuticals labeled with Samarium-153, I-124, I-131, Y-90, and Ga-66 have the highest absorbed dose per unit administered activity (cGy/mCi) values.

Table 9.9 Residence times (Hr) of CSF compartments and source organs for intralumbar injection models

Residence time (hr)	Physical T1/2	Lower CSF	Upper CSF	Cranial CSF	Adrenals	Brain	LL bowel	Sm bowel	Stomach	UL bowel	Heart	Kidneys	Liver	Red marrow	Cort. bone	Trab bone	Spleen	Lungs	Thyroids	Urin bladder	Remainder
Sm-153 EDTMP	46.7	9.5	8.6	3.2								0.0290	0.0210		5.2000	5.2000		0.0200		2.6000	7.4000
Sm-153 EDTMP LS	46.7	44.6	3.3	1.2																	
Ga-66 citrate	9.49	5.65	2.93	0.51	0.0020		0.1040	0.0940	0.0365	0.1550		0.0365	0.2160	0.2330	0.2150	0.3500	0.0320			0.0275	3.2200
Ga-67 citrate LS	78.3	10.6	10.4	4.5	0.0360		1.2000	0.2700		0.7800		0.5800	3.4000	3.7000	7.1000	1.8000	0.5100			0.2700	51.0000
Ga-67 citrate	78.3	61	5.2	2.2																	
Ga-68 citrate	1.1	1.3	0.2	0.01	0.0001		0.0003	0.0067		0.0025		0.0009	0.0053	0.0057	0.0110	0.0027	0.0008			0.0005	0.0790
Ga-68 citrate LS	1.1	1.57	0.01	0																	
In-111 Pentetreotide	67.9	10.3	9.9	4.11			0.2900	0.0660		0.1900		2.7000	0.9500				0.9600			2.2000	7.4000
In-111 Pentetreotide LS	67.9	56.4	4.6	1.9																	
Tl-201 Chloride	73.1	10.4	10.2	4.3		1.4200	2.0600	8.4000	1.6700	2.7500	1.9300	3.0700	2.7600					0.6100	0.3300	0.0700	39.3500
I-123 sodium iodide	13.2	6.52	3.95	0.84								0.0340							0.0048	0.4500	2.5000
I-124 sodium iodide	100.32	11.16	11.14	5.04								0.1000							0.1000	1.4000	8.5000
I-125 sodium iodide	1443.36	20.33	17.76	11.23								0.1300							1.1000	1.8000	9.9000
I-131 sodium iodide LS	193	12.9	12.9	6.6								0.1100							0.2100	1.6000	9.5000
I-131 sodium iodide	193	90.5	9.1	4.62																	
F-18 (FDG)	1.83	1.94	0.42	0.02		0.0218					0.0119	0.0030	0.0138				0.0010	0.0059		0.0129	0.1650
Y-90 chloride	64	10.2	9.7	3.9									10.3100		13.0600	21.2100				0.6300	6.8500
Y-90 DTPA	64	10.2	9.7	3.9																	
Y-90 Zevalin	64	10.2	9.7	3.9																	

Table 9.10 Simulated radiation dosimetry to organs and CSF from intralumbar injection of 14 radiopharmaceuticals

cGy/mCi	Ilumb	Ilumb	Ilumb	Ilumb	Ilumb	Ilumb	Ilumb	Ilumb	Ilumb	Ilumb	Ilumb	Ilumb	Ilumb	Ilumb
Organ	Sm-153	Ga-67	Ga-68	In-111	Tl-201	I-123	I-124	I-125	I-131	Y-90 Cl	Y-90 DTPA	Y-90 Aby	F-18 FDG	Ga-66
Adrenals	0.080	0.570	0.100	0.660	0.330	0.120	1.700	0.075	0.730	0.200	0.059	0.820	0.160	1.500
Brain	0.061	0.300	0.013	0.370	0.270	0.046	1.600	0.240	0.540	2.300	2.100	2.900	0.033	0.750
Breasts	0.009	0.150	0.009	0.068	0.097	0.012	0.230	0.013	0.120	0.200	0.059	0.820	0.014	0.260
Eyes	0.029	0.220	0.008	0.180	0.200	0.021	0.420	0.056	0.240				0.011	0.290
Lens of eyes	0.022	0.210	0.007	0.150	0.180	0.016	0.360	0.033	0.200				0.010	0.270
Gallbladder wall	0.007	0.240	0.004	0.150	0.280	0.029	0.450	0.019	0.100	0.200	0.059	0.820	0.035	0.470
LLI wall	0.019	0.600	0.009	0.260	0.860	0.020	0.320	0.021	0.160	0.200	0.059	13.000	0.013	1.100
Small intestine	0.025	0.280	0.037	0.240	1.200	0.037	0.530	0.024	0.260	0.200	0.059	3.800	0.040	0.700
Stomach	0.017	0.240	0.020	0.200	0.500	0.028	0.420	0.018	0.210	0.200	0.059	0.820	0.031	0.410
ULI wall	0.020	0.390	0.029	0.250	0.880	0.030	0.450	0.019	0.220	0.200	0.059	9.900	0.032	1.200
Heart wall	0.024	0.260	0.028	0.200	0.730	0.037	0.560	0.021	0.260	0.200	0.059	7.700	0.069	0.500
Kidneys	0.083	0.450	0.061	1.800	1.300	0.081	1.200	0.065	0.580	0.200	0.400	0.270	0.100	1.000
Liver	0.018	0.370	0.024	0.280	0.280	0.029	0.450	0.019	0.220	11.000	0.059	13.000	0.039	0.590
Lungs	0.029	0.230	0.027	0.190	0.170	0.036	0.520	0.025	0.250	0.200	0.059	5.500	0.046	0.470
Muscle	0.019	0.200	0.017	0.150	0.140	0.024	0.390	0.023	0.190	0.200	0.059	0.820	0.026	0.360
Ovaries	0.020	0.260	0.012	0.170	0.280	0.023	0.370	0.020	0.180	0.200	0.059	1.100	0.018	0.380
Pancreas	0.039	0.330	0.046	0.410	0.270	0.060	0.850	0.030	0.390	0.200	0.059	0.820	0.079	0.720
Red marrow	0.770	0.550	0.330	0.630	0.300	0.130	2.100	0.170	1.000	12.000	1.500	5.000	0.180	2.600
Bone surfaces	2.800	1.000	0.065	0.520	0.510	0.150	1.100	0.490	0.510	13.000	0.059	2.500	0.088	1.900
Skin	0.011	0.150	0.009	0.075	0.094	0.012	0.250	0.014	0.130	0.200	0.059	0.820	0.013	0.250
Spleen	0.020	0.450	0.028	1.100	0.190	0.031	0.480	0.019	0.230	0.200	0.059	26.000	0.040	0.740
Testes	0.011	0.170	0.004	0.078	2.100	0.011	0.200	0.016	0.110	0.200	0.059	25.000	0.005	0.210
Thymus	0.014	0.210	0.016	0.120	0.140	0.022	0.360	0.016	0.180	0.200	0.059	0.820	0.026	0.360
Thyroid	0.020	0.220	0.018	0.150	1.600	0.042	2.800	3.200	4.400	0.200	0.059	0.820	0.030	0.390
Urin bladder wall	2.500	0.240	0.007	1.000	0.140	0.130	2.300	0.350	1.800	3.100	7.300	2.500	0.030	0.360
Uterus	0.030	0.250	0.012	0.220	0.240	0.030	0.450	0.033	0.220	0.200	0.059	1.100	0.019	0.350
Total body	0.093	0.240	0.021	0.200	0.200	0.037	0.490	0.074	0.230	1.400	0.068	1.400	0.046	0.670
ED	0.350	0.360	0.065	0.460	0.820	0.049	0.720	0.260	0.600	2.500	0.430	8.800	0.047	0.790
EDE	0.260	0.340	0.055	0.310	0.940	0.060	1.000	0.190	0.590	3.000	0.810	12.000	0.065	0.900
Ventricle CSF	**0.00**	**0.00**	**0.00**	**0.00**	**0.00**	**0.00**	**0.00**	**0.00**	**0.00**	**0.00**	**0.00**	**0.00**	**0.00**	**0.00**
C-Spine CSF	**74.00**	**14.00**	**4.10**	**16.00**	**4.40**	**4.60**	**61.00**	**15.00**	**83.00**	**200.00**	**200.00**	**200.00**	**3.70**	**49.00**
L-Spine CSF	**170.00**	**32.00**	**60.00**	**37.00**	**9.70**	**17.00**	**160.00**	**38.00**	**180.00**	**550.00**	**550.00**	**550.00**	**38.00**	**280.00**
Convexity CSF	**26.00**	**6.30**	**0.10**	**5.70**	**7.20**	**0.93**	**15.00**	**9.22**	**39.00**	**43.00**	**43.00**	**43.00**	**0.14**	**3.70**
Skull	0.46	0.20	0.01	0.57	0.21	0.07	2.30	0.82	1.00	4.30	4.30	4.30	0.01	0.92
Vertebra	1.00	0.79	0.50	2.40	0.23	0.76	6.50	2.40	2.30	7.70	7.70	7.70	0.52	9.20
Red marrow	0.77	0.55	0.33	0.63	0.30	0.13	2.10	0.17	1.00	12.000	1.500	5.000	0.18	2.600
Ratios (Therapeutic windows)														
Ventricle CSF to BM	**0.0**	**0.0**	**0.0**	**0.0**	**0.0**	**0.0**	**0.0**	**0.0**	**0.0**	**0.0**	**0.0**	**0.0**	**0.0**	**0.0**
C-Spine CSF to BM	**96.1**	**25.5**	**12.4**	**25.4**	**14.7**	**35.4**	**29.0**	**88.2**	**83.0**	**16.7**	**133.3**	**40.0**	**20.6**	**18.8**
L-Spine CSF to BM	**220.8**	**58.2**	**181.8**	**58.7**	**32.3**	**130.8**	**76.2**	**223.5**	**180.0**	**45.8**	**366.7**	**110.0**	**211.1**	**107.7**
Convex CSF to BM	**33.8**	**11.5**	**0.3**	**9.0**	**24.0**	**7.2**	**7.1**	**54.2**	**39.0**	**3.6**	**28.7**	**8.6**	**0.8**	**1.4**

Absorbed Dose Vs. Depth

Absorbed dose vs. depth over the cerebral convexity and the cervical spine are listed in Tables 9.11 and 9.12, respectively. Absorbed dose as a function of depth in the cerebral convexity shows rapid decline with the half-dose range being at 0.15 cm in the convexity. In the cervical spinal cord, the half-dose range varies between 0.01 and 0.10 cm, except for Ga-66 (Table 9.12).

In the spinal cord (Table 9.12) radiation absorbed doses also showed rapid decline over distance from the CSF interface. Except for Ga-66, half-dose range occurs at 50% at the shell that is 0.10 cm from the CSF interface.

Table 9.11 Cerebral convexity absorbed dose vs. depth from CSF to 3 cm after intralumbar injection of 14 radiopharmaceuticals plus 5 under lumbar stasis (LS). Range parameters include distance (cm) to the shell that receives less than 50% of CSF radiation dose and distance to the shell that receives more than 90% of total radiation dose including CSF

cGy/mCi	Ilumb	Ilumb	Ilumb	Ilumb	Ilumb	Ilumb	Ilumb	Ilumb	Ilumb	Ilumb	Ilumb	Ilumb	Ilumb	Ilumb	Ilumb	Ilumb	Ilumb	Ilumb	Ilumb
Distance (cm)	Sm-153	Ga-67	Ga-68	In-111	Tl-201	I-123	I-124	I-125	I-131	Y-90 Cl	Y-90 DTPA	Y-90 Aby	Sm-153 LS	Ga-67 LS	Ga-68 LS	In-111 LS	I-131 LS	F18 FDG	Ga-66
0.00	26.00	6.30	0.10	5.70	7.20	0.93	15.00	9.22	39.00	43.00	43.00	43.00	9.90	3.20	0.00	2.65	27.00	0.14	3.70
0.05	3.30	0.36	0.05	0.80	0.28	0.08	7.90	0.54	5.10	23.00	23.00	23.00	1.30	0.18	0.00	0.37	3.60	0.03	2.40
0.15	0.15	0.18	0.02	0.47	0.13	0.05	4.10	0.42	0.63	11.00	11.00	11.00	0.06	0.09	0.00	0.22	0.44	0.01	1.60
0.25	0.06	0.15	0.01	0.43	0.11	0.04	2.40	0.36	0.55	6.40	6.40	6.40	0.02	0.08	0.00	0.20	0.38	0.00	1.30
0.35	0.05	0.13	0.01	0.39	0.09	0.04	1.60	0.32	0.50	3.40	3.40	3.40	0.02	0.07	0.00	0.18	0.35	0.00	0.97
0.45	0.05	0.13	0.00	0.38	0.09	0.04	1.30	0.31	0.49	1.70	1.70	1.70	0.02	0.06	0.00	0.18	0.34	0.00	0.78
0.55	0.05	0.12	0.00	0.35	0.08	0.03	1.10	0.28	0.46	0.74	0.74	0.74	0.02	0.06	0.00	0.16	0.32	0.00	0.62
0.65	0.05	0.11	0.00	0.33	0.08	0.03	0.95	0.28	0.44	0.27	0.27	0.27	0.02	0.06	0.00	0.16	0.31	0.00	0.50
0.75	0.05	0.11	0.00	0.33	0.07	0.03	0.92	0.26	0.43	0.08	0.08	0.08	0.02	0.06	0.00	0.15	0.30	0.00	0.40
0.85	0.05	0.11	0.00	0.31	0.07	0.03	0.86	0.24	0.42	0.02	0.02	0.02	0.02	0.05	0.00	0.15	0.29	0.00	0.32
0.95	0.04	0.10	0.00	0.30	0.07	0.03	0.84	0.22	0.40	0.01	0.01	0.01	0.02	0.05	0.00	0.14	0.28	0.00	0.27
1.05	0.04	0.10	0.00	0.29	0.07	0.03	0.82	0.22	0.40	0.00	0.00	0.00	0.02	0.05	0.00	0.14	0.28	0.00	0.23
1.15	0.04	0.10	0.00	0.29	0.07	0.03	0.78	0.21	0.38	0.00	0.00	0.00	0.02	0.05	0.00	0.13	0.27	0.00	0.20
1.25	0.04	0.10	0.00	0.28	0.07	0.03	0.78	0.21	0.38	0.00	0.00	0.00	0.02	0.05	0.00	0.13	0.27	0.00	0.19
1.35	0.04	0.10	0.00	0.27	0.06	0.03	0.75	0.20	0.37	0.00	0.00	0.00	0.02	0.05	0.00	0.13	0.26	0.00	0.17
1.45	0.04	0.09	0.00	0.26	0.06	0.03	0.72	0.18	0.36	0.00	0.00	0.00	0.02	0.05	0.00	0.12	0.26	0.00	0.16
1.55	0.04	0.09	0.00	0.25	0.06	0.03	0.71	0.18	0.35	0.00	0.00	0.00	0.02	0.05	0.00	0.12	0.25	0.00	0.15
1.65	0.04	0.09	0.00	0.25	0.06	0.02	0.70	0.17	0.35	0.00	0.00	0.00	0.02	0.05	0.00	0.12	0.24	0.00	0.15
1.75	0.04	0.09	0.00	0.25	0.06	0.03	0.67	0.16	0.35	0.00	0.00	0.00	0.02	0.05	0.00	0.12	0.25	0.00	0.14
1.85	0.04	0.09	0.00	0.25	0.06	0.03	0.72	0.16	0.34	0.00	0.00	0.00	0.02	0.05	0.00	0.12	0.24	0.00	0.14
1.95	0.04	0.09	0.00	0.24	0.06	0.02	0.71	0.16	0.33	0.00	0.00	0.00	0.02	0.04	0.00	0.11	0.23	0.00	0.14
2.05	0.04	0.09	0.00	0.23	0.06	0.02	0.66	0.14	0.33	0.00	0.00	0.00	0.01	0.04	0.00	0.11	0.23	0.00	0.14
2.15	0.04	0.08	0.00	0.23	0.06	0.02	0.65	0.13	0.32	0.00	0.00	0.00	0.01	0.04	0.00	0.11	0.22	0.00	0.14
2.25	0.04	0.08	0.00	0.23	0.06	0.02	0.66	0.14	0.32	0.00	0.00	0.00	0.01	0.04	0.00	0.11	0.22	0.00	0.14
2.35	0.04	0.08	0.00	0.23	0.06	0.02	0.68	0.13	0.32	0.00	0.00	0.00	0.01	0.04	0.00	0.11	0.22	0.00	0.14
2.45	0.04	0.08	0.00	0.23	0.06	0.02	0.65	0.13	0.32	0.00	0.00	0.00	0.01	0.04	0.00	0.11	0.22	0.00	0.14
2.55	0.04	0.08	0.00	0.22	0.06	0.02	0.67	0.13	0.31	0.00	0.00	0.00	0.01	0.04	0.00	0.10	0.22	0.00	0.14
2.65	0.04	0.08	0.00	0.22	0.06	0.02	0.63	0.12	0.31	0.00	0.00	0.00	0.01	0.04	0.00	0.10	0.22	0.00	0.13
2.75	0.04	0.08	0.00	0.22	0.06	0.02	0.59	0.13	0.31	0.00	0.00	0.00	0.01	0.04	0.00	0.10	0.21	0.00	0.13
2.85	0.04	0.08	0.00	0.22	0.06	0.02	0.56	0.12	0.30	0.00	0.00	0.00	0.01	0.04	0.00	0.10	0.21	0.00	0.13
2.95	0.04	0.08	0.00	0.21	0.06	0.02	0.57	0.11	0.30	0.00	0.00	0.00	0.01	0.04	0.00	0.10	0.21	0.00	0.12
CSF % of Total	84.92	65.87	43.55	38.88	75.95	51.32	29.62	59.25	70.69	47.96	47.96	47.96	84.59	66.18		38.78	70.42	54.50	23.30
Range at layer (cm)																			
50% Dose	0.05	0.05	0.15	0.05	0.05	0.05	0.15	0.05	0.05	0.15	0.15	0.15	0.05	0.05		0.05	0.05	0.05	0.15
90% Total dose	0.05	1.85	1.05	2.35	1.35	2.15	2.15	1.85	1.35	0.25	0.25	0.25	0.05	1.85		2.35	1.75	1.75	1.85
Red marrow	0.770	0.550	0.330	0.630	0.300	0.130	2.100	0.170	1.000	12.000	1.500	5.000	0.920	0.820	0.340	1.700	3.300	0.180	2.600
CSF to marrow	33.77	11.45	0.30	9.05	24.00	7.15	7.14	54.24	39.00	3.58	28.67	8.60	10.76	3.90	0.00	1.56	8.18	0.78	1.42

Table 9.12 Cervical spine depth radiation absorbed dosimetry from CSF interface to 0.44 cm after intralumbar injection of 14 radiopharmaceuticals plus 5 under lumbar stasis (LS). Range parameters include distance (cm) to the shell that receives less than 50% of CSF radiation dose and distance to the shell that receives more than 90% of total radiation dose including CSF

cGy/mCi	Ilumb	Ilumb	Ilumb	Ilumb	Ilumb	Ilumb	Ilumb	Ilumb	Ilumb	Ilumb	Ilumb	Ilumb	Ilumb	Ilumb	Ilumb	Ilumb	Ilumb	Ilumb	Ilumb
(cm)	Sm-153	Ga-67	Ga-68	In-111	Tl-201	I-123	I-124	I-125	I-131	Y-90 Cl	Y-90 DTPA	Y-90 Aby	Sm-153 LS	Ga-67 LS	Ga-68 LS	In-111 LS	I-131 LS	F18 FDG	Ga-66
0.00	74.00	14.00	4.10	16.00	4.40	4.60	61.00	15.00	83.00	200.00	200.00	200.00	29.00	7.40	0.27	7.91	59.00	3.70	49.00
0.01	21.00	2.30	2.80	5.70	0.54	1.20	43.00	3.10	25.00	140.00	140.00	140.00	8.20	1.40	0.23	3.38	19.00	1.50	45.00
0.04	8.50	1.60	2.30	4.00	0.31	0.81	36.00	2.90	11.00	120.00	120.00	120.00	3.60	0.97	0.20	2.51	8.20	0.81	42.00
0.06	4.00	1.40	1.90	3.70	0.28	0.80	32.00	2.80	5.80	110.00	110.00	110.00	1.70	0.94	0.19	2.47	4.90	0.55	40.00
0.09	1.90	1.30	1.70	3.60	0.26	0.76	28.00	2.70	4.00	95.00	95.00	95.00	0.84	0.90	0.19	2.45	3.70	0.42	38.00
0.11	1.10	1.20	1.40	3.60	0.25	0.75	24.00	2.70	3.50	84.00	84.00	84.00	0.53	0.81	0.19	2.39	3.40	0.36	36.00
0.14	0.78	1.10	1.20	3.40	0.24	0.74	22.00	2.60	3.30	75.00	75.00	75.00	0.41	0.78	0.17	2.28	3.20	0.35	35.00
0.16	0.62	1.10	1.10	3.60	0.23	0.73	20.00	2.60	3.30	68.00	68.00	68.00	0.35	0.87	0.16	2.54	3.10	0.35	34.00
0.19	0.55	1.00	0.93	3.50	0.22	0.72	18.00	2.60	3.30	61.00	61.00	61.00	0.32	0.78	0.16	2.46	3.20	0.35	33.00
0.21	0.53	1.00	0.81	3.30	0.22	0.72	17.00	2.50	3.20	55.00	55.00	55.00	0.31	0.80	0.16	2.37	3.30	0.35	32.00
0.24	0.52	0.96	0.71	3.40	0.21	0.70	15.00	2.40	3.10	50.00	50.00	50.00	0.32	0.68	0.16	2.27	3.00	0.34	32.00
0.26	0.53	1.00	0.64	3.30	0.20	0.70	14.00	2.50	3.20	45.00	45.00	45.00	0.32	0.77	0.16	2.18	3.00	0.34	31.00
0.29	0.50	0.97	0.55	3.20	0.20	0.69	13.00	2.40	3.10	41.00	41.00	41.00	0.30	0.81	0.14	2.20	3.10	0.33	31.00
0.31	0.49	0.93	0.48	3.30	0.20	0.69	13.00	2.40	3.00	38.00	38.00	38.00	0.31	0.75	0.12	2.41	2.90	0.33	30.00
0.34	0.53	0.92	0.42	3.20	0.19	0.69	12.00	2.40	3.10	36.00	36.00	36.00	0.35	0.67	0.11	2.20	3.10	0.33	30.00
0.36	0.49	0.89	0.40	3.30	0.20	0.70	11.00	2.40	3.10	33.00	33.00	33.00	0.31	0.61	0.12	2.24	3.00	0.33	29.00
0.39	0.49	1.00	0.37	3.40	0.21	0.70	11.00	2.50	3.00	32.00	32.00	32.00	0.29	0.81	0.12	2.21	3.00	0.33	29.00
0.41	0.55	1.00	0.36	3.30	0.20	0.68	11.00	2.50	3.00	31.00	31.00	31.00	0.37	0.86	0.12	2.40	3.10	0.34	30.00
0.44	0.51	0.94	0.36	3.30	0.20	0.72	11.00	2.40	2.90	30.00	30.00	30.00	0.31	0.96	0.14	2.05	3.30	0.35	30.00
Top CSF	74.00	14.00	4.10	16.00	4.40	4.60	61.00	15.00	83.00	200.00	200.00	200.00	29.00	7.40	0.27	7.91	59.00	3.70	49.00
Bottom CSF	170.00	32.00	60.00	37.00	9.70	17.00	160.00	38.00	180.00	550.00	550.00	550.00	820.00	180.00	74.00	202.00	1300.00	38.00	280.00
CSF % of Total dose	62.93	40.45	18.20	19.98	50.23	25.41	14.81	24.43	48.00	14.88	14.88	14.88	60.24	32.79	8.68	15.53	42.60	31.46	7.47
Range (cm)																			
50% Dose	0.01	0.01	0.06	0.01	0.01	0.01	0.11	0.01	0.01	0.09	0.09	0.09	0.01	0.01	0.31	0.01	0.01	0.01	>0.44
90% Total dose	0.06	0.36	0.31	0.39	0.34	0.39	0.36	0.39	0.31	0.34	0.34	0.34	0.09	0.39	0.39	0.39	0.34	0.36	0.39
Red marrow	0.770	0.550	0.330	0.630	0.300	0.130	2.100	0.170	1.000	12.000	1.500	5.000	0.920	0.820	0.340	1.700	3.300	0.180	2.600
Top CSF to BM	96.10	25.45	12.42	25.40	14.67	35.38	29.05	88.24	83.00	16.67	133.33	40.00	31.52	9.02	0.79	4.65	17.88	20.56	18.85

Lumbar Stasis (LS)

Simulation of lumbar stasis of 5 selected radiopharmaceuticals results in organ dosimetry as shown in Table 9.13. Absorbed dose vs. depth with the assumption of lumbar stasis is listed in Tables 9.11 and 9.12. Lumbar stasis markedly increases the

Table 9.13 Simulated radiation dosimetry of organs after intralumbar injection of 5 radiopharmaceuticals with and without lumbar stasis (LS)

cGy/mCi	Ilumb	Ilumb	Ilumb	Ilumb	Ilumb	Ilumb	Ilumb	Ilumb	Ilumb	Ilumb
Organ	Sm-153	Ga-67	Ga-68	In-111	I-131	Sm-153 LS	Ga-67 LS	Ga-68 LS	In-111 LS	I-131 LS
Adrenals	0.080	0.570	0.100	0.660	0.730	0.190	0.820	0.100	1.600	2.500
Brain	0.061	0.300	0.013	0.370	0.540	0.034	0.200	0.009	0.280	0.550
Breasts	0.009	0.150	0.009	0.068	0.120	0.010	0.110	0.007	0.110	0.210
Eyes	0.029	0.220	0.008	0.180	0.240	0.015	0.130	0.005	0.130	0.250
Lens of eyes	0.022	0.210	0.007	0.150	0.200	0.012	0.120	0.004	0.097	0.200
Gallbladder wall	0.007	0.240	0.004	0.150	0.100	0.003	0.120	0.000	0.070	0.076
LLI wall	0.019	0.600	0.009	0.260	0.160	0.013	0.330	0.006	0.180	0.220
Small intestine	0.025	0.280	0.037	0.240	0.260	0.045	0.270	0.024	0.410	0.640
Stomach	0.017	0.240	0.020	0.200	0.210	0.029	0.210	0.018	0.310	0.490
ULI wall	0.020	0.390	0.029	0.250	0.220	0.033	0.290	0.019	0.350	0.510
Heart wall	0.024	0.260	0.028	0.200	0.260	0.046	0.270	0.027	0.430	0.710
Kidneys	0.083	0.450	0.061	1.800	0.580	0.120	0.550	0.060	1.600	1.600
Liver	0.018	0.370	0.024	0.280	0.220	0.033	0.290	0.020	0.380	0.540
Lungs	0.029	0.230	0.027	0.190	0.250	0.049	0.260	0.026	0.410	0.680
Muscle	0.019	0.200	0.017	0.150	0.190	0.028	0.180	0.015	0.240	0.420
Ovaries	0.020	0.260	0.012	0.170	0.180	0.019	0.180	0.009	0.190	0.310
Pancreas	0.039	0.330	0.046	0.410	0.390	0.086	0.420	0.046	0.790	1.200
Red marrow	0.770	0.550	0.330	0.630	1.000	0.920	0.820	0.340	1.700	3.300
Bone surfaces	2.800	1.000	0.065	0.520	0.510	1.400	0.900	0.063	1.200	1.400
Skin	0.011	0.150	0.009	0.075	0.130	0.011	0.100	0.007	0.100	0.210
Spleen	0.020	0.450	0.028	1.100	0.230	0.036	0.340	0.022	0.770	0.580
Testes	0.011	0.170	0.004	0.078	0.110	0.005	0.086	0.001	0.042	0.091
Thymus	0.014	0.210	0.016	0.120	0.180	0.022	0.170	0.014	0.220	0.400
Thyroid	0.020	0.220	0.018	0.150	4.400	0.029	0.200	0.017	0.270	3.600
Urin bladder wall	2.500	0.240	0.007	1.000	1.800	0.980	0.140	0.003	0.510	1.400
Uterus	0.030	0.250	0.012	0.220	0.220	0.023	0.170	0.009	0.210	0.330
Total body	0.093	0.240	0.021	0.200	0.230	0.082	0.240	0.019	0.360	0.550
ED	0.350	0.360	0.065	0.460	0.600	0.250	0.360	0.064	0.640	1.200
EDE	0.260	0.340	0.055	0.310	0.590	0.200	0.300	0.055	0.470	1.000
Ventricle CSF	**0.00**	**0.00**	**0.00**	**0.00**	**0.00**	**0.00**	**0.00**	**0.00**	**0.00**	**0.00**
C-Spine CSF	**74.00**	**14.00**	**4.10**	**16.00**	**83.00**	**29.00**	**7.40**	**0.27**	**7.91**	**59.00**
L-Spine CSF	**170.00**	**32.00**	**60.00**	**37.00**	**180.00**	**820.00**	**180.00**	**74.00**	**202.00**	**1300.00**
Convexity CSF	**26.00**	**6.30**	**0.10**	**5.70**	**39.00**	**9.90**	**3.20**	**0.00**	**2.65**	**27.00**
Skull	0.46	0.20	0.01	0.57	1.00	0.18	0.10	0.00	0.27	0.72
Vertebra	1.00	0.79	0.50	2.40	2.30	2.60	2.40	0.49	6.90	8.70
Red marrow	0.77	0.55	0.33	0.63	1.00	0.92	0.82	0.34	1.70	3.30
Ratios (Therapeutic windows)										
Ventricle CSF to BM	**0.0**	**0.0**	**0.0**	**0.0**	**0.0**	**0.0**	**0.0**	**0.0**	**0.0**	**0.0**
C-Spine CSF to BM	**96.1**	**25.5**	**12.4**	**25.4**	**83.0**	**31.5**	**9.0**	**0.8**	**4.7**	**17.9**
L-Spine CSF to BM	**220.8**	**58.2**	**181.8**	**58.7**	**180.0**	**891.3**	**219.5**	**217.6**	**118.8**	**393.9**
Convex CSF to BM	**33.8**	**11.5**	**0.3**	**9.0**	**39.0**	**10.8**	**3.9**	**0.0**	**1.6**	**8.2**

radiation absorbed doses and therapeutic windows in lumbar CSF space and to a lesser degree in the cervical spine. Such increase if planned or known may allow for a planned increase to the ablation radiation dose to the region if needed. Alternatively, it may also allow lowering of injected activities to avoid systemic therapy. However, it may also cause increased toxicity if stasis was unexpended or not intended. These quantitative values of the effects on absorbed dose of ventricular stasis in the CSF and in the surrounding tissues may provide valuable guidance to manage LM treatment strategies when stasis is encountered.

Conclusion

Simulation of biokinetics using compartmental models, and Monte Carlo radiation transport using anthropomorphic models, along with published models of systemic administration dosimetry models, provides a basis for estimation of radiation absorbed dose in normal organs and in CSF compartments after intrathecal injection of radiopharmaceuticals either by intraventricular or intralumbar routes. The profiles of absorbed dose vs depth also allow estimation of radiation exposure in neural tissues adjacent to

CSF interface in the ventricle, cerebral convexity, and spinal canal. Dosimetric parameters of organ doses, CSF doses, half-dose ranges, and 90% total dose ranges allow evaluation of potential choices of radiopharmaceuticals, dosing schemes, and combination with other interventional modalities. These models also provide preliminary assessment of the potential effects of ventricular and/or lumbar stasis in the CSF.

It should be noted that since the conclusion of this modeling work roughly 20 years ago, continued advancement of CSF biokinetic models, radiation transport anthropomorphic models, and dosimetry software has occurred. However, the modeling utilized in this work should still give approximations to absorbed doses adequate for the evaluation of the *relative* merits of the prospective agents.

Discussion

Limitations of Dosimetric Models

The complicated admixture of anatomy and physiology is indeed difficult to model. Mathematical models provide conceptual representation that is subject to limitations of actual anatomy, physiology, pathology, and pharmacologic intervention. Standardized anthropomorphic models are used to represent body organs. While the 5-compartment biokinetic model in Fig. 9.3 is an attempt to address physiologic CSF flow, the simplified 4-compartment IRCP 53 model in Fig. 9.4 has been used more commonly. Elevated cranial residence times in Table 9.2 and increased convexity doses in Table 9.4 are noted with 4-compartment IRCP 53 model. The choice of 5-compartment model in Fig. 9.3 versus 4-compartment Fig. 9.4 could be arbitrated by image-derived residence times from serial imaging of patients. Further refinement of parameters in these biokinetic models (Figs. 9.3 and 9.4) may be another worthwhile exercise when image-derived residence times of the study radiopharmaceuticals become available for calibration.

Spinal fluid flow could be altered by pathology including LM [20]. Radiopharmaceutical retention or residence time in the CSF could be increased by binding to macromolecules inside spinal fluid or binding to the meninges. Active excretion from the meninges will decrease residence time and radiation absorbed doses. Intervention from radiation therapy, drug treatment, or surgical intervention may also alter CSF flows and dosimetry. With rational and reasonable models, CSF flow changes from pathologic alteration and /or treatment changes could be objectively assessed and quantified.

This study of dosimetric models also provides objective and rational common platforms to compare and choose candidate radiopharmaceuticals.

Prediction of Potential Toxicities and Efficacy in LM

Dosimetry results in Tables 9.3, 9.4, and 9.10 demonstrated the high radiation doses to the CSF compartments by Y-90 compounds necessary to ablate LM. However, Y-90 chloride would also have unacceptably high red marrow toxicity (12 cGy/

mCi) which manifests in low therapeutic windows. Because of the low model-based red marrow uptake and fast renal clearance, Y-90 DTPA has the lowest bone marrow dose (1.5 cGy/mCi). Conversely, Y-90 Zevalin would result in high radiation doses to the large bowel, liver, spleen, and testis (13, 13, 25, and 24 cGy/mCi, respectively). Based on either 4- or 5-compartment models, Y-90 DTPA would be a good candidate for LM therapy. Gallium 66 citrate may also be a good candidate, considering the high radiation doses to CSF compartments, but given the long range of increased absorbed doses vs. depth in the adjacent neural tissues, brain and spinal cord toxicity could be a limiting factor. Judicious use of modeling data presented in this study, along with empirical image data collection, will enable rational choice of radiopharmaceuticals for LM.

Dosing Considerations: An Example with Y-90 DTPA

The choice of dosing schemes with radiopharmaceuticals would consider potential toxicity to the critical organs (which would likely involve bone marrow), potential efficacy, dosing intervals, and cumulative toxicity from prior radiation or chemotherapy.

To design a single treatment session, high radiation dose to the target (CSF and meninges) and low radiation dose to critical organs are desirable. For instance, based on a red marrow dose of 1.5 cGy/mCi for Y-90 DTPA and a lethal dose of radiation to the marrow at 400 cGy [21] the intraventricular dose of Y-90 DTPA would reach the lethal red marrow radiation absorbed dose at 267 mCi. To set a safety zone of 50%, the maximum intraventricular dose of Y-90 DTPA will be 133 mCi. If this dose is fractionated into 6 weekly treatment sessions, it would be 22 mCi for each injection. The total radiation absorbed doses in the ventricle, cervical spine, lumbar spine, convexity, and red marrow would be 1386, 4400, 8800, 1474, and 33 cGy, respectively. Based on depth dosimetry in Tables 9.5, 9.6, and 9.7, radiation absorbed dose at 0.2 cm from the CSF interface will be 242, 1210, and 286 cGy for the ventricle, cervical spine, and convexity for each treatment session.

Furthermore, comparison of biologic half-lives in Tables 9.14 and 9.15 by simulation with those from image-based calculations will allow justification or modification of the models. Comparison of the biologic half-lives from radiopharmaceuticals of the same molecule labeled with different radionuclides may also determine whether biologic pathways are similar as null hypothesis.

Additional Dosimetric Considerations: CSF Blockage, Postsurgical Cavity Therapy

Ventricular stasis and lumbar stasis are worrisome conditions that may be encountered during intrathecal therapy. Modeling of these conditions provides insight and allows analysis of the loculated radiopharmaceuticals in the brain or spinal cord.

Table 9.14 Residence times (Table 9.2) and biologic half-lives (Tb) of intraventricular radiopharmaceuticals. VS indicates simulated ventricular stasis

Half-lives		Residence T (h)				Biologoic half-life (Tb)			
IVent radiopharmaceuticals	Physical Tp	Ventricle	Lower CSF	Upper CSF	Cranial CSF	Ventricle	Lower CSF	Upper CSF	Cranial CSF
Sm-153 EDTMP	46.70	1.27	7.43	8.66	5.20	0.90	5.80	6.90	3.91
Sm-153 EDTMP VS	46.70	39.90	2.60	3.00	1.80	68.13	1.88	2.18	1.28
Ga-66 citrate	9.49	1.31	4.09	2.94	1.33	1.01	4.05	2.60	1.02
Ga-66 citrate ICRP M	9.49	1.31	0.46	0.96	8.17	1.01	0.33	0.72	14.11
Ga-67 citrate	78.30	1.28	8.37	10.40	6.78	0.90	6.28	7.96	5.01
Ga-67 citrate VS	78.30	54.40	3.94	4.90	3.20	73.00	2.84	3.56	2.29
Ga-67 citrate ICRP M	78.30	1.42	3.08	6.37	22.05	1.00	2.20	4.69	19.04
Ga-68 citrate	1.10	0.69	0.55	0.18	0.09	0.85	0.59	0.14	0.07
Ga-68 citrate VS	1.10	1.45	0.01	0.00	0.00	11.90	0.01		
In-111 Pentetreotide	67.90	1.28	8.11	9.95	6.35	0.90	6.14	7.69	4.72
In-111 Pentetreotide VS	67.90	50.30	3.50	4.34	2.80	71.94	2.52	3.15	2.00
Tl-201 Chloride	73.10	1.42	8.24	10.18	6.57	1.00	6.21	7.83	4.87
I-123 sodium iodide	13.20	1.20	4.85	3.97	1.89	0.89	4.52	3.48	1.46
I-124 sodium iodide	100.32	1.29	8.84	11.16	7.54	0.90	6.54	8.40	5.52
I-125 sodium iodide	1443.36	1.30	16.25	17.76	15.80	0.90	11.37	12.44	11.06
I-131 sodium iodide	193.00	1.29	10.26	12.96	9.53	0.90	7.40	9.44	6.85
I-131 sodium iodide VS	193.00	79.70	7.03	8.90	6.50	77.60	5.01	6.39	4.62
I-131 sodium iodide ICRP M	193.00	1.44	4.39	9.09	26.56	1.01	3.10	6.53	20.39
F-18 flurodeoyglucose FDG	1.83	0.93	1.00	0.37	0.17	1.00	1.12	0.30	0.13
F-18 FDG ICRP M	1.83	0.93	0.02	0.05	1.55	1.00	0.01	0.04	2.61
Y-90 chloride	64.00	1.42	8.00	9.75	6.16	1.00	6.08	7.57	4.58
Y-90 DTPA	64.00	1.42	8.00	9.75	6.16	1.00	6.08	7.57	4.58
Y-90 DTPA ICRP M	64.00	1.42	2.78	5.76	20.91	1.00	1.99	4.27	18.78
Y-90 Zevalin	64.00	1.42	8.00	9.75	6.16	1.00	6.08	7.57	4.58

Table 9.15 Residence times (Table 9.9) and biologic half-lives (Tb) of intralumbar radiopharmaceutical. LS indicates simulated lumbar stasis

Half-lives	Physical Tp	Residence T(h)			Biologoic half-life (Tb)		
ILumb radiopharmaceuticals		Lower CSF	Upper CSF	Cranial CSF	Lower CSF	Upper CSF	Cranial CSF
Sm-153 EDTMP	46.70	9.50	8.60	3.20	7.68	6.85	2.33
Sm-153 EDTMP LS	46.70	44.60	3.30	1.20	91.96	2.41	0.85
Ga-66 citrate	9.49	5.65	2.93	0.51	6.69	2.59	0.37
Ga-67 citrate	78.30	10.60	10.40	4.50	8.12	7.96	3.25
Ga-67 citrate LS	78.30	61.00	5.20	2.20	92.29	3.79	1.56
Ga-68 citrate	1.10	1.30	0.20	0.01	5.04	0.16	0.01
Ga-68 citrate LS	1.10	1.57	0.01		90.61	0.01	
In-111 Pentetreotide	67.90	10.30	9.90	4.11	7.99	7.65	2.98
In-111 Pentetreotide LS	67.90	56.40	4.60	1.90	92.56	3.35	1.35
Tl-201 Chloride	73.10	10.40	10.20	4.30	8.01	7.84	3.11
I-123 sodium iodide	13.20	6.52	3.95	0.84	6.89	3.46	0.61
I-124 sodium iodide	100.32	11.16	11.14	5.04	8.40	8.38	3.63
I-125 sodium iodide	1443.36	20.33	17.76	11.23	14.26	12.44	7.84
I-131 sodium iodide	193.00	12.90	12.90	6.60	9.39	9.39	4.69
I-131 sodium iodide LS	193.00	90.50	9.10	4.62	93.19	6.53	3.26
F-18 flurodeoyglucose FDG	1.83	1.94	0.42	0.02	5.11	0.35	0.01
Y-90 chloride	64.00	10.20	9.70	3.90	7.96	7.53	2.83
Y-90 DTPA	64.00	10.20	9.70	3.90	7.96	7.53	2.83
Y-90 Zevalin	64.00	10.20	9.70	3.90	7.96	7.53	2.83

Such modeling in the ventricle (a cylinder of 1.6 cm in diameter and 9 cm in length) and in the lumbar spine (a cylinder of 22 cm and diameter of 0.9 cm) may allow application to understand focal CSF blockade. These models may also be applied to understand dosimetry of postsurgical cavities with which innovative radiopharmaceutical therapies have been designed and reported.

Appendix: Dosimetry Methods for Brain Dose as a Function of Depth

Anthropomorphic Model for Brain

Depth dose profiles in the brain from activity in the cranial CSF excluding the ventricles were calculated by determining absorbed fractions for the brain margins using Monte Carlo simulation of the radiation transport in a mathematical model of the head. This model was based on the model contained in Evans et al. [Evans 1995]. The general model was modified by removing all spinal parts, along with the eyes, tumor, and facial skeleton. The remaining model consisted of brain, cranial CSF, cranial skeleton, and soft tissue of the head and neck. The following equations were used for this modeling: (Note: Units of all of the following equations are in cm.)

Outer Surface of Brain:

$$\left(\frac{x}{6.51}\right)^2+\left(\frac{y}{8.51}\right)^2+\left(\frac{z-16.85}{5.66}\right)^2=1$$

Outer Surface of Cranial CSF:

$$\left(\frac{x}{6.6}\right)^2+\left(\frac{y}{8.6}\right)^2+\left(\frac{z-16.85}{5.75}\right)^2=1$$

Outer Surface of Cranial Skeleton:

$$\left(\frac{x}{7.5}\right)^2+\left(\frac{y}{9.5}\right)^2+\left(\frac{z-16.85}{6.65}\right)^2=1$$

Outer Surface of Soft Tissue of Neck:

$$\left[\frac{x}{8}\right]^2+\left[\frac{y}{10}\right]^2=1 \quad \text{and} \quad 0\le z\le 16.85$$

Outer Surface of Soft Tissue of Head:

$$\left[\frac{x}{8}\right]^2+\left[\frac{y}{10}\right]^2+\left[\frac{z-16.85}{7.15}\right]^2=1 \quad \text{and} \quad z\succ 16.85$$

Brain Margins were modeled as concentric ellipsoidal shells starting on the inside surface of the CSF going inward into the brain and each having a thickness of 1 mm. The inner and outer surface of each brain margin is described by the following set of equations:

Outer Surfaces 1 to 30:

$$\left(\frac{x}{6.61-(i\cdot 0.1)}\right)^2+\left(\frac{y}{8.61-(i\cdot 0.1)}\right)^2+\left(\frac{z-16.85}{5.76-(i\cdot 0.1)}\right)^2=1 \quad \text{i = 1 to 30}$$

Inner Surfaces 1 to 30:

$$\left(\frac{x}{6.51-(i\cdot 0.1)}\right)^2+\left(\frac{y}{8.51-(i\cdot 0.1)}\right)^2+\left(\frac{z-16.85}{5.66-(i\cdot 0.1)}\right)^2=1 \quad \text{i = 1 to 30}$$

Model For Ventricles

To calculate the dose to the brain from activity in the ventricles, the ventricles were modeled as two separate 1.57cm diameter cylinders running from anterior to posterior as defined by the equations below. For photon dose contributions to other organs, the cranial CSF results from Evans et al. [Evans 1995] were used.

$$\left(\frac{x+1.3}{0.7867}\right)^2+\left(\frac{z-16.85}{0.7867}\right)^2=1 \qquad -4.5\le y\le 4.5$$

$$\left(\frac{x-1.3}{0.7867}\right)^2+\left(\frac{z-16.85}{0.7867}\right)^2=1 \qquad -4.5\le y\le 4.5$$

Depth dose around the ventricles was determined by modeling 19 cylindrical shells around a single ventricle. Thickness of the shells ranged from 1 mm to 5 mm. These shells were modeled using the following equation where t_i is the thickness of the shell i.

$$\left(\frac{x-1.3}{0.7867+t_i}\right)^2+\left(\frac{z-16.85}{0.7867+t_i}\right)^2=1 \qquad -4.5\le y\le 4.5$$

Anthropomorphic Model For Spine

Depth dose profiles in the spinal cord were calculated by determining absorbed fractions for the spinal cord margins using Monte Carlo simulation of the radiation transport in a mathematical model of the spine, based on the model contained in Evans et al. [Evans 1995]. The model consisted of the spinal cord, the spinal CSF, and the surrounding bone, all contained in a soft tissue trunk as defined in the Cristy Eckerman phantom [Cristy 1987]. The following equations were used for this modeling: (Note: Units of all of the following equations are in cm.)

Soft Tissue Trunk:

$$\left(\frac{x}{20}\right)^2+\left(\frac{y}{10}\right)^2\leq 1 \qquad 0\leq z\leq 70$$

Spinal Cord:

$$\left(\frac{x}{0.45}\right)^2+\left(\frac{y-5.5}{0.45}\right)^2\leq 1 \qquad 25.97\leq z\leq 70$$

Spinal cord depth dose profiles were determined by using margins modeled as concentric ellipsoidal shells starting on the inside surface of the CSF going inward into the spinal cord and each having a thickness of 0.25 mm. The surfaces of the spinal cord margins are described by the following set of equations:

Spinal Cord Margin Surfaces:

$$\left(\frac{x}{0.45-(i\cdot 0.025)}\right)^2+\left(\frac{y-5.5}{0.45-(i\cdot 0.025)}\right)^2=1 \qquad i=1 \text{ to } 18$$

Spinal CSF:

$$\left(\frac{x}{0.8}\right)^2+\left(\frac{y-5.5}{0.8}\right)^2\leq 1 \qquad 11.46\leq z\leq 70$$

Exclusive of the spinal cord. The spinal CSF was split into two regions corresponding to the ICRP-53 (3) CSF kinetic model with a bounding plane located at z=25.97 cm.

Vertebral Bone:

$$\left(\frac{x}{2.0}\right)^2+\left(\frac{y-5.5}{2.5}\right)^2\leq 1 \qquad 11.46\leq z\leq 70$$

Exclusive of the spinal cord and spinal CSF.

References

1. Sakka L, Coll G, Chazal J. Anatomy and physiology of cerebrospinal fluid. Eur Ann Otorhinolaryngol Head Neck Dis. 2011;128(6):309–16.
2. Dreha-Kulaczewski S, et al. Respiration and the watershed of spinal CSF flow in humans. Sci Rep. 2018;8(1):5594.
3. Enzmann DR, Pelc NJ. Normal flow patterns of intracranial and spinal cerebrospinal fluid defined with phase-contrast cine MR imaging. Radiology. 1991;178(2):467–74.

4. Levy LM, Di Chiro G. MR phase imaging and cerebrospinal fluid flow in the head and spine. Neuroradiology. 1990;32(5):399–406.
5. Radiation dose to patients from radiopharmaceuticals (addendum 2 to ICRP publication 53). Ann ICRP. 1998;28(3):1–126.
6. ICRP. Radiation dose to patients from radiopharmaceuticals. Addendum 3 to ICRP Publication 53. ICRP Publication 106. Approved by the Commission in October 2007. Ann ICRP. 2008;38(1–2):1–197.
7. Stabin M, et al. Radiation dosimetry for technetium-99m-MAG3, technetium-99m-DTPA, and iodine-131-OIH based on human biodistribution studies. J Nucl Med. 1992;33(1):33–40.
8. Eary JF, et al. Samarium-153-EDTMP biodistribution and dosimetry estimation. J Nucl Med. 1993;34(7):1031–6.
9. Stabin MG, et al. Radiation dosimetry for indium-111-pentetreotide. J Nucl Med. 1997;38(12):1919–22.
10. Hays MT, et al. MIRD dose estimate report no. 19: radiation absorbed dose estimates from (18)F-FDG. J Nucl Med. 2002;43(2):210–4.
11. ICRP. ICRP publication 30, part 1. Ann ICRP. 1979.
12. Wiseman GA, et al. Radiation dosimetry results for Zevalin radioimmunotherapy of rituximab-refractory non-Hodgkin lymphoma. Cancer. 2002;94(4 Suppl):1349–57.
13. MCNP Manual. Monte Carlo N-particle transport code system. RSIC; 1994.
14. Weber DA, et al. MIRD radionuclide data and decay schemes. Society of Nuclear Medicine; 1989.
15. Loevinger R, Budinger T, Watson EE, editors. MIRD primer for absorbed dose calculations. New York: S.o.N. Medicine; 1991.
16. Evans JF, Stabin MG, Stubbs JB. Specific absorbed fractions of energy from internal photon sources in brain tumor and cerebrospinal fluid. Med Phys. 1995;22(3):331–40.
17. Cristy M, Eckerman K. Specific absorbed fractions of energy at various ages from internal photon sources. In: ORNL/TM-8381/V1. Oak Ridge National Laboratory; 1987.
18. ICRP Publication 60. 1990 recommendations of the international commission on radiological protection. Ann ICRP 21, vol. 1–3. Pergamon Press; 1991.
19. Wong FSR. Simulation of radiation dosimetry of intraventricular injection of commercially available radiopharmaceuticals for intrathecal radionuclide therapy. Radiology. 2021;165: p. Abstract accepted and presented in RSNA 2021.
20. Glantz MJ, et al. A randomized controlled trial comparing intrathecal sustained-release cytarabine (DepoCyt) to intrathecal methotrexate in patients with neoplastic meningitis from solid tumors. Clin Cancer Res. 1999;5(11):3394–402.
21. Chang DS, et al. Basic radiotherapy physics and biology. Cham: Springer; 2014. p. 1. Online resource (XIX, 348 pages 158 illustrations, 147 illustrations in color.

Chapter 10
Human Radiation Dosimetry from Imaging: Guidance for Therapy

Richard E. Wendt III

Introduction

The fundamental concept of internal dosimetry is that sources of ionizing radiation within the body irradiate targets of that radiation within the body into which energy is deposited. Typically, the rate at which the radiation absorbed dose (i.e., the energy per unit mass) is delivered is low compared to that in external beam radiotherapy, and the primary consideration has thus been the dose delivered and not the rate at which it was delivered. This helps to explain why the biological effect of doses from radionuclide therapies may differ from that delivered by external beam therapy [1].

The Medical Internal Radiation Dose Committee (MIRD) schema [2, 3] is widely used for internal dosimetry. It has matured from relatively simplistic models of human anatomy at its inception to much more sophisticated and realistic ones today. In its simpler forms, the MIRD approach considers whole organs containing a uniform spatial distribution of a radionuclide as the sources and whole organs as the targets in which the average energy per unit mass of the target is determined. The passage of radiation from the source to the target and its absorption in the target is characterized by sets of representative phantoms in which the radiation transport has been simulated by Monte Carlo techniques. Although the word dosimetry implies that a dose is being measured, in fact, the vast majority of internal doses are estimated rather than being truly measured.

The disintegration of the radionuclides that are most commonly encountered in Nuclear Medicine might release penetrating radiation in the form of gamma rays or X-rays and non-penetrating radiation in the form of conversion electrons, Auger

R. E. Wendt III (✉)
Department of Imaging Physics, The University of Texas MD Anderson Cancer Center, Houston, TX, USA
e-mail: rwendt@mdanderson.org

F. C. L. Wong (ed.), *Radiopharmaceuticals in the Management of Leptomeningeal Metastasis*, https://doi.org/10.1007/978-3-031-14291-8_10

electrons, beta particles, alpha particles, or positrons. The charged particles in non-penetrating radiation might subsequently produce penetrating radiation through the bremsstrahlung effect or the annihilation of a positron with an electron. While the non-penetrating radiation delivers most of the therapeutic effect in close proximity to the site of the disintegration, the penetrating radiation delivers a dose to more distant targets and is also the means by which the spatial distribution of the radionuclide within the body and the changes in that distribution over time are detected and measured from outside of the patient's body.

The customary approach to making these measurements is to take images of the patient at a number of times after the administration of the radionuclide. Ideally, these images would be quantitative so that they would reflect the actual radioactivity that is present in various regions of the image. From these images, the radioactivity in the source regions may be determined. The time series of these measurements then can be viewed as a time–activity curve in which the measured radioactivity is plotted as a function of time. If the temporal measurements are sufficient in number and in temporal distribution, the underlying continuous–time curve may be estimated with high fidelity. Because radioactivity is the rate of disintegration, i.e., disintegrations per unit time, the integral of the time–activity curve, which is the area under that curve, gives the number of disintegrations that are represented by the curve. The number of disintegrations, which is known as the cumulated activity or the time-integrated activity, is related to the energy that is absorbed in a target region by a factor that is known as the S-value or the dose conversion factor. This factor, which is the dose in the target region per disintegration in the source region, embodies the radiation transport between the source and target through the specific model of the patient that is being used. These factors are typically pre-computed for specific radionuclides and patient models for the sake of efficiency. A patient-specific calculation would be ideal but would require supporting data such as a whole-body CT scan that might not be available. In order to get such an estimate in a clinically useful time would require more computational resources than many clinics currently have. However, the future ability to perform practical patient-specific dosimetry is foreseeable as technology advances.

Radionuclide and Radiopharmaceutical Properties

A number of different radionuclides have been used in the diagnosis, treatment planning, or treatment of leptomeningeal conditions. Their salient features for quantitative imaging are given in Table 10.1. These features have been abstracted for the most part from the MIRD radionuclide data [4].

The pharmaceutical to which the radionuclide is bound affects how the administered activity is distributed within the leptomeningeal space and how the portion of the administered activity that leaves that space passes through the rest of the body.

Table 10.1 Salient imaging features of relevant radionuclides

Radionuclide	Major photon emissions energy (abundance[a])	Physical half-life
Tc-99m	119.5 keV (8.92%) 140.5 keV (89.1%)	6.015 h
I-124	511 keV[b] (45.7%) 602.7 keV (62.9%) 722.8 keV (10.4%) 1.691 MeV (10.9%)	4.176 days
I-125	~27 keV (115%) 31 keV (13%)	59.4 days
I-131	364.5 keV (81.7%) 637 keV (7.17%) 722.9 keV (1.77%)	8.0207 days
In-111	171.3 keV (90.6%) 245.4 keV (94.1%)	2.8047 days
Au-198	411.8 keV (95.6%)	2.69517 days
Y-90	511 keV[b] (32 ppm) Bremsstrahlung X-rays	2.671 days
Y-86	511 keV[b] (63.8%) 443.1 keV (16.9%) 627.7 keV (32.6%) 703.3 keV (15.4%) 777.4 keV (22.4%) 1.077 MeV (82.5%) 1.153 MeV (30.5%) 1.921 MeV (20.8%)	14.74 h
Zr-89	511 keV[b] (45.5%) 909.2 keV (99.0%)	3.267 days
F-18	511 keV[b] (193%)	109.77 min

[a]The abundance is also called the branching ratio
[b]Co-incidence photons

The effective half-life in various compartments may well vary among the radiopharmaceuticals and thus the times at which images are acquired must be chosen consistently with these different effective half-lives.

Quantitative Imaging of Radionuclides

In most cases, especially when a radiopharmaceutical is distributed widely throughout the body, imaging is superior to probe-based measurements for dosimetric purposes. Gamma cameras that are based upon single, large scintillation crystals of sodium iodide doped with thallium backed by an array of photomultiplier tubes that are read out using Anger logic [5] are most commonly employed.

When a choice is available, a camera with a thicker crystal should be used for I-131 and In-111. A camera with a 5/8″ thick sodium iodide crystal is about 1.55 times as sensitive as one with a 3/8″ thick crystal to the 364 keV photopeak of I-131. It is about 1.3 times as sensitive to the 173 keV photopeak and 1.48 times as sensitive to the 247 keV photopeak of In-111. Newer gamma camera technology that employs cadmium zinc telluride (CZT) detectors is optimized for the 140 keV photopeak of Tc-99m and lower energies. It is less well-suited to the imaging of medium and high energy radionuclides such as In-111 and I-131, although medium energy collimators are offered for most CZT-based cameras.

The parallel-hole collimator of the gamma camera detector absorbs photons that are not normally incident upon the face of the detector. Parallel-hole collimators have the desirable property that their sensitivity does not vary substantially with the distance of the source from the collimator. There are trade-offs among sensitivity, spatial resolution, and septal penetration in the design of a collimator. Typically, higher performance in one aspect, such as spatial resolution, implies lower performance in the others, such as sensitivity. Most gamma camera manufacturers supply only a single design for a high energy collimator that is suitable for I-131. Because of the very high energy 637 and 723 keV gamma emissions of I-131, there is visible septal penetration even with a collimator that is well-designed to handle the 364 keV gamma rays that dominate the spectrum of the source in air and are used for image formation.

It is possible to purchase after-market collimators with characteristics that are different than those of the original equipment manufacturers' collimators, as well as ones that are specially built to the customer's specifications. With these, the user must be prepared to incorporate such a collimator's non-standard characteristics into the subsequent data processing, especially in tomographic reconstruction algorithms that incorporate a model of the collimator response.

The most commonly employed scintigraphy for dosimetry consists of opposed-view, whole-body scans using large, rectangular field of view detectors. The patient is translated with respect to the detectors so that over the course of the image acquisition time, the entire body is imaged. The data are presented as a rectangular, static image even though the data were not all acquired during the same time interval and thus there could be biodistribution during the acquisition of the overall image.

Scintigraphy is subject to the effects of the absorption of some of the emitted photons by the patient and the scattering of photons within the patient (and to a lesser extent, within the detector). These effects give rise to the attenuation of the counts from the patient and the mislocation of some of them within the image. As a consequence, the calibration of counts in a pixel of the image to the radioactivity within the corresponding volume of the patient requires that these effects be minimized if not corrected for.

Attenuation correction can be accomplished in several ways. The long-standing approach in whole-body imaging is to make a transmission scan of the patient prior to the administration of the radiopharmaceutical. This is done by positioning the patient on the scanner table in the same way that the post-administration scans will be performed, placing a sheet source beneath the patient (often on the bottom detector of the camera) and acquiring a whole-body scan using the other detector. This scan will resemble a low spatial resolution whole-body X-ray. A scan of the sheet source in the absence of the patient, which is called the "blank scan," is needed for the calibration of the transmission scan. Unless the radionuclide in the sheet source is the same as that of the radiopharmaceutical, the transmission scan must be corrected for the different attenuation by the patient's body of the photons from the different radionuclides [6]. Since this transmission scan is affected by the entire projected thickness of the patient at a particular point in the image, it cannot be used to correct the subsequently acquired radiopharmaceutical images from each of the two opposing views. However, if those two views are combined in a geometric mean by taking the square root of the product of the counts in each image, then the resulting data can be corrected for attenuation by applying the square root of the ratio of the blank scan to the transmission scan to the geometric mean data.

Another approach to attenuation correction is to exploit the fact that many patients receive computed tomography scans as part of their overall workups. Unfortunately, the topogram or scout view, which looks like a whole-body X-ray and is used for prescribing the coverage of the transaxial slices, has spatial distortions that arise from the fan-beam geometry of modern CT scanners. However, the actual transaxial CT slices can be reprojected in the same orientation as the geometric mean whole-body radiopharmaceutical image, which is typically an anterior–posterior view, to give a geometrically accurate X-ray. With proper corrections for different energies, which are well-understood in the attenuation correction of SPECT/CT and PET/CT data, the transmission correction could also be determined in this manner.

Ideally, since the gamma emissions of radionuclides are mono-energetic, any photon that was detected at an energy below the photopeak energy could be considered to have scattered and one would use a very narrow energy window centered on the photopeak energy. In practice, the energy resolution of the NaI(Tl) detector, which is on the order of 10%, and the variation in energy response across the face of the gamma camera detector mean that an energy window width of 15–20% of the photopeak energy is needed in order to capture all of the unscattered photons from the photopeak. As a consequence, there are also many scattered photons that fall within the photopeak energy window. The imaging of the bremsstrahlung X-rays from Y-90 is unusual in that there is no photopeak but rather a broad continuous spectrum. Rong et al. found that the best energy window for their experimental conditions was from 100 to 160 keV [7], and others have come to a similar conclusion for P-32, another pure beta-emitter [8].

Correction for scattering of photons within the body is based upon the loss of energy that scattering photons undergo [5]. One can place an energy window below the photopeak window and acquire counts that could not have arisen from unscattered photons. These can then be used to estimate the number of counts in the photopeak window that have arisen from scattered photons and thereby to correct the counts in the photopeak window to reflect those only from unscattered photons.

Referring to Table 10.1, Tc-99m has a minor photon emission at about 122 keV, which should be taken into account when ascribing the number of counts in an energy window below the 140.5 keV photopeak window to scatter. Although the photopeak of I-131 at 364 keV is the one that is used for imaging, gamma emissions at 637 and 723 keV will scatter down into the 364 keV photopeak window. Thus, for I-131, a triple energy window approach is used in which an energy window about the 364 keV photopeak window is used to estimate down-scatter from the higher energy emissions, while an energy window below the 364 keV photopeak window is used to estimate the scattering of the 364 keV emissions within the photopeak window [9]. For the imaging of In-111, a triple-window approach that combines 20% photopeak windows at 171 and 245 keV with a single 10% scatter window between them at 209 keV was found to produce the best clinical results [10]. Other investigators have used additional energy windows [11].

It should be noted that CZT detectors have much better energy resolution than do NaI(Tl)-based detectors and thus may be capable of more accurate scatter correction of their images.

The standard approach to calibration is to include a source of known activity within the image. It should be about 1% of the activity that was administered to the patient. After all of the desired corrections have been applied to the image, the counts in a region of interest that surrounds the standard source, the duration of the image acquisition, and the activity of the source at the time that the image was acquired can be used to compute a calibration factor in terms of counts per unit time per unit activity (e.g., cpm/uCi or cpm/kBq). When a single standard source is used, it is commonly placed in air. In some protocols, another standard source is placed in a device such as a block or cylinder of acrylic plastic that introduces both scatter and attenuation of that source. If this is the case, that device should be included in the transmission scan so that its attenuation properties can be measured. It is important that the source be positioned far enough away from the patient that there be little scatter of photons from the source that interact with the patient and then reach the detector and thus appear in the image. A separation of 2–3″ (5–8 cm) is sufficient in most cases. If the standard cannot be placed in the patient scan, a separate scan of the standard alone should be obtained using the same camera settings. One of the uses of the standard source information besides calibration is verification that the camera is working properly from day to day. The imaged activity in the standard source should decay with the physical half-life of the radionuclide if the camera is set up the same (e.g., with the same energy window settings) for each image and if the corrections for possibly different scanning speeds in different images have been properly applied.

Whether administered via the lumbar route as illustrated in Fig. 10.1 of Hesterman et al. [12] or through an intra-cranial port as illustrated in Figs. 2 and 3 of Wong and Kim [13] and in Fig. 2 of Larson et al. [14], the biodistribution of an intrathecal radiopharmaceutical is complicated. It can take several hours for the radioactivity to reach the opposite end of the CSF space. The concentration of the radiopharmaceutical at a particular point will vary depending upon its location and

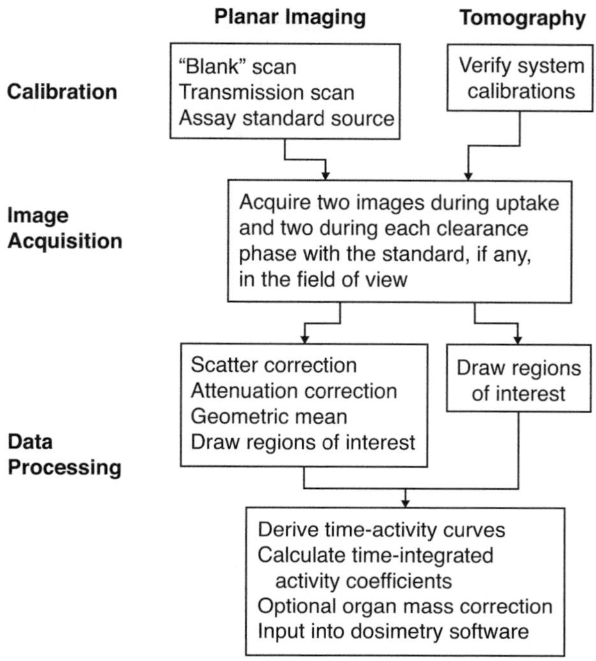

Fig. 10.1 Workflow for the use of quantitative imaging in dosimetry

the time since the administration. The model of Stabin and Evans [15] assumed just a lumbar injection site CSF compartment, a spinal CSF compartment, and a brain CSF compartment.

When one is considering a simple situation in which there is an uptake phase and then a clearance phase, it is recommended to acquire a very early image and another image close to the peak of the uptake. At least two images should be acquired for each clearance phase (e.g., two for a single exponential clearance and four for a bi-exponential clearance) during the interval when that phase dominates the time–activity curve. These measurements should ideally span five effective half-lives of the radiopharmaceutical, although as a practical matter, much more than a week of imaging (e.g., one physical half-life of I-131) may be prohibitively difficult both for the patient from a logistical perspective and for the clinical need to proceed with treatment in a timely manner.

The positron emitters in Table 10.1 are typically imaged by positron emission tomography (PET). Modern PET includes a low-dose CT scan for attenuation correction. The calibration and quality assurance of a PET scanner ensures that the resulting images are quantitative, often in units of kBq/cc. Most commercially available PET scanners have axial fields of view of 15–25 cm and thus require that the patient be translated with respect to the scanner over the course of the image acquisition, just as is done in whole-body gamma camera imaging.

Yttrium-90 is a particularly challenging radionuclide to image. It is generally considered to be a pure beta-emitter, although those emissions produce bremsstrahlung X-rays that can be imaged with a gamma camera, and there are also very low abundance co-incidence photons arising from pair production that can be imaged with a PET scanner. The bremsstrahlung images have low spatial resolution and are difficult to quantify, whereas the co-incidence images take an impractically long time to acquire. The use of Y-86 as a surrogate has been proposed because of its 63.8% abundant co-incidence photons. The use of Zr-89 as a surrogate when the chemistry is propitious has been proposed because of the complicated decay scheme of Y-86.

Both I-124 and Y-86 have many photon emissions in addition to the annihilation photons that arise from their proton emissions. These other photons give rise to a relatively high singles rate and the prompt gammas can elevate the false co-incidence rates in PET images [16, 17]. Appropriate, radionuclide-specific corrections should be applied.

An important factor in the accuracy of dosimetric imaging is the reproducibility of the patient positioning. With the longer-lived radionuclides, several separate imaging sessions are required. The patient immobilizers that are used in radiotherapy can be effective for this application. One common immobilizer technology is an airtight bag that is filled with small plastic beads. The bag is placed on the scanner table and the patient lies upon it in the imaging position. A vacuum is drawn on the bag, which evacuates the air within it and causes it to become firm and to conform to the patient's contours. As long as the vacuum is maintained, the patient can arise from the table and lie down again on the immobilizer and be able to feel when he or she is properly positioned. This also can make the patient more comfortable during long acquisitions because the patient can relax instead of actively having to hold still in a particular position. It is also a good idea to make an indentation in the immobilizer for each standard source so that it can be positioned consistently in each image.

Data Processing for Dosimetry

Several software packages for internal dosimetry are reaching the stage of commercial availability. These automate some of the processing steps that are described below, and they potentially interface their outputs with other tools and picture archiving and communication systems (PACS).

Regions of interest are outlines of organs in the images. In most software systems, they may be drawn by hand. Some software has automated tools that detect the boundaries between organs and produce the outline. Subsequent manual editing of automatically defined boundaries can usually be performed if necessary. Volumes of interest are three-dimensional extensions of regions of interest. The simplest ones are simply stacks of the two-dimensional regions of interest from the slices of a tomographic acquisition. In the case of SPECT/CT, PET/CT, and PET/MR, the CT or MR is usually well-aligned with the SPECT or PET and thus one can use the CT or MR images for the definition of the regions of interest for various organs.

The usual steps in processing whole-body, opposed-view planar images are to compute a scatter-corrected image if multiple energy windows were acquired for that purpose. At this point, one can continue with a pixel-by-pixel processing or analyze composite data from regions of interest. The author has found that the two approaches give very similar results on the same data sets.

The transmission image must be converted to attenuation correction factors, and it might need to be adjusted for the difference in photopeak energy between the sheet source radionuclide, which is often Co-57, and the radionuclide of interest. If the radionuclide is the same, the attenuation correction factor is the square root of the ratio of the unobstructed counts in the so-called blank scan (C_B) to the counts in the transmission scan (C_T), $\mathrm{ACF} = \sqrt{C_B / C_T}$. If the radionuclides are different, then the attenuation correction factor is the square root of the ratio of the blank scan to the transmission scan raised to the power of the ratio of the mass attenuation coefficient of the radionuclide of interest (μ_{Em}) to the mass attenuation coefficient of the radionuclide with which the transmission scan was made (μ_{Tm}), $\mathrm{ACF} = \sqrt{\left(C_B / C_T\right)^{(\mu_{Em}/\mu_{Tm})}}$.

In the pixel-by-pixel analysis, a geometric mean image is calculated by reversing the posterior image left for right, multiplying together the corresponding pixels in each scatter-corrected image and taking the square root of each resulting pixel. This geometric mean image is then multiplied, pixel-by-pixel, by the attenuation correction factor image.

There are two approaches to calibrating the resulting image. One is to use the known activity of the standard and the number of counts in a region of interest surrounding it to yield the counts per unit activity. Each pixel in the image can be divided by this sensitivity factor to yield an image in units of activity. The other approach is to assume that all of the administered activity is present in the image that is made at the first time point. For this to be valid, the patient should not have urinated since the administration of the radiopharmaceutical.

Regions of interest are drawn around the whole body, the standard source, and particular organs or areas in which there is a visible concentration of radioactivity. If the images are not well-registered spatially, then the regions might have to be moved on individual images. In planar images, there can be counts within a region of interest that come from overlying and underlying tissues rather than the organ or tumor itself. One way to correct this, at least approximately, is to draw a so-called background region near the region in question and over an area that appears to have typical uptake in it. The counts in that region represent the tissues surrounding the region of interest and if subtracted from those in the region of interest would leave only the counts that came from the actual source. Sometimes the best image in which to visualize a source region is not the initial image but rather one of the later ones after there has been uptake in the source region and clearance from the non-targeted tissues.

A time–activity curve is constructed for each region by plotting the total activity in a region in each image against the time at which each of the images was acquired. If the radionuclide in the dosimetric images is the same as the radionuclide in the therapeutic radiopharmaceutical, then these data points may be fit directly so that the area under the curve, which is the number of disintegrations that took place within that region of interest, may be determined. If this area is divided by the administered activity, the result will have the dimension of time. In the older literature, this is called the residence time, whereas the current term is time-integrated activity coefficient [3]. There is a special source called the remainder of the body which has a time-integrated activity coefficient that is equal to that of the whole body minus those of each of the identified source organs.

PET is, for all practical purposes, quantitative. SPECT is becoming so, as several manufacturers have introduced combinations of hardware and software that produce images with voxels having units of activity per unit volume. A variety of corrections, most notably attenuation correction using CT or MR, are incorporated into these products. One can build the source time–activity curves from the activity in volumes of interest. Since tomographic imaging solves the problem of overlying and underlying tissues, no background correction is necessary. Constructing volumes of interest is more labor-intensive than planar regions of interest, but there is a growing number of tools that are available to help.

The time-integrated activity coefficients can be entered into a MIRD-style dosimetry program such as OLINDA/EXM [18] in order to obtain estimates of the dose in the target organs. One chooses a human model that most nearly resembles the patient in size. However, since radiation absorbed dose is energy per unit mass, it is possible to improve the dosimetric estimate by adjusting the target organ masses in the calculation. To obtain the mass of most organs, one can estimate their volumes from a CT or MR scan and multiply by the nominal densities of the tissues [19]. An exception is the lungs, in which the density varies with the degree of inflation. An approach that is based upon the Hounsfield Units of the CT scan has proven to be effective in estimating individual patients' lung masses [20]. Software such as OLINDA contains the quantity that in MIRD dosimetry is called the S-value, which is the mean energy deposited in the target for each disintegration in the source, for the standard models. A few S-values or specific absorbed fractions [21–25] for more specialized models of the central nervous system may be found in the literature, but when using them, the dosimetry calculations must be done by hand. The dose to a specific region of the spinal cord from a concentrated accumulation of the radiopharmaceutical at a particular location might need to be assessed using Monte Carlo simulation [26].

Summary

The workflow for the use of quantitative imaging in the dosimetry of intrathecal radiopharmaceutical therapy is illustrated in Fig. 10.1.

Internal dosimetry using the MIRD schema requires information about the time-course of the radioactivity concentrations within the patient. Quantitative imaging provides that information in a form from which the time-integrated activity coefficients that are used by software such as OLINDA/EXM can be determined.

References

1. Hall EJ, Giaccia AJ. Radiobiology for the radiologist. 6th ed. Philadelphia, PA: Lippincott Williams & Wilkins; 2006.
2. Loevinger R, Budinger TF, Watson EE. MIRD primer for absorbed dose calculations. Revised edition. New York: Society of Nuclear Medicine; 1991.
3. Bolch WE, Eckerman KF, Sgouros G, Thomas SR. MIRD pamphlet no. 21: a generalized schema for radiopharmaceutical dosimetry—standardization of nomenclature. J Nucl Med. 2009;50(3):477–84.
4. Eckerman KF, Endo A. MIRD radionuclide data and decay schemes. 2nd ed. Reston, VA: Society of Nuclear Medicine; 2008.
5. Cherry SR, Sorenson JA, Phelps ME. Physics in nuclear medicine. 4th ed. Philadelphia: Elsevier Saunders; 2012.
6. Ficaro EP, Fessler JA, Rogers WL, Schwaiger M. Comparison of americium-241 and technetium-99m as transmission sources for attenuation correction of thallium-201 SPECT imaging of the heart. J Nucl Med. 1994;35(4):652–63. [cited 2020 Jan 23]. http://jnm.snmjournals.org/content/35/4/652.long.
7. Rong X, Du Y, Frey EC. A method for energy window optimization for quantitative tasks that includes the effects of model-mismatch on bias: application to Y-90 bremsstrahlung SPECT imaging. Phys Med Biol. 2012;57(12):3711–25. https://doi.org/10.1088/0031-9155/57/12/3711.
8. Clarke LP, Cullom SJ, Shaw R, Reece C, Penney BC, King MA, et al. Bremsstrahlung imaging using the gamma camera: factors affecting attenuation. J Nucl Med. 1992;33(1):161–6. http://jnm.snmjournals.org/content/33/1/161.short.
9. Macey DJ, Grant EJ, Bayouth JE, Giap HB, Danna SJ, Sirisriro R, et al. Improved conjugate view quantitation of I-131 by subtraction of scatter and septal penetration events with a triple energy window method. Med Phys. 1995;22(10):1637–43. [cited 2019 Aug 31]. https://doi.org/10.1118/1.597423.
10. Holstensson M, Hindorf C, Ljungberg M, Partridge M, Flux GD. Optimization of energy-window settings for scatter correction in quantitative 111In imaging: comparison of measurements and Monte Carlo simulations. Cancer Biother Radiopharm. 2007;22(1):136–42. [cited 2019 Aug 31]. https://doi.org/10.1089/cbr.2007.307.
11. Penney BC, Rajeevan N, Bushe KS, Hademenos G, King MA, de Vries DJ, et al. A scatter reduction method for In-111 scintigrams using five energy windows. In: Conference record of the 1991 IEEE nuclear science symposium and medical imaging conference, vol. 3; 1991. p. 1866–73.
12. Hesterman JY, Kost SD, Holt RW, Dobson H, Verma A, Mozley PD. Three-dimensional dosimetry for radiation safety estimates from intrathecal administration. J Nucl Med. 2017;58(10):1672–8. http://jnm.snmjournals.org/content/58/10/1672.abstract.
13. Wong FC, Kim EE. Nuclear medicine in neuro-oncology. In: Levin VA, editor. Cancer in the nervous system. 2nd ed. New York: Oxford University Press; 2002. p. 60–72. [cited 2019 Aug 18]. https://www.soc-neuro-onc.org/UploadedFiles/Levin/Levin_ch02_p60-72.pdf.
14. Larson SM, Carrasquillo JA, Cheung N-KV, Press OW. Radioimmunotherapy of human tumors. Nat Rev Cancer. 2015;15:347–60.
15. Stabin MG, Evans J. The radiation dosimetry of intrathecally administered radionuclides. In: Schalfke-Stelson AT, Stabin MG, Sparks RB, editors. Proceedings of the sixth international radiopharmaceutical dosimetry symposium. Gatlinburg, TN: Oak Ridge Associated Universities; 1999. p. 500–12.
16. Lubberink M, Herzog H. Quantitative imaging of 124I and 86Y with PET. Eur J Nucl Med Mol Imaging. 2011;38(Suppl 1):10. [cited 2019 Sep 8]. https://www.ncbi.nlm.nih.gov/pmc/articles/PMC3098993/.

17. Conti M, Eriksson L. Physics of pure and non-pure positron emitters for PET: a review and a discussion. Eur J Nucl Med Mol Imaging Phys. 2016;3:8. [cited 2019 Sep 8]. https://www.ncbi.nlm.nih.gov/pmc/articles/PMC4894854/.
18. Stabin MG, Sparks RB, Crowe E. OLINDA/EXM: the second-generation personal computer software for internal dose assessment in nuclear medicine. J Nucl Med. 2005;46(6):1023–7. http://jnm.snmjournals.org/cgi/content/abstract/46/6/1023.
19. International Commission on Radiological Protection. ICRP publication 89: basic anatomical and physiological data for use in radiological protection: reference values. Ann ICRP. 2002;32(3–4):1–265. [cited 2018 Apr 5]. http://www.icrp.org/publication.asp?id=icrp%20publication%2089.
20. Busse N, Erwin W, Pan T. Evaluation of a semiautomated lung mass calculation technique for internal dosimetry applications. Med Phys. 2013;40(12):122503 . [cited 2019 Jun 10]. https://doi.org/10.1118/1.4830433.
21. Bouchet LG, Bolch WE, Weber DA, Atkins HL, Poston JW Sr. MIRD pamphlet no. 15: radionuclide S values in a revised dosimetric model of the adult head and brain. J Nucl Med. 1999;40(3):62S–101. [cited 2019 Sep 14]. https://www.snmmi.org/files/docs/MIRD15.pdf.
22. Villoing D, McMillan D, Kim KP, Park IL, Lee A-K, Choi H, et al. Korean pediatric and adult head computational phantoms and application to photon specific absorbed fraction calculations. Radiat Prot Dosimetry. 2017;176(3):294–301. [cited 2019 Sep 14]. https://doi.org/10.1093/rpd/ncx009.
23. Fallahpoor M, Abbasi M, Parach AA, Bitarafan Rajabi A, Kalantari F. Image-based versus atlas-based patient-specific S-value assessment for Samarium-153 EDTMP cancer palliative care: a short study. Iran J Nucl Med. 2018;26(2):76–81. http://irjnm.tums.ac.ir/article_31621.html.
24. Johansson L, Nosslin B. Dosimetry of intrathecally administered radiopharmaceuticals. In: Watson EE, Schalfke-Stelson AT, editors. Proceedings of the fifth international radiopharmaceutical dosimetry symposium. Oak Ridge, TN: Oak Ridge Associated Universities; 1992. p. 188–210. [cited 2019 Sep 15]. https://inis.iaea.org/collection/NCLCollectionStore/_Public/23/071/23071441.pdf?r=1&r=1.
25. Reynoso-Mejía CA, Delfin-Loya A, Kerik-Rotenberg N, Moranchel M. S-values of cortical and subcortical structures calculated from a voxelized head phantom. AIP Conf Proc. 2019;2090(1):030006. [cited 2019 Sep 15]. https://aip.scitation.org/doi/abs/10.1063/1.5095901.
26. Wong F, Sparks R. Radiation dosimetry models of intralumbar injection of 14 radiopharmaceuticals. J Nucl Med. 2009;50(Suppl 2):1871. http://jnm.snmjournals.org/content/50/supplement_2/1871.abstract.

Chapter 11
Regulatory Oversight of Radiopharmaceuticals

Dao Le

Introduction

Radiopharmaceuticals, as compounds that contain a drug labeled with a radioactive isotope, are primarily under the regulatory control of two central agencies: the Nuclear Regulatory Commission (NRC) and the Food and Drug Administration (FDA). The principal role of the FDA is to regulate the safety and efficacy of the radioactive drugs as they are used in medical practice, whereas the mission of the NRC is to "ensure the safe use of radioactive materials for beneficial civilian purposes while protecting people and the environment [1]." Beyond these two federal agencies, oversight of the production, preparation, handling, transport, and use of radiopharmaceuticals is also governed by other regulatory authorities such as Environmental Protection Agency (EPA), Occupational Safety and Health Administration (OSHA), and the Department of Transportation (DOT).

The regulations set forth by these federal agencies may be administered at the state level. For example, State Boards of Pharmacy govern the practice of pharmacy; State Departments of Health Services may oversee matters relating to radiation exposure to the public; and State Departments of Environmental Quality manage the radioactive waste programs. Figure 11.1 depicts a typical paradigm of regulatory authority over radioactive material use for a specific state like Texas. Additionally, for most large hospitals there also exists an additional internal or local regulatory layer to ensure compliance with appropriate federal and state regulations. For instance, hospitals that use radioactive materials often have a

D. Le (✉)
The University of Texas, MD Anderson Cancer Center, Houston, TX, USA

F. C. L. Wong (ed.), *Radiopharmaceuticals in the Management of Leptomeningeal Metastasis*, https://doi.org/10.1007/978-3-031-14291-8_11

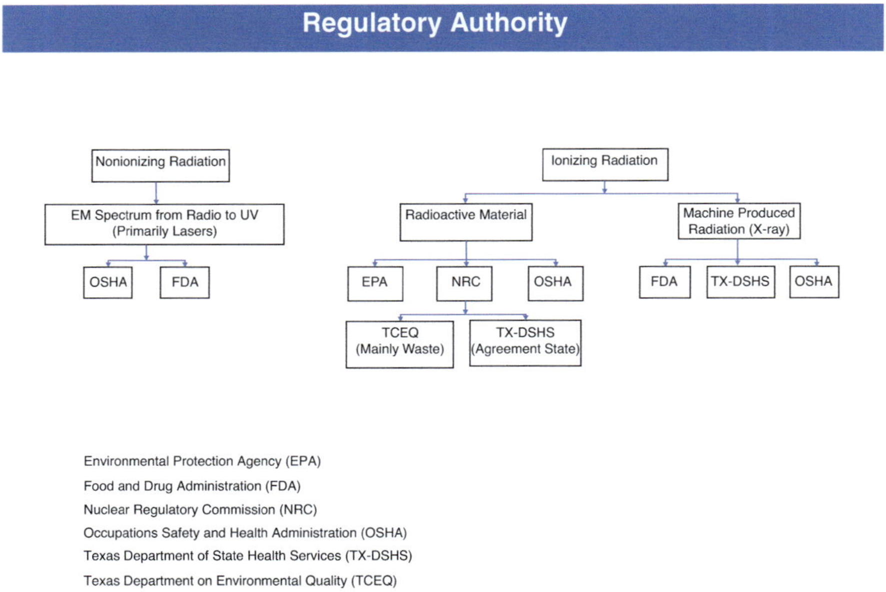

Fig. 11.1 A typical paradigm of regulatory authority over radioactive material use for a specific state like Texas

Radiation Safety (RS) group to oversee the institution's radiation program, facilities, and procedures. Typically, RS group works with the institutional Radiation Safety Committee (RSC), in compliance with Federal/State regulations, to oversee all uses of radioactive material, as permitted by the radioactive material (RAM) license, in the institution. Consequently, no one may order, possess, receive, or administer RAM until he/she has been approved as an Authorized User by the local RSC.

The purpose of this chapter is to offer a basic understanding of the regulations that govern the preparation, handling, and use of radiopharmaceuticals in a hospital nuclear medicine (NM) department. The aim is to assist healthcare providers to better navigate the steadily increasing regulatory oversight around the use of radioactive materials. There is a high level of expectation from these oversight organizations and full compliance is mandatory in order to continue the necessary nuclear medicine procedures. The chapter provides an overview of the regulations related to both the use of FDA-approved radiopharmaceuticals and investigational radiopharmaceuticals in a clinical nuclear medicine practice. It is important to note that detailed discussion on all regulations pertaining to radiopharmaceuticals is beyond the scope of this chapter. This chapter cannot be a substitute for an in-depth understanding of specific regulations. It is advised that health care providers always obtain up-to-date information regarding federal, state, and local regulations pertaining to your specific practice.

Federal Regulatory Authority of Radiopharmacuticals

Nuclear Regulatory Commission

Because radioactive pharmaceuticals are comprised of ionizing radiation, there are legal restrictions as to who is permitted to transport, obtain, handle, and use these agents. At the federal level, the NRC was created by Congress to protect the patients, public, and workers from unnecessary exposure to radiation.

Today's NRC is very focused on reactor licensing and safety, but the agency also has oversight over radioactive materials licensing for a variety of purposes, including medical use of radioisotopes. The NRC issues specific licenses to medical, industrial, and academic centers for possession and use of byproduct, source, and special nuclear materials. Once issued, the radioactive materials (RAM) license can be changed during renewal or by submission of an amendment. Many facilities are in a constant state of amendment submissions in order to stay current with both authorized users listed and radionuclides being used [2].

Food and Drug Administration

Historically, the use of radioactive materials was solely under the auspices of the NRC. It was not until 1975 that the Food and Drug Administration (FDA) assumed authority over the approval and licensing of radiopharmaceuticals. Currently, it is well established that the FDA regulates radiopharmaceutical use in terms of their chemical toxicity and efficacy.

In 1975, FDA issued a final rule that placed all radiopharmaceuticals, both established radioactive drugs and investigational radioactive drugs, under the regulatory authority of the FDA. The FDA would regulate radiopharmaceuticals the same way as traditional pharmaceuticals, thus evaluating new radiopharmaceuticals through the investigational new drug applications (IND). For new drugs, the FDA regulatory process comes into effect when the drug has proven to be safe and effective in preclinical studies (animal data) and now is ready to be tested on human patients. At this point, the researcher would submit an IND application to the FDA.

According to the Agency, there are three pathways for conducting research studies involving an investigational new radioactive drug or biological product:

1. Under an approved Investigational New Drug Application (IND).
2. Exempt from IND requirements (i.e. protocol involving placebo).
3. Under the authority of an FDA-approved Radioactive Drug Research Committee (RDRC) [3].

The IND is an exemption granted to the study sponsor from the FDA allowing for the shipment of drugs across state lines for distribution. Recall that FDA requires that only drugs that have submitted an NDA and obtained approval can be transported across state lines. Since investigational drugs have not gained NDA approval status, the only way for commercial distribution is by obtaining IND approval. The IND application must contain three main components:

1. Animal pharmacology and toxicology studies to show safety.
2. Manufacturing information ensuring that the new drug will be available for the study.
3. The clinical protocol which contains details of the study [4].

There are three types of IND applications:

- *Investigator IND*, also known as physician-sponsored IND, is when a physician who is conducting the study submits the application. Under this type of IND, the physician is held responsible for all aspects of the study including preparation, dispensing, and administration of the drug.
- *Emergency Use IND* can be used when a physician determines that the use of the experimental agent is needed for urgent medical conditions to benefit the patient. Due to the time sensitivity, the physician was unable to go through the traditional submission and approval process. Further, this type of IND can also be used in circumstances where the patient does not meet the requirements for existing studies or if an approved study protocol does not exist.
- *Treatment IND*, also known as expanded access protocols, is submitted when an experimental agent has shown to be safe and effective. While it is being reviewed by the FDA, the experimental agent can be used for treatment of patients with immediate life-threatening conditions or serious diseases where there is no alternative therapy.

Once the IND has been submitted, the investigator must wait 30 calendar days before initiating the clinical study [4]. The goal of the IND is to gather information for submission of the New Drug Application (NDA), which allows for the marketing of a new drug in the USA. Since 1938, the regulation and control of new drugs by the FDA have been based on the NDA.

For the purpose of data collection, clinical trials are conducted in phases which build on top of one another. There are five phases: Phase 0 through Phase IV, wherein each phase has a different aim. For instance, the goal of Phase 0 is to investigate how a drug is processed in the body, while in Phase III, the purpose is to demonstrate that the new radiopharmaceutical is at least as safe and effective as existing options. Typically, the FDA requires completion of Phase I, II, and III prior to submission of the NDA. The documentation required in the NDA must convey the entire developmental history of the drug product from drug discovery, preclinical, clinical, and post-marketing safety surveillance commitments to ensure continued efficacy and safety. Once approved, the new radiopharmaceutical is marketed and becomes a standard of care in the clinical practice [4].

Other Pertinent Regulatory Agencies

There are five regulatory agencies that have direct regulatory authority over radiopharmaceuticals at the federal level. Beyond the first two, NRC and FDA, which have been discussed, the list also includes the Occupational Safety and Health Administration (OSHA), Environmental Protection Agency (EPA), and the Department of Transportation (DOT).

Occupational Safety and Health Administration (OSHA)

OSHA is an agency under the United States Department of Labor with the charge to ensure the safe and healthy working conditions for working individuals [5]. OSHA enforces standards that focus on worker safety by monitoring and limiting exposure to workers. To comply with set regulations, radiation workers are required to wear radiation dosimeters in order to monitor radiation exposure. Radiation dosimeters are issued based on the workers use of radioactive materials. For instance, personnel monitoring for radiation exposure is required for personnel who have the potential to reach 10% of the applicable limits: annual Deep Dose Equivalent (DDE) limit is 5000 mrem (50 mSv) per year to a radiation worker and 100 mrem (1 mSV) per year to a member of the public. An annual report of radiation exposure must be provided by the employer to any radiation worker who received a measure exposure of 100 mrem (1 mSv) or greater during the previous calendar year [6].

Environmental Protection Agency (EPA)

The EPA is an independent agency with a mandate from the federal government to protect human health and the environment [7]. In regard to radiation, the EPA has regulations governing the levels of radioactive materials in the general environment and outside of the boundaries that are under the control of persons possessing or using radioactive materials under a RAM license such as a nuclear medicine clinic or a nuclear pharmacy. Examples of outside boundaries include radioactive materials released into the air or into the water supply. It is important to point out that the EPA does not regulate radioactive material that enters the environment from patients. Therefore, patient release of radiation after administration of a radioactive agent via urination or defecation into public sewer systems does not count toward effluent release into the environment. Conversely, in an academic research hospital setting, besides patient release, there can be release of radioactive material down the drain. Generally, the hospital radiation safety group or the radiation safety officer (RSO) works to ensure that the amount of radioactive material released into the water is within regulatory limits by performing an annual calculation. Keep in mind that individual states may set more stringent effluent release standards.

Department of Transportation (DOT)

In a Nuclear Medicine Department audit, an NRC or State Radiation Inspector could inquire about the training documents for shippers and transporters of radiopharmaceuticals. The NRC and DOT share responsibilities of regulating radioactive transport. The transfer and/or shipment of packages that contain radioactive materials are considered hazardous material (hazmat) shipments and are governed by the United States Department of Transportation (USDOT/DOT). The DOT issues most of the regulations regarding transportation in Title 49: 49CFR Part 107-Hazardous Materials Program Procedures and 49CFR Parts 171–180, 390–397-Hazardous Materials Regulations-Department of Transportation. In the same way, the NRC regulations relating to the transport of hazmat are found in 10CFR Part 30.34(c) and Part 30.41-Nuclear Regulatory Commission (NRC) and 10CFR Part 71-Nuclear Regulatory Commission-Packaging and Transportation of Radioactive Material. The NRC is most concerned with high level quantities of radiation and advises licensees in 10CFR 71.5 to comply with DOT regulations when NRC regulations do not apply [8]. In a hospital nuclear medicine department, typically the foremost concern is the documentation and maintenance of training documents.

The US DOT under 49CFR. 172.700 stipulates general training in the safe handling of hazmat for all employees who: prepare packages of hazmat for shipment, operate a vehicle to transport hazmat, and are responsible for the safety of transporting hazmat. In a nuclear medicine department, where radiopharmaceuticals are supplied by an outside nuclear pharmacy vendor, generally, nuclear medicine technologists (NMT) are responsible for preparing return shipments, of either unused doses or used doses with residual activity, to the pharmacy vendor. Therefore, according to 49CFR 172.404, a RAM licensee must provide certificate of training for all employees involved with packaging, marking, labeling, measuring, loading, transporting, and storage of packages containing RAM. This training must be completed within 90 days of employment and every 3 years thereafter [9]. The DOT training must address the following topics:

- General awareness and knowledge of radioactive materials.
- Function-specific training on tasks that the employee will perform such as packaging or labeling.
- Safety considerations of radioactive materials.
- Security awareness training.

The DOT requires that the employee is tested in the four topic areas and documentation of successful completion is usually in the form of a certificate. Many hospitals either have an in-house DOT training program or subscribe to outside vendors for either live or web-based DOT training.

State Regulatory Control

Federal regulatory agencies generally have a memorandum of understanding with different state agencies and give States the right to ensure compliance through enforcement of laws governing the use of radioactive materials.

For a clinical NM practice, the day-to-day regulatory scrutiny is experienced more on a state and local level. In a NM clinic, the inspectors that come through the facility are often from either the local State Health Radiation Control group (if the state is an Agreement State) or from the State Board of Pharmacy (if the hospital has a nuclear pharmacy operation). Additionally, the State Medical Board would handle issues related to physicians' use of radiopharmaceuticals, but an inspection of the facility from the State Medical Board is not common.

Although not tied to either federal or state regulatory agencies, accreditation organizations have surveyors to evaluate hospital compliance to set standards which are reflective of federal and state regulations. Generally, the difference between a regulatory agency inspection and an accreditation assessment is that the regulator focuses on exactly what is in the regulations, whereas the accreditation inspector looks at the institutions overall standard of operation. One such organization is The Joint Commission (TJC), an independent, not-for-profit group that accredits and certifies health care organizations [10].

For state inspections, well-established laws and regulations are enforceable and if violated, civil and criminal enforcement is warranted. More often than not, the result is an issuance of monetary penalties but in extreme cases, the right to use RAM can be revoked. Whereas, in the case of an accreditation body such as TJC, standards issued by accrediting bodies do not have a force of law but carry a symbol of quality. Typically, accreditation is voluntary but is often tied to monetary reimbursement for the institution or program. Another example of an accreditation body is the American College of Radiology (ACR) where accreditation is a recognition that the facility operates at a high level in medical imaging [11].

NRC/State Health Radiation Control: RAM Inspection

As noted previously, there are currently 38 States that have entered into Agreement with the NRC. Commonly, the Agreement States have their own equivalent regulations to the NRC regulations found in Title 10 CFR. Texas is an example of an Agreement State and Fig. 11.2 illustrates a comparison of the NRC Title 10 CFR and Texas Title 25 of Texas Administrative Code. For the State of Texas, the rules and regulations that govern the use of RAM are enforced by the Texas Department of State Health Services (TXDSHS), Radiation Control Program. The mission of the TXDSHS, Radiation Control Program is to "protect and promote the physical and environmental health of the people of Texas. The goal of the program is to prevent unnecessary radiation exposure to the public through licensing, registration, inspection, enforcement, and managing emergency response [12]." In Texas, for

Radiation Regulations – Radioactive Material

- NRC regulations found in Title 10 CFR
  - Part 19 – Notices, instructions and reports to workers: inspection and investigations
  - Part 20 – Standards for Protection Against Radiation
  - Part 30 – General Provisions for Byproduct Material
  - Part 33 – Specific domestic licenses of broad scope for byproduct material
  - Part 35 – Medical Use
- Texas equivalent regulations found in Title 25 of Texas Administrative Code
  - §289.203 – Notices, Instructions, and Reports To Workers; Inspections
  - §289.202 – Standards for Protection Against Radiation
  - §289.201 – General Licensing of Byproduct Material
  - §289.252 – licensing of Radioactive Material
  - §289.256 – Medical Use

Fig. 11.2 Comparison of the NRC Title 10 CFR and Texas Title 25 of the Texas Administrative Code

hospitals with broad scope RAM licenses, RAM inspections are performed at least every 2 years. The number one compliance tip offered by the State is to read the RAM license carefully and know what the license authorizes in terms of isotope, quantity (millicurie vs Curie levels), make/model of devices and their use.

State Boards of Pharmacy (BOP): Pharmacy Inspection

For hospitals that have an in-house nuclear pharmacy, or a hot lab listed under the hospital Pharmacy Department, BOP inspections can be expected. Depending on your state, inspections can occur on an annual or biennial schedule. However, if the nuclear medicine department uses a centralized commercial nuclear pharmacy for all their radiopharmaceutical products, then hospital BOP inspections are typically an uncommon occurrence. There are only a small number of hospitals or imaging centers that have their own nuclear pharmacies to prepare and dispense radiopharmaceuticals for on-site use. In general, only academic hospitals have on-site nuclear pharmacies.

State Boards of Pharmacy are responsible for establishing regulations for pharmacy practice. In an inspection, the inspector could ask for a variety of documentation to ensure compliance to set regulations such as licensing and registration, appropriate training documents for pharmacy personnel, and prescription files. Additionally, State BOP expect pharmacies to have policies and procedures that adhere to guidelines that apply to their unique practice settings. The United States Pharmacopeia (USP) is a nonprofit organization that sets standards for drug quality and thus influences medicine and pharmacy practice. USP General Chapter <825>

Pharmaceuticals-Preparation, Compounding, Dispensing and Repackaging is a general chapter that provides guidance for the preparation, compounding, dispensing, and repackaging of compounded sterile and nonsterile radiopharmaceuticals [13]. However, it is important to note that USP is a nongovernmental, nonprofit organization, and standards issued are only legally enforceable when a regulatory agency, such as State BOP or FDA, with authority requires compliance. However, according to USP, almost all states have laws governing pharmaceutical compounding. In August of 2016, the National Association of Boards of Pharmacy (NABP) adopted the Model State Pharmacy Act and Model Rules which provides guidance to state BOP on developing state rules which incorporate USP guidelines [14]. Besides state BOP, the FDA has included provisions of USP standards into the Federal Food, Drug, and Cosmetic Act, mandating USP standards for compounding sterile products [15].

Accreditation Organizations: The Joint Commission Inspection

USP works closely with State legislatures, State BOPs, and different accrediting organizations, such as TJC, to ensure quality compounding of drugs for patients. Although accreditation bodies do not have a force of law, hospitals strive to establish compliance with accreditation standards to demonstrate commitment to providing the highest quality of patient care. Moreover, hospitals are required to be in compliance with the Federal requirements stated in the Medicare Conditions of Participation (CoP), set forth in 42 CFR Part 482, in order to receive reimbursement from the Centers for Medicare and Medicaid Services (CMS) [16]. CMS acknowledges that the standards of certain accrediting organizations meet or exceed CMS's expectations, therefore will accept the certification from these accreditation organizations. For hospitals, achieving certification status from CMS accepted accreditation organizations ensures that the facility also meets CMS standards. Keep in mind that in order to validate an organization's accreditation process, CMS can come and perform a validation survey and typically these validation surveys can be performed shortly after an accreditation visit [17].

In a hospital nuclear medicine setting, a common accreditation organization encountered is The Joint Commission (TJC). A compliance checklist for diagnostic imaging can be found on the TJC website [18]. Additionally, TJC defines medication as any product designated by the FDA as a drug. Consequently, radiopharmaceuticals have the same level of supervision as other medications in terms of prescribing, dispensing, storage, security, administration, and monitoring of adverse events. For a nuclear medicine clinic and hospital nuclear pharmacy, the primary difference between a NRC and a BOP inspection is that the regulatory agencies focus exactly on their regulations, whereas the accreditation inspection is all-encompassing, covering any aspects that may affect the quality of health care. Questions from TJH auditors can include radiation safety (similar to NRC) matters and encompass the preparation of a radiopharmaceutical (similar to BOP).

Internal/Local Regulatory Authority

Radiation Safety Committee/Radiation Safety Office

The Radioactive Materials License (RAML) is a legal document that grants the user permission to possess and use radioactive materials. Typically, the RAML sets forth the types and quantities of materials that are allowed and specific conditions under which the material may be used. Additionally, it lists names of the Radiation Safety Officer (RSO) and the members of the Radiation Safety Committee (RSC). For the NRC, facilities (typically hospitals) that are authorized for two or more different types of uses of byproduct materials are required to establish a RSC. The RSC is charged with supervision over all uses of radioactive materials permitted by the RAML [12].

The responsibilities of the RSC may include:

- Evaluating and approving any applicant requesting authorization to use radioactive materials at the facility.
- Reviewing the overall compliance status of clinical authorized users.
- Developing criteria to evaluate the training and experience of new research and clinical authorized user applicants.
- Evaluating new uses of radioactive material and of machines that produce radiation as necessary.
- Reviewing overexposures and significant incidents including spills, contamination, unsafe practices, and medical events.
- Reviewing items of non-compliance following an inspection.
- Handle all concerns or issues related to radiation use.

More often than not, large hospitals/academic hospitals possess a Broad Scope License. In this setting, the approval by the RSC is required for ANY individual to use radioactive material. When an individual has been given approval, the person is referred to as an Authorized User (AU). In some hospitals, authorization is granted to individuals (in a specific department) by modality; diagnostic studies, unsealed therapy, and special uses and emerging technologies fall under Nuclear Medicine authority, whereas the use of sealed sources for therapy is under the authority of individuals in Radiation Oncology. The RSC reserves the right to change or revoke any authorization [19].

Radioactive Drug Research Committee

As discussed previously under FDA regulatory control, there are three pathways for conducting research studies involving an investigational new radioactive drug or biological product. One mechanism for conducting human research involving a radioactive drug is through the approval of a local Radioactive Drug Research Committee (RDRC). The Committee allows investigators to conduct research studies using radiotracers in human subjects to establish feasibility prior to committing to the significant expense and effort of filing an IND application.

This arrangement is similar to the agreement between NRC and Agreement States. Here, the FDA is allowing the RDRC to approve radioactive drug research studies if, and only if, the RDRC commits to upholding FDA regulations.

FDA regulations (21 CFR Sec. 361.1) allow for the research use, in human subjects, of radioactive drugs that are not currently under an FDA-accepted IND or NDA application, provided that certain specified conditions outlined in 21 CFR Sec. 361.1 are met:

- The research is considered basic science research and is done for the purpose of advancing scientific knowledge.
- The research study is approved by an FDA-approved RDRC based on certain requirements.
- The pharmacologic dose of the radioactive drug to be administered is known not to cause any clinically detectable pharmacologic effect in humans.
- The radiation dose to be administered is justified by the quality of the study being undertaken and the importance of the information it seeks to obtain and is within the limits specified [20].

The RDRC, established under such authority and in accordance with the stated regulations, serves to initially and continually review such research investigations to ensure compliance with the provisions of FDA guidelines.

FDA regulations require that the RDRC work together with hospital's Institutional Review Board (IRB). The function of the IRB is to protect the rights and welfare of human research. Furthermore, all protocols approved by RDRC must also be approved by the IRB. With the proposed structure of the RDRC, competitive advances in radioactive drug research studies can be performed while remaining within the continual purview of the IRB [21].

Although the FDA has given the RDRC authority over these types of research, the Agency has continuous oversight over these studies through mandated scheduled report submission on all approved RDRC studies to the FDA. The FDA will also perform inspections of all RDRCs. The Office of Regulatory Affairs (ORA) field investigators handle these types of inspections and will generate an inspection report [22]. If the report indicates failure of the Institutional RDRC to comply with FDA regulations, then the FDA could withdraw approval of the RDRC.

Institutional Review Board

The protection of human research patients is addressed in 45 CFR 46, which contains the provisions for the requirement and establishment of an Institutional Review Board (IRB). The IRB is an administrative body established to protect the rights and welfare of human research subjects recruited to participate in research activities conducted under the auspices of the institution with which it is affiliated [23].

The IRB is charged with the responsibility to review and have oversight of all research involving human participants. The function of the IRB is to protect the welfare, rights, and privacy of human subjects. The IRB has the authority to approve, disapprove, and monitor all research activities that fall within its jurisdiction as specified by both the federal regulations and institutional policy. In addition, for many hospitals, the Scientific Research Committee (SRC) is another committee that works with the IRB. The SRC is charged with the responsibility of overseeing all aspects of the scientific research that is in the protocol such as the methods used to validate the scientific questions, the relevance of the biostatistical analysis, and the pertinence of the proposed procedures.

Many hospitals have an elaborate research infrastructure, built around the charge of the IRB, in order to maintain high ethical standards and ensure strict compliance with all regulatory policies. In instances where hospital research programs are disbanded, the cause is often due to regulatory deficiencies. When there is research conducted at the hospital, the FDA holds the sponsor-investigators (i.e. hospital) to the same standards as industry (i.e. large pharmaceutical companies). The responsibility, the liability, and the funding are immense; thus, it is vital that the hospital has a clinical research infrastructure that is robust.

As previously mentioned, for research studies that involve a radiopharmaceutical, there is an extra layer of oversight due to the risks associated with radiation. This chapter focuses primarily on issues related to the regulation of radiopharmaceuticals; thus, the focus will be on radiopharmaceutical research in an academic hospital setting. The rules and regulations surrounding human research in each academic hospital vary but the end goal is the same, to maintain high ethical standards and full compliance with all regulatory agencies. Figure 11.3 is an illustration of one internal research infrastructure and is the basis for the following discussion.

In this research pathway, most of the steps are applicable to all research protocols. However, there are two review committees that are specific to studies that

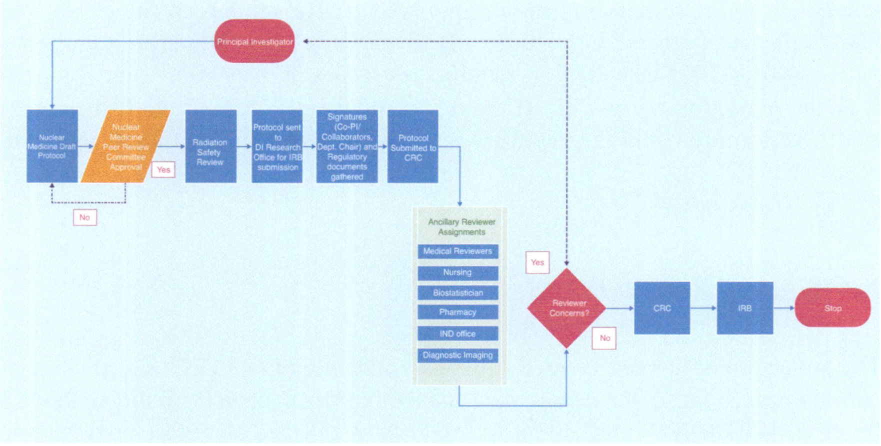

Fig. 11.3 Illustration of one research pathway

involve radiopharmaceuticals: the Nuclear Medicine Peer Review Committee (NMPRC) and the Radiation Safety Committee (RSC). At this particular institution, the purpose of the NMPRC is to allow for the review of all aspects related to nuclear medicine by the experts in this field. The standard operating procedure (SOP) requires that all studies involving radioactive materials must list a faculty in the Department of NM as a principal investigator (PI), co-PI, or collaborator. Additionally, the clinical research protocol must be submitted and presented to the NMPRC for review and approval prior to review by the IRB. The NMPRC would typically include NM physicians and technologists, health physicists, nuclear pharmacists, and other key experts. Similar to the RDRC, the NMPRC allows for additional subject matter experts when warranted. The committee members evaluate the clinical protocol on matters to include, but not limited to, need and feasibility of the study, eligibility criteria, imaging parameters, safety and safety monitoring plans, and procurement of the investigational radiopharmaceutical. Once the clinical study has been approved by the NMPRC, it will then proceed to the next review committee which, according to the research pathway illustration, is the RSC. Figure 11.4 is an example of the standard of operation for a NMPRC.

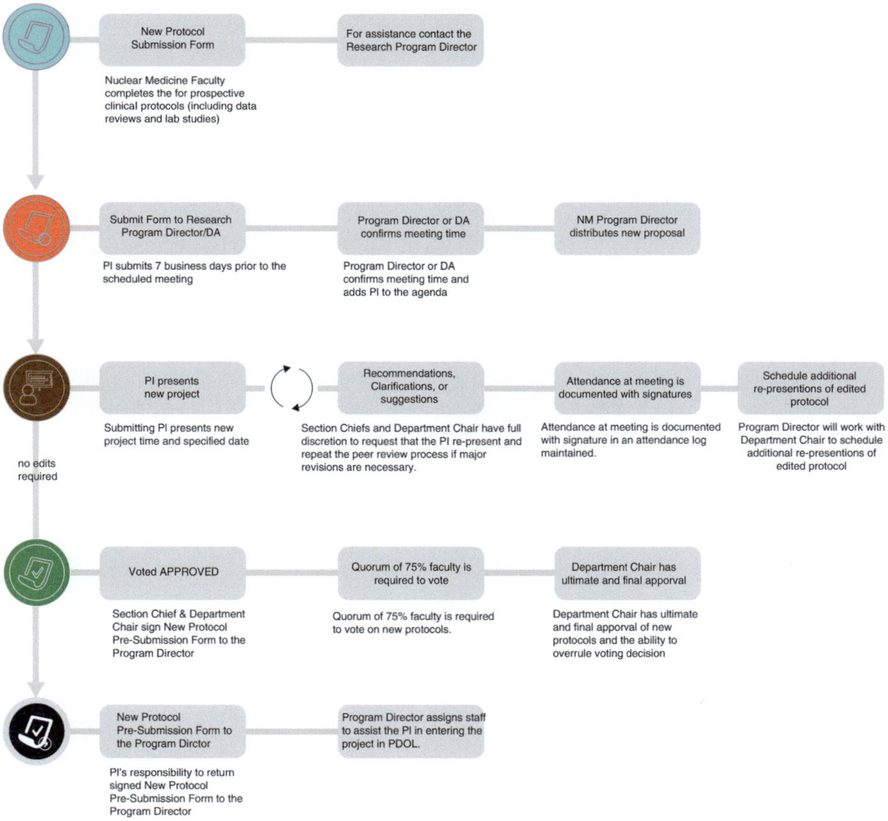

Fig. 11.4 An example of Nuclear Medicine Peer Review Committee pathway

The RSC, as discussed previously, will review and approve all aspects related to the radioisotopes, including uses under a clinical study. The RSC grants the researcher AU status for the investigational radioisotope and this allows the investigator to use the isotope for the clinical research study. To be eligible for clinical authorization under this structure, the applicant must be a physician who is certified by a medical specialty board under a certification process recognized by the NRC or Agreement State. Furthermore, before the hospital (Dept. of NM) can order and receive the isotope, it must be on the hospital RAM license. If the isotope is not on the RAM license, the RS group will submit an amendment to the NRC/Agreement State to add the isotope. A typical amendment would include an outline of the use, user qualification, maximum amount, storage, preparation details, and waste disposal. When the amendment is approved, the hospital must put processes and procedures in place that adhere strictly to the commitments made to the NRC/State regarding the isotope.

Regulatory Outlook of Radiopharmaceuticals

For those practicing clinical NM, dealing with regulations can be a daunting task. A common challenge is to comply with the regulations and not have the regulations dictate the practice. For a hospital NM clinical practice, the rules and regulations of internal committees act as a safeguard or a checkpoint of compliance for users. Ideally, all violations can be identified at the local level before progression into state and federal infractions.

The future of radiopharmaceuticals is promising. Many believe that nuclear medicine has experienced an exponential resurgence of interest. In the last few years, we have seen a rapid increase in FDA approvals for radiopharmaceuticals. The excitement is beyond individual diagnostic imaging or single therapeutic agents but rather theragnostic radionuclides that offer low dose imaging followed by high dose therapy such as the agents used for neuroendocrine tumors (NETS): gallium Ga-68 dotatate and lutetium Lu-177 dotatate. With tremendous growth in the use of radiopharmaceuticals, governing agencies will have increased involvement in the regulation of nuclear medicine. However, due to the complexity of the regulations, there are many published guidances available to assist with implementing programs that will comply with all the different regulations. As nuclear medicine professionals, it is our responsibility to provide the most safe and effective care to our patients. To honor this obligation, we must continually work to increase our knowledge of the regulations and find ways for seamless integration into our daily practice.

References

1. United States Nuclear Regulatory Commission. About NRC. https://www.nrc.gov/about-nrc.html. Accessed Nov 2019.
2. United States Nuclear Regulatory Commission. Licensing. https://www.nrc.gov/about-nrc/regulatory/licensing.html. Accessed Nov 2020.

3. United States Food and Drug Administration. Guidance for industry and researchers: the Radioactive Drug Research Committee: human research without an investigational new drug application. 2010. https://www.fda.gov/downloads/Drugs/Guidances/UCM163892.pdf. Accessed Jan 2019.
4. United States Food and Drug Administration. Investigational new drug (IND) application. https://www.fda.gov/drugs/developmentapprovalprocess/howdrugsaredevelopedandapproved/approvalapplications/investigationalnewdrugindapplication/default.htm. Accessed Jan 2019.
5. United States Department of Labor. About OSHA. https://www.osha.gov/about.html. Accessed Jan 2019.
6. 25 Texas Administrative Code §289.256. Medical and veterinary use of radioactive material. Texas regulations for control of radiation. Sept 2020.
7. United Stated Environmental Protection Agency. Our mission and what we do. https://www.epa.gov/aboutepa/our-mission-and-what-we-do. Jan 2019.
8. United State Nuclear Regulatory Commission. Transportation of radioactive material. https://www.nrc.gov/reading-rm/basic-ref/students/for-educators/11.pdf. Accessed Jan 2019.
9. Electronic Code of Federal Regulations e-CFR. Title 49-transportation. https://ecfr.io/Title-49/.
10. The Joint Commission. About the Joint Commission. https://www.jointcommission.org/about_us/about_the_joint_commission_main.aspx. Accessed Jan 2019.
11. American College of Radiology. The gold standard in accreditation. https://www.acr.org/Clinical-Resources/Accreditation. Accessed Jan 2019.
12. Texas Department of State Health Services. Radioactive materials licensing and radiation control program. Radioactive materials program authorization and scope. https://www.dshs.texas.gov/radiation/ram/. Accessed Nov 2020.
13. United States Pharmacopeia. Developing USP general chapter <825>. http://www.usp.org/chemical-medicines/general-chapter-825. Accessed 2020–2021.
14. National Association of Boards of Pharmacy. Model pharmacy act/rules. https://nabp.pharmacy/publications-reports/resource-documents/model-pharmacy-act-rules/. Accessed Feb 2019.
15. United States Pharmacopeia. Recognition of USP compounding standards. http://www.usp.org/compounding/legal-considerations. Accessed Jan 2021.
16. Centers for Medicare & Medicaid Services. Conditions for coverage (CfCs) & conditions of participations (CoPs). https://www.cms.gov/Regulations-and-Guidance/Legislation/CFCsAndCoPs/index.html?redirect=/CFCsAndCoPs/16_ASC.asp. Accessed Dec 2020.
17. Centers for Medicare & Medicaid Services. CMS to strengthen oversight of Medicare's accreditation organizations. https://www.cms.gov/newsroom/press-releases/cms-strengthen-oversight-medicares-accreditation-organizations. Accessed Feb 2019.
18. The Joint Commission. Compliance checklist: diagnostic imaging. https://www.jointcommission.org/assets/1/18/imaging_checklist-June-2016.pdf.
19. Texas Department of State Health Services. Radiation control program. How to avoid compliance problems relating to radioactive materials licenses. https://www.dshs.texas.gov/radiation/ram/compliance-tips.aspx.
20. United States Federal Food and Drug Administration. Radioactive Drug Research Committee (RDRC) program. https://www.fda.gov/drugs/scienceresearch/ucm574871.htm. Accessed Dec 2018.
21. United States Food and Drug Administration. Information sheet guidance for IRBs, clinical investigators, and sponsors FDA inspections of clinical investigators. https://www.fda.gov/downloads/regulatoryinformation/guidances/ucm126553.pdf. Accessed Jan 2019.
22. United States Federal Food and Drug Administration. Compliance program. https://www.fda.gov/downloads/ICECI/ComplianceManuals/ComplianceProgramManual/UCM244484.pdf. Accessed Jan 2019.
23. United States Department of Health & Human Services. 45 CFR 46. https://www.hhs.gov/ohrp/regulations-and-policy/guidance/faq/45-cfr-46/index.html. Accessed Feb 2019.

Chapter 12
Radionuclides in the Management of Leptomeningeal Metastasis: Framework and Opportunities

Franklin C. L. Wong

Introduction: Radiopharmaceuticals in LM Management

Leptomeningeal metastasis (LM) is a refractory and progressive lethal cancer complication involving the arachnoids and the CSF space surrounding the brain and spinal cord. There are unique biologic barriers to overcome for assessment of CSF flow and for LM therapy, both in technical and logistic realms. There have been increasing uses of radiopharmaceuticals in the care of cancer patients including those with LM.

This chapter follows the description of LM in humans, physiology and pathology, and state-of-the-art of diagnosis in LM as well as therapeutic interventions in earlier chapters. Imaging and dosimetry could provide guidance for the use of radionuclide to manage LM but they have their own limitations. Radiation dosimetry of radiopharmaceuticals in treating LM and dosimetry simulation has been illustrated in earlier chapters. Their uses in the design of potentially efficacious LM trials are further explored in this chapter based on known trials and existing preclinical data. This chapter surveys the framework under which radiopharmaceuticals are developed for diagnosis and therapy of LM. Special issues are identified for more detailed discussion and for opportunities of development.

F. C. L. Wong (✉)
Department of Nuclear Medicine, University of Texas M. D. Anderson Cancer Center, Houston, TX, USA
e-mail: fwong@mdanderson.org

F. C. L. Wong (ed.), *Radiopharmaceuticals in the Management of Leptomeningeal Metastasis*, https://doi.org/10.1007/978-3-031-14291-8_12

Intrathecal Radiopharmaceuticals for Assessment of CSF Flow

In the USA, In-111 DTPA (physical half-life of 67.2 h) is the only one FDA-approved radiopharmaceutical for intrathecal diagnostic use. In-111 DTPA is a good diagnostic surrogate of CSF flow of small molecules because it is relatively inert and not bound to components of the meninges or CSF proteins nor transported by carriers across meninges. In times of interrupted supply, Tc99m- DTPA is often used but has the limitation of short physical half-life of 6 h that would not allow effective scan beyond 1 day.

Since biochemical properties of a radiopharmaceutical may alter its CSF transit, retention or dosimetry of a molecule, the spatial and temporal intrathecal distribution and radiation dosimetry of each candidate intrathecal radiopharmaceutical need to be ascertained before clinical applications. Radiolabeled colloids may precipitate to the dependent area. Tumor-specific monoclonal antibodies are designed to bind to tumors for targeting. Halide anions are often extracted by spinal iodide/halide transporters with active transport to effect a prompt return to the general circulation as illustrated in our in vivo studies of rats (Fig. 12.1). Accelerated excretion of intrathecal halides from the CSF has been reported in rabbits [1], sheep [2], dogs [3], and monkeys [4] and is expected to occur in humans.

Heavy metal cations may bind to proteins in the subarachnoid space (SAS) resulting in prolonged retention as demonstrated by in vitro protein binding experiments in Fig. 12.2. Increasing radioactivities (0.1–1.0 uCi) of Y-90 or In-111 chlorides were incubated with aliquots of diluted CSF (1:2 and 1:4) in total volumes of 0.4 mL. After the bound and free fractions of radionuclides were separated by Amico Ultra Millipore filters under centrifugation, dose-dependent serum protein binding with In-111 and Y-90 chloride is confirmed, in the same manner as with diluted serum (1:2 and 1:8) (Fig. 12.2). The low dilutions of CSF and serum assure the findings may approximate in vivo binding. Such protein binding may increase the in vivo residence time. Comparison is made between intrathecal Ga-67

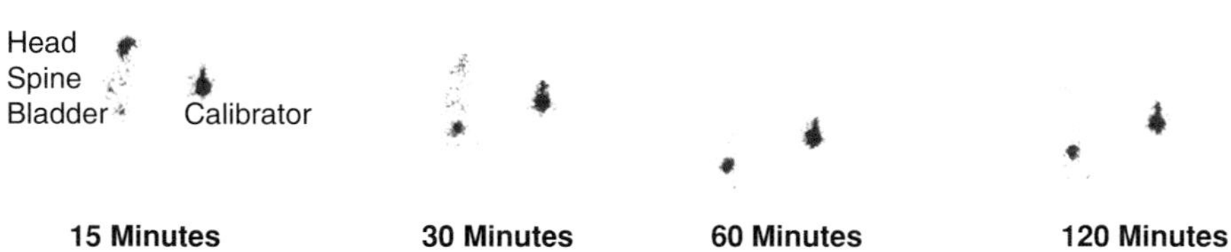

Fig. 12.1 Prompt clearance of I-131 NaI after cisternal injection with effective half-life <0.5 h. Whole-body images after intrathecal injection of 20 μCi of ^{131}I-NaI in a rat which had been pretreated with 0.2 g of oral non-radioactive NaI. Lateral images were taken at 15, 30, 60 and 120 min after injection. A calibrator of 20 μCi of ^{131}I-NaI was also placed in the field of view for quantification. Radioactivity in the head and spine were found to be 948, 272, 68 and 60 counts for the four images respectively indicating prompt clearance of ^{131}I-NaI from CSF. There was also prompt renal clearance of ^{131}I to the urinary bladder without retention in other organs

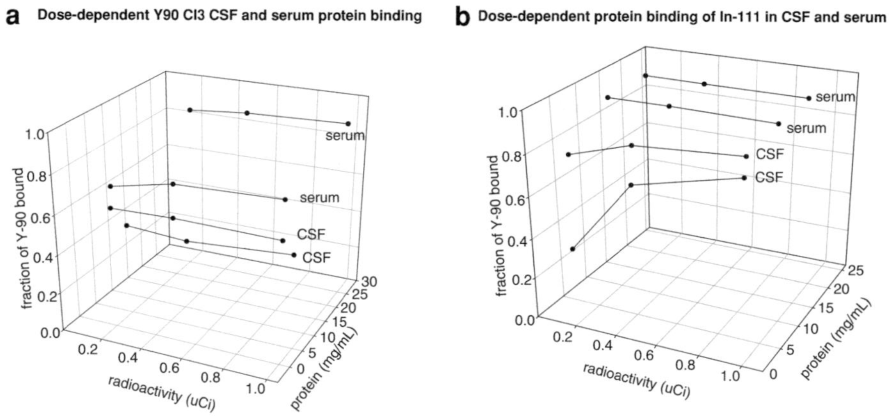

Fig. 12.2 Dose-dependent protein binding of free Y-90 and In-111 cations in CSF and serum. In vitro binding studies using Y-90 chloride (**a**) and In-111 chloride (**b**) with diluted CSF (protein = 0.71 mg/mL) and diluted serum (protein = 68 mg/mL) from a patient with LM. After incubation in volumes of 0.4 mL and centrifugation through Amico filters, radioactivities in filtrates were counted. Retention of radioactivity is noted by diluted CSF having protein at 0.089 and 0.355 mg/mL and by diluted serum having protein at 4.25 and 25.5 mg/mL for Y-90 (8.50 and 17 mg/mL for In-111). Fractions of radionuclide bound are dose-dependent on radioactivity and protein concentration and increase with less dilution. It can be inferred that free Y-90 and In-111 are mostly protein-bound in the undiluted CSF or undiluted serum

dosimetry values from patient image with Te of 20 h (Chap. 4, Fig. 4.8) versus from modeling which assumes no binding to LM (1–7 h in Chap. 9, Table 9.2). In addition to demonstrating patent CSF pathways in the first 24 h, that in vivo imaging study also reveals significant delayed retention of Ga-67 resulting in increases in CSF dosimetry and in therapeutic window (column 4 of Table 12.1).

Commercially available radiopharmaceuticals such as Ga-67 citrate (half-life of 78.3 h) and Tl-201 chloride (half-life of 73.1 h) may be candidate for alternatives to In-111 DTPA as alternative flow tracers. In fact, from a purely technical point of review, most commercially available diagnostic radiopharmaceuticals such as those described in Chap. 3 may be used for intrathecal evaluation of CSF flow because they only need to illustrate the bulk flow of CSF. A radionuclide such as Ga-67 citrate with longer physical half-life (78.3 h) is preferred to provide more prolonged visualization of the CSF beyond 1 day in contrast to the more commonly used off-label agent Tc99m DTPA. Certainly, the radiation dosimetry to organs and CSF compartments should also be considered for each potential candidate.

Many other radiopharmaceuticals in Chap. 3 (Tables 3.2 and 3.3) may be interesting intrathecal diagnostic agents to detect LM because of high sensitivity of detection from direct exposure to LM deposits bypassing the many biologic barriers encountered if administered by intravenous injection. However, it will take several days to clear the radiopharmaceutical in the CSF enough to reveal underlying tumor deposits because of the relatively slow CSF flow turnover (only five times per day). As reported by multiple intrathecal radiolabeled tumor-specific monoclonal

Table 12.1 Comparative intrathecal radiation dosimetry of Ga-66, Ga-67, and Ga-68 citrate

(cGy/mCi) Injection	Ventricular	Ventricular	Ventricular	Ventricular	Ventricular	Ventricular	Ventricular	Ventricular	Ventricular
Organ/radionuclide	Ga-67	Ga67	Ga67/Ga67	Ga-68	Ga68	Ga68/Ga68	Ga-66	Ga66	Ga66/Ga66
Pharmaceuticals	Citrate	Citrate	Vitrate	Citrate	Citrate	Citrate	Citrate	Citrate	Citrate
Source	Simulation	Image	Image/simulation	Simulation	Derived	Derived/simulation	Simulation	Derived	Derived/simulation
Adrenals	0.540	0.270	0.500	0.049	0.043	0.878	1.200	0.630	0.525
Brain	0.420	0.930	2.214	0.200	0.180	0.900	2.900	5.700	1.966
Breasts	0.150	0.072	0.480	0.005	0.004	0.755	0.230	0.099	0.430
Eyes	0.250	0.260	1.040	0.038	0.051	1.342	0.410	0.520	1.268
Lens of eyes	0.220	0.190	0.864	0.030	0.039	1.300	0.360	0.430	1.194
Gallbladder wall	0.240	0.130	0.542	0.002	0.002	1.158	0.400	0.220	0.550
LLIWall	0.590	0.100	0.169	0.004	0.005	1.023	0.940	0.120	0.128
Small intestine	0.270	0.140	0.519	0.018	0.011	0.611	0.600	0.200	0.333
Stomach	0.230	0.120	0.522	0.010	0.008	0.832	0.350	0.170	0.486
ULI wall	0.380	0.130	0.342	0.014	0.008	0.600	1.000	0.170	0.170
Heart wall	0.250	0.130	0.520	0.014	0.012	0.857	0.420	0.220	0.524
Kidneys	0.430	0.610	1.419	0.030	0.097	3.233	0.850	2.100	2.471
Liver	0.360	0.280	0.778	0.012	0.029	2.417	0.510	0.640	1.255
Lungs	0.230	0.130	0.565	0.014	0.012	0.857	0.400	0.210	0.525
Muscle	0.200	0.110	0.550	0.010	0.010	0.960	0.320	0.170	0.531
Ovaries	0.260	0.110	0.423	0.006	0.006	0.983	0.330	0.140	0.424
Pancreas	0.320	0.190	0.594	0.022	0.020	0.909	0.600	0.330	0.550
Red marrow	0.520	0.300	0.577	0.170	0.057	0.335	2.400	1.700	0.708
Bone surfaces	1.000	0.370	0.370	0.048	0.043	0.896	1.800	1.500	0.833
Skin	0.140	0.087	0.621	0.008	0.009	1.060	0.240	0.150	0.625
Spleen	0.440	0.130	0.295	0.014	0.010	0.707	0.639	0.200	0.313
Testes	0.160	0.075	0.469	0.002	0.002	1.059	0.180	0.073	0.406
Thymus	0.200	0.100	0.500	0.009	0.007	0.828	0.311	0.150	0.482
Thyroid	0.220	0.160	0.727	0.019	0.022	1.158	0.396	0.310	0.783
Urin bladder wall	0.240	0.300	1.250	0.004	0.200	57.143	0.317	2.000	6.309
Uterus	0.240	0.120	0.500	0.006	0.008	1.474	0.300	0.170	0.567
Total body	0.240	0.160	0.667	0.016	0.018	1.125	0.668	0.590	0.883
ED	0.360	0.150	0.417	0.080	0.022	0.275	0.752	0.630	0.838
EDE	0.330	0.150	0.455	0.030	0.025	0.833	0.930	1.000	1.075
Ventricle CSF	3.500	11.000	**3.143**	30.000	10.000	**0.333**	52.000	80.000	**1.538**
C-Spine CSF	14.000	15.000	**1.071**	3.400	11.000	**3.235**	49.000	50.000	**1.020**
L-Spine CSF	25.000	18.000	**0.720**	25.000	4.200	**0.168**	200.000	65.000	**0.325**
Convexity CSF	9.600	30.000	**3.125**	0.900	5.900	**6.556**	9.800	28.000	**2.857**
Skull	0.310	0.960	**3.097**	0.093	0.610	**6.559**	1.800	6.900	**3.833**
Vertebra	0.710	0.630	**0.887**	0.260	0.320	**1.231**	7.600		**0.000**
Red marrow (BM)	0.520	0.300	**0.577**	0.170	0.057	**0.335**	2.400	1.700	**0.708**
Dose ratios (RX window)									
Ventricle CSF to BM	6.731	36.667	**5.448**	176.471	175.439	**0.994**	21.667	47.059	**2.172**
C-Spine CSF to BM	26.923	50.000	**1.857**	20.000	192.982	**9.649**	20.417	29.412	**1.441**
L-Spine CSF to BM	48.077	60.000	**1.248**	147.059	73.684	**0.501**	83.333	38.235	**0.459**
Convex CSF to BM	18.462	100.000	**5.417**	5.294	103.509	**19.552**	4.083	16.471	**4.034**

antibodies studies, discrete intrathecal tumor deposits are visualized only after adequate clearance of the radioactivity from the CSF that takes 5 days [5, 6]. The well-known tumor seeking PET radiopharmaceutical F-18 FDG may be an interesting intrathecal diagnostic agent to depict LM deposits. However, its short physical half-life of 2 h may limit its sensitivity because of the long duration required for clearing the free tracer from the CSF.

CSF Radionuclide Imaging and Radiation Dosimetry

Conventional scintigraphy has limitation of low spatial resolution (greater than 1 cm), limited temporal resolution (20-min per scan), and limited field of views (15–20 cm) of gamma camera in static imaging. The use of whole-body scanner has enabled scanning of the entire neural axis in 20 min of the entire CSF space as one compartment as reported in Chap. 4. Because of patient comforts, our prior Ommayograms and cisternogram have been limited to four sessions of 20 min each in 24 h to produce four-time points of observation. Advances in instrumentation have resulted in shorter imaging time and larger field-of-view in commercially available gamma cameras, SPECT-CT and PET/CT scanners for clinical use. Spatial resolution of below 0.5 cm is possible nowadays. Whole-body PET-CT scanner can complete a whole-body PET scan in one session as short as 18–30 s [7]. These capabilities would allow studying human physiology and pathology in uniform manners (in one session) and in shorter duration to minimize patient discomfort and resultant artifacts from patient motions.

As demonstrated in Chaps. 8 and 9, radiation dosimetry is a tool of common languages between radiation therapy and molecular imaging to describe and correlate with toxicity and efficacy with the use of therapeutic radiopharmaceuticals. Standardized radionuclide radiation dosimetry schemes and software are available to derive radiation absorbed doses from imaging. While standardized radiation dosimetry report can be generated from the gamma camera, SPECT scanner, or PET/CT scanner, meticulous input of clinical data and physiologic parameters are important to produce reliable and repeatable dosimetry reports. Intrathecal radiation dosimetry needs additional attention because of the intricate anatomy and physiology and there have not been standardized imaging schemes. Large variations are noted in image-based calculations, blood or CSF sampling dosimetry as reported with I-124 Omburtamab PET-CT dosimetry study [8]. Large magnitude of variation is common with earlier dosimetry reports with I-131 labeled immunoconjugates [9, 10]. The current precision of radiation dosimetry from image-based calculation is in the range of 20%. Nevertheless, image-based radiation dosimetry provides a means of reconciliation and refinement for theoretic dosimetry models. Conventional radiation dosimetry methods can be further enhanced by newer three-dimensional schemes with voxel-based assessment such as GEANT4 and VIDA software [11].

There are important concerns and efforts to address radiation dosimetry at depths of meninges and brain tissues for more refined safety and efficacy assessment. An earlier study reported radiation dosimetry estimates at depths from I-131 and Ga-67 compounds under the same model [12]. Similar reports in the literature are mostly for individual compounds or with various models. Our simulations of Chap. 9 report the depths in which 50% dose rate occurs and in which 90% of total radiation dose deposited in the tissue. In Table 9.7 in Chap. 9, Ga-66 has the longest range with 50% dose rate at >0.44 cm in the cervical spine CSF. Radiation dosimetry at depths would be relevant consideration when treating LM plaques on meninges and when there is concern of toxicity to neural tissues underlying CSF.

The advantage of using one common set of simulation models (as in Chap. 9) is that multiple potential radiopharmaceutical candidates can be compared to serve as the first step in the design of intrathecal radiopharmaceutical trials. Accordingly, dosimetry of different isotopes of the same element (Gallium) can be derived as in Table 12.1. The physiologic models can be revised, and the residence times can be further refined to test hypothetical residence times from altered physiology and calibrated from patient imaging. As in Table 12.2, radiation dosimetry from simulation, hypothetical model, or image-based measurement can be tabulated for direct comparison for trial design of novel radiopharmaceuticals and novel schemes of therapy.

Table 12.2 Intrathecal radiation dosimetry of In-111 DTPA, In-111 Octreotide, Y-90 Zevalin, I-131 NaI, 131 HSA, I-124 NaI, and I-124 Omburtamab from simulation and image-calculation

(cGy/mCi) Injection	Intraventricular	Intraventricular	Intraventricular	Intraventricular	Intraventricular	Intraventricular	Intraventricular	Intraventricular	Intraventricular	Intraventricular	Intraventricular
Organ/radionuclide	In-111	In-111	Y-90	I-131	I-131	I-131	I-131 HSA cGy/mCi	I-131/I-131	I-131/I-131	I-124	I-124
Pharmaceuticals	DTPA	Octreotide	Zevalin	NaI	NaI	NaI	Human serum albumin	HSA/NaI	HSA/NaI	NaI	Omburtamab OM
Source	ICRP53 + simulation	Simulation	Simulation	Simulation	Hypothetical	Hypothetical/simulate	ICRP53 + simulate	ICRP53/hypothetical	ICRP53/simulation	Simulation	Image
Adrenals	0.241	0.600	0.810	0.420	0.097	0.231	2.960	30.515	7.048	1.500	1.480
Brain	2.405	0.690	4.400	2.500	0.137	0.055	4.070	29.622	1.628	2.700	3.737
Breasts	0.036	0.065	0.810	0.094	0.057	0.610	1.480	25.829	15.745	0.220	
Eyes		0.250		0.610	0.044	0.072				0.580	
Lens of eyes		0.200		0.490	0.033	0.068				0.480	
Gallbladder wall		0.140	0.810	0.160	0.079	0.494				0.420	1.702
LLIWall	0.056	0.250	13.000	0.130	0.136	1.047	1.591	11.690	12.238	0.310	1.258
Small intestine	0.085	0.220	3.800	0.170	0.096	0.564	1.739	18.133	10.229	0.500	1.406
Stomach	0.100	0.190	0.810	0.140	0.421	3.007	1.739	4.131	12.421	0.390	2.627
ULI wall	0.070	0.230	9.700	0.150	0.106	0.709	1.702	16.011	11.347	0.420	1.443
Heart wall		0.190	7.500	0.180	0.078	0.436	6.290	80.230	34.944	0.520	1.369
Kidneys	0.185	1.700	0.270	0.370	0.334	0.902	2.997	8.976	8.100	1.100	1.406
Liver	0.063	0.260	13.000	0.150	0.074	0.496	2.368	31.828	15.787	0.420	5.994
Lungs	0.081	0.180	5.400	0.170	0.204	1.199	4.810	23.602	28.294	0.490	1.258
Muscle		0.140	0.810	0.160	0.079	0.492				0.370	1.147
Ovaries	0.074	0.170	1.100	0.140	0.119	0.846	1.591	13.426	11.364	0.350	
Pancreas	0.130	0.380	0.810	0.240	0.101	0.420	1.961	19.474	8.171	0.780	1.628
Red marrow (BM)	0.518	0.590	4.900	0.670	0.118	0.176	2.664	22.615	3.976	1.900	1.110
Bone surfaces		0.530	2.400	0.620	0.115	0.186				1.100	2.183
Skin		0.077	0.810	0.140	0.061	0.435				0.260	0.999
Spleen	0.070	1.000	25.000	0.160	0.084	0.526	4.810	57.126	30.063	0.440	2.035
Testes	0.031	0.076	24.000	0.095	0.093	0.974	1.443	15.600	15.189	0.190	
Thymus		0.110	0.810	0.140	0.069	0.492				0.350	1.184
Thyroid	0.144	0.160	0.810	4.000	2.779	0.695	2.368	0.852	0.592	2.800	1.480
Urin bladder wall		0.980	2.400	1.500	2.950	1.967	1.554	0.527	1.036	2.300	1.258
Uterus	0.107	0.210	1.100	0.170	0.178	1.047	1.628	9.146	9.576	0.430	
Total body	0.063	0.200	1.300	0.480	0.115	0.240	2.000	17.376	4.167	0.490	1.665
ED		0.460	8.600	0.490	0.441	0.900	3.108	7.048	6.343	0.700	1.739
EDE	0.444	0.290	12.000	0.590	0.412	0.698	5.180	12.573	8.780	1.000	1.961
Ventricle CSF	4.200	4.200	63.000	16.000	11.870	**0.742**	16.000	**1.348**	**1.000**	16.000	2.294
C-Spine CSF	16.000	16.000	200.000	56.000	4.789	**0.086**	56.000	**11.694**	**1.000**	62.000	1.665
L-Spine CSF	29.000	29.000	440.000	59.000	1.831	**0.031**	59.000	**32.221**	**1.000**	130.000	2.072
Convexity CSF	8.750	8.750	67.000	150.000	7.760	**0.052**	150.000	**19.330**	**1.000**	23.000	
Dosimetry ratio to BM (Therapeutic window):											
Ventricle CSF to BM	8.108	7.119	12.857	23.881	100.927	**4.226**	6.006	**0.060**	**0.252**	8.421	2.067
C-Spine CSF to BM	30.888	27.119	40.816	83.582	36.233	**0.434**	21.021	**0.580**	**0.252**	32.632	1.500
L-Spine CSF to BM	55.985	49.153	89.796	88.060	13.662	**0.155**	22.147	**1.621**	**0.252**	68.421	1.867
Convex CSF to BM	16.892	14.831	13.673	223.881	67.350	**0.301**	56.306	**0.836**	**0.252**	12.105	

Considerations in Intrathecal Radiopharmaceuticals Therapy

Molecular Targeting Versus Geographic Targeting

Delayed visualization of LM by tumor-seeking intrathecal radiopharmaceuticals also raises the question of how much fraction of the targeting radiopharmaceutical is bound to and retained by the LM. That leads to the issue of how important the radiation dose contribution from LM binding of radiopharmaceuticals is. It will be crucial to ascertain the contribution in radiation dose from target-binding (molecular targeting) compared with radiation dose from adjacent CSF flow without binding (geographic targeting).

With intrathecal injection of tumor seeking radiopharmaceuticals, the fraction of radionuclide bound could be relatively low because meningeal barriers may prevent direct binding and cell surface antigens may not be available for binding at the time of tracer exposure. Furthermore, the constant dilution and flowing CSF may dislodge bound radionuclide resulting in decreased exposure of LM to irradiation. In the case of I-131 labeled 81C6 studies, delayed visualization of tumor deposit in the spine at day 5 is suggestive of low retention by binding to LM. The radiation absorbed dose contribution from radiolabeled pharmaceuticals in the flowing CSF may indeed contribute to more than from bound radiopharmaceutical. In fact the CSF clearance rate of intrathecal radiolabeled monoclonal antibody I-131 antitenascin [9, 10] is similar to that of I-131 labeled HSA [13] at 13 h.

With specific binding of tumor-seeking radiopharmaceutical to LM on meninges (molecular targeting), the contribution to total radiation absorbed dose from binding needs to be determined because there is also contemporaneous radiation exposure from neighboring free flowing radiopharmaceuticals in the CSF (geographic targeting). An indirect evaluation of contribution from LM binding may be derived from the reported clearance half-times after intraventricular injection of I-124 Omburtamab (8H9) [8]. The median clearance half-times are 8.19, 6.86, 7.83, and 7.02 h (average of 7.43 h for all CSF compartments) from PET corresponding to contribution from both bound and free I-124 8H9 in the ventricle, cervical, thoracic, and lumbar spine, respectively. The serial CSF samples from the Ommaya reservoir have a clearance time of 6.3 h indicating faster loss of unbound I-124 8H9. One likely explanation for the faster clearance time from CSF sampling is that there is significant binding of I-124 8H9 to LM on meninges. Therefore, clearance half-times may be translated into residence time and hence in radiation absorbed dose based on exposure. The grossly simplified estimates of contribution are 85% (6.3 h/7.43 h) in radiation absorbed dose from free flowing I-124 8H9 (geographic targeting) and 15% (1–6.3 h/7.43 h) from bound I-124 8H9 (molecular targeting).

Meticulous patient preparation and image processing as well as precise radiation dosimetry are needed for such analysis. Image-based clearance time/residence times of CSF compartments and simplified parameters such as geometric-mean images for calculation of Te in Chap. 4 may also be utilize to estimate contribution from molecular targeting. With CSF sampling and comparison to dosimetry models assuming bulk flow only, gross estimates of contribution from binding to LM may be possible for other tumor-targeting radiopharmaceuticals.

The level of gain in radiation absorbed dose from molecular targeting may need to be balanced with the cost of manufacturing and delivery of radiolabeled monoclonal antibody, which is subject to technical and regulatory requirements of both radiopharmaceutical and biologic categories. Concerns of relatively low radiation absorbed dose contribution from molecular targeting versus geographic targeting also lead to the notion of using intrathecal radiopharmaceuticals without tumor affinity to ablate LM nonspecifically.

Since the turn of the millennium, multiple therapeutic radiopharmaceuticals have been developed and many approved for intravenous injection to treat human tumors and neuro-oncologic applications as in Chap. 3 (Tables 3.4 and 3.5). They may also be candidates for intrathecal use. Potential alternative intrathecal therapeutic radiopharmaceuticals may involve small molecules, anions, cations, anions, monoclonal antibodies, peptides, alpha emitter. Several radiopharmaceuticals in Tables 9.1 and 9.2 have been studied using the common models in Chap. 9. Applying radiopharmaceuticals approved by FDA for system use to intrathecal use has the advantage that the manufacturing processes and systemic toxicity and efficacy profiles have been established. Certainly, compliance with regulations of use in alternative route is still needed. After thorough considerations of scientific merits and logistics, candidate radiopharmaceuticals still need to go through clinical trials to establish specific safety and efficacy before approval by authorities in procedures outlined in Chap. 11.

Novel Intrathecal Use of Radiopharmaceuticals with Therapeutic Potentials

Other than the sole FDA-approved In111- DTPA, radiopharmaceuticals including I-131 labeled HSA, Tc99m- labeled DTPA, and Tc99m- labeled EDTA have been used as CSF bulk flow surrogate in cisternograms. Preclinical studies have demonstrated that radiopharmaceuticals may encounter unique molecular events inside the CSF before excretion through the bulk flow pathways.

One example is spinal active transport of halide anions outside of the CSF as reported with animal experiments, dogs and rabbits [1, 3] and illustrated in Fig. 12.1. Another example is in vivo protein binding inside the CSF (typically with heavy metal cations), as exemplified by Fig. 12.2. These processes may accelerate or delay exit of radiopharmaceuticals from the CSF resulting in diminished or increased radiation absorbed dose, compared with that of the bulk flow (typically evaluated by In-111 DTPA cisternograms).

In the following non-exhaustive list of available radiopharmaceuticals, their intrathecal radiation dosimetry from simulation, imaging, hypothetic guesses, and derivation by substitution of different radioisotopes of the same element of available radiopharmaceuticals are examined for potential use in LM therapy:

Radioactive Cations

Radioactive isotopes of gallium (Ga-67, Ga-68, and perhaps Ga-66) in the form of citrate or chloride are commercially available for intravenous use. Simulated radiation dosimetry from intraventricular injection of Ga-67, Ga-68, and Ga-66 is listed in Table 12.1, along with estimates from imaging of Ga-67 (Chap. 4, Fig. 4.8) and derived estimates of Ga-68 and Ga-66 (based on Ga-67 imaging pharmacokinetics but incorporated with individual radiogallium emission characteristics). Comparison between (imaging or derived) dosimetry to that of simulation for Ga-67 citrate demonstrates significant gains in CSF radiation absorbed doses and therapeutic windows (columns 4, 7, and 10). This is likely related to protein binding (as demonstrated in Fig. 12.2) resulting in increased clearance time and hence dosimetry values in the CSF compartments.

Conversely, Ga-67 has affinity to tumors, inflammation, and infection sites for which it approved by the FDA. The Ga-67 binding to LM may be similar or different from protein binding in the CSF. As such, the extent of its intrathecal binding to LM on meninges from intrathecal injection has not been studied. The extent of radiopharmaceutical binding to LM may be grossly estimated from serial measurement of total radiogallium in CSF (in vitro) and serial imaging revealing the total radiogallium in the CSF plus those bound to meninges and LM (in vivo). An example of such calculation is illustrated with I-124 8H9 in section "Radiolabeled Monoclonal Antibodies and Proteins" below.

It would be a worthwhile imaging trial to assess the temporal and spatial biodistribution in CSF, meninges, and whole body of Ga-67, Ga-68, and Ga-66 to establish their radiation dosimetry profiles. Then contributions from free radiogallium, protein-bound radiogallium, and radiogallium bound to LM can be determined to compare with simulation findings (Table 12.1) to assess whether each of them would be good intrathecal therapy candidate.

Radioactive Anions (Halides- I-131, I-124 NaI, and Perhaps At-211)

Based on simulation assuming thyroid blockade and normal CSF flow without active transport, radiation dosimetry to the CSF compartments is favorable for I-131 sodium iodide, I-124 sodium iodide, and I-131 HSA (Table 12.2 columns 5, 8, and 11) to serve as therapeutic agents. However, because of the concern of active transport outside of the CSF as revealed in Fig. 12.1, a hypothetical dosimetry profile is construed by decreasing residence times for all compartments to below 1 h to construct a hypothetical dosimetry (Table 12.2 column 6). This set of hypothetical radiation dosimetry indeed shows diminished radiation to the CSF compartments compared with simulation (Table 12.2 column 7) and with I-131 HSA (Table 12.2 column 9). The above exercise demonstrates the utility of using one common model to compare multiple compounds with different physiology. It also provides target values (Table 12.2 column 5) for interventional schemes to inhibit active transport carriers and recover efficacy.

Since active transport carriers of iodide can be blocked by digoxin, perchlorate, or iodide [1], the effectiveness of blockade may be estimated from repeating dosimetry study under the treatment with active transport inhibitor. Successful blockade of intrathecal outward active transport of halide will result in moving the values in column 6 towards column 5 (or column 10 for I-124 NaI) in Table 12.2 to recover efficacy.

Inspection of Table 12.2 columns 9 and 10 shows the disadvantages of using I-131 HSA as intrathecal radiopharmaceuticals because of the higher radiation absorption doses to the kidneys, ovaries, pancreas, testis, and total body when comparison is made with those of I-131 sodium iodide, whether from simulation or from the hypothetical case. However, I-124 sodium iodide has remained a good candidate for intrathecal therapy. Conversely, intrathecal outward active transport may render the radiation dosimetry to the CSF tool only fractions of simulated values in Table 12.2 column 10. Then active transport inhibition may be needed to recover efficacy.

Radiolabeled Monoclonal Antibodies and Proteins

Y-90 labeled anti-CD20 monoclonal antibody (Zevalin) was marketed in the USA to treat refractory lymphoma. Even though no LM molecular targeting is assumed for Zevalin, simulations in Table 12.2 indeed reveal high radiation doses to the CSF compartments and high therapeutic window (column 4). It is also associated with high radiation dose to the bone marrow, liver, spleen, and testis that may limit its use.

I-131-labeled human serum albumin (HSA) of radioiodine serum albumin (RISA) was used extensively to study vascular flow as well as CSF flow. Although high radiation doses to the spinal fluid compartments may be used for treating LM, high dose to the heart wall, spleen, lungs, and bone marrow (Table 12.2 column 8) may limit its use.

Radiolabeled monoclonal antibodies have been used in oncologic diagnosis and therapy. The main advantage is the specificity to the targeted malignancy. When applied to intrathecal LM therapy, hematotoxicity is usually the dose-limiting toxicity (DLT) because of the circulating radioactivity after the radiopharmaceutical leaves the CSF. With I-131 labeled monoclonal antibodies such as 81C6, the injected dose is usually limited to 80 mCi, in adult and in children [14].

Because of favorable imaging characteristic and emission profile, Lu-177 labeled compounds including monoclonal antibodies have the potential advantage of serving as diagnostic agent at low radioactivity and then as therapeutic agent at high radioactivity. One of such intrathecal trial uses Lu-177 Omburtamab (9H8) with which a first-in-human study has been conducted in our institution (2021–2022, more description in Chap. 8).

Radio-Labeled Peptides (In-111 Octreotide, Cu-67 Sartate, Lu-177 Lutathera)

In-111 labeled Octreotide is an FDA approved diagnostic agent to detect neuroendocrine tumors. Lu-177 Lutathera (Dotatate) is an FDA approved therapeutic agent to treat neuroendocrine tumors. Cu-67 Sartate [15, 16] is an experimental therapeutic agent to treat neuroendocrine tumors that can be detected by gamma imaging and SPECT-CT. These radiopharmaceuticals have somatostatin receptor affinity and may also be considered for intrathecal use. While tumor targeting may be only for neuroendocrine tumors, geographic targeting and perhaps nonspecific somatostatin receptor binding to LM and meninges may be sufficient to render additional ablative effects to suppress or eradicate LM. These commercially available radiopharmaceuticals still need additional considerations before intrathecal therapeutic trials are designed and conducted.

One of the considerations would be intrathecal radiation dosimetry. Preliminary findings in Table 12.2 column 3 suggest that In111-octreotide may deliver sufficient radiation dose to the CSF compartments for therapeutic effects. Similar inspection of the diagnostic agent In111 in Table 12.2 column 2 suggests that In-111 DTPA may serve similar therapeutic function at higher activities (e.g., >30 mCi). The advantage of studying In-111 DTPA is that it has been approved for intrathecal use at radioactivity at 1 mCi. Extension from simulation studies as in Table 12.2 to clinical practice will require trial confirmation of safety and efficacy. Meticulous serial imaging, radioactivity measurements in vitro and in vivo will be important to derive the requisite radiation dosimetry to support use of these candidate intrathecal therapeutic agents.

Potential Use of Alpha Emitters (Radium-223)

Radium 223 chloride with half-life of 11.4 days has been used as an FDA-approved radiopharmaceuticals to treat osseous metastasis from prostate cancer. Because of the heavy alpha particles, the radiation payload to the target is high but its range is only three cell layers (<0.6 mm). Therefore, it has to be in very close proximity to the tumor or LM to be effective in delivering the radiation payload. The bystander effect (or geographic targeting) from alpha emitters in the circulating CSF has little contribution to ablate LM. If direct binding to LM deposits and no binding to the normal meninges are confirmed, Ra-223 labeled compounds would be good intrathecal candidate therapeutics.

Another alpha emitter Astatine 211 (At-211) is the halide member with the largest atomic number. Its biological behavior closely resembles that of iodide. Its production requires a cyclotron but the feasibility At-211 generator has been reported.

There are no intrathecal radiation dosimetric models for alpha emitters because of the very powerful radiation but short range that requires different models and processing. Substantial intellectual investment will be needed to harness the advantages of alpha emitter to treat LM.

Conclusion

Leptomeningeal metastasis has remained a lethal cancer complication, despite progresses in oncology, chemotherapy, targeted therapy, and radiation therapy. A plethora of new promising radiopharmaceuticals are available for human use against LM. Advances in instrumentation and radiation dosimetry algorithms and software have made possible detection and quantification as well as personalized dosimetry to allow assessment and prediction of efficacy as well as toxicity.

We are in a fortune a time with cumulative experience learned from treating cancer by oncologic colleagues, the advancement in radiopharmaceuticals and scanners as well as dosimetry algorithms and LM monitoring electrophysiology and the pending standardized RANO-LM criteria. Earlier chapters have outlined progresses and challenges on each of the above aspects as well as the regulatory matters. We are well equipped to tackle LM and to push the Kaplan–Meier curves to the right. Nevertheless, the use of radiopharmaceuticals to diagnose and to treat LM still needs to go through clinical trials and follow regulatory guidelines as well as local oversights, preferably in efficient, wise, succinct, and passionate manners.

Acknowledgement The author also thanks Dr. E. Edmund Kim of the University of California, Irvine for serving as collaborator on protocol DR10-0344 to evaluate patient studies while in M.D. Anderson Cancer Center.

References

1. Becker B. Cerebrospinal fluid iodide. Am J Phys. 1961;201:1149–51.
2. Madsen JR, et al. Cerebrospinal fluid anion transport: studies of pertechnetate in unanesthetized sheep. Neurosurgery. 1985;17(5):778–83.
3. Coben LA, Smith KR. Iodide transfer at four cerebrospinal fluid sites in the dog: evidence for spinal iodide carrier transport. Exp Neurol. 1969;23(1):76–90.
4. Post RM, Allen FH, Ommaya AK. Cerebrospinal fluid flow and iodide 131 transport in the spinal subarachnoid space. Life Sci. 1974;14(10):1885–94.
5. Lashford LS, et al. A pilot study of 131I monoclonal antibodies in the therapy of leptomeningeal tumors. Cancer. 1988;61(5):857–68.
6. Bigner DD, et al. Phase I studies of treatment of malignant gliomas and neoplastic meningitis with 131I-radiolabeled monoclonal antibodies anti-tenascin 81C6 and anti-chondroitin proteoglycan sulfate Me1–14 F (ab')2—a preliminary report. J Neurooncol. 1995;24(1):109–22.
7. Zhang X, et al. Subsecond total-body imaging using ultrasensitive positron emission tomography. Proc Natl Acad Sci U S A. 2020;117(5):2265–7.
8. Pandit-Taskar N, et al. Biodistribution and dosimetry of intraventricularly administered (124)I-omburtamab in patients with metastatic leptomeningeal tumors. J Nucl Med. 2019;60(12):1794–801.
9. Moseley RP, Papanastassiou V, Zalutsky MR. Immunoreactivity, pharmacokinetics and bone marrow dosimetry of intrathecal radioimmunoconjugates. Int J Cancer. 1992;52(1):38–43.
10. Moseley RP, et al. Intrathecal administration of 131I radiolabelled monoclonal antibody as a treatment for neoplastic meningitis. Br J Cancer. 1990;62(4):637–42.
11. Hesterman JY, et al. Three-dimensional dosimetry for radiation safety estimates from intrathecal administration. J Nucl Med. 2017;58(10):1672–8.
12. van Dieren EB, et al. A dosimetric model for intrathecal treatment with 131I and 67Ga. Int J Radiat Oncol Biol Phys. 1994;30(2):447–54.
13. Stabin MEJ. The radiation dosimetry of intrathecally administered radionuclides. In: Sixth international radiopharmaceutical dosimetry symposium. ORISE; 1999. 99-0164. p. 5–514.
14. Brown MT, et al. Intrathecal 131I-labeled antitenascin monoclonal antibody 81C6 treatment of patients with leptomeningeal neoplasms or primary brain tumor resection cavities with subarachnoid communication: phase I trial results. Clin Cancer Res. 1996;2(6):963–72.
15. Hicks RJ, et al. (64)Cu-SARTATE PET imaging of patients with neuroendocrine tumors demonstrates high tumor uptake and retention, potentially allowing prospective dosimetry for peptide receptor radionuclide therapy. J Nucl Med. 2019;60(6):777–85.
16. Laffon E, de Clermont H, Marthan R. An abbreviated therapy-dosimetric equation for the companion diagnostic/therapeutic [(64/67)Cu]Cu-SARTATE. EJNMMI Res. 2021;11(1):75.

Index

F. C. L. Wong (ed.), *Radiopharmaceuticals in the Management of Leptomeningeal Metastasis*, https://doi.org/10.1007/978-3-031-14291-8

MIX
Papier aus verantwortungsvollen Quellen
Paper from responsible sources
FSC® C105338

If you have any concerns about our products,
you can contact us on
ProductSafety@springernature.com

In case Publisher is established outside the EU,
the EU authorized representative is:
Springer Nature Customer Service Center GmbH
Europaplatz 3, 69115 Heidelberg, Germany

Printed by Libri Plureos GmbH
in Hamburg, Germany